Psychology and Sociology Applied to Medicine

AN ILLUSTRATED COLOUR TEXT

Psychology and Sociology Applied to Medicine

AN ILLUSTRATED COLOUR TEXT

Fourth Edition

Edwin Roland van Teijlingen MA MEd PhD

Professor, Bournemouth University, Bournemouth, UK

Honorary Professor, School of Health Sciences, University of Nottingham, UK

Visiting Professor, Nobel College, Pokhara University, Kathmandu, Nepal

Visiting Professor, Manmohan Memorial Institute of Health Sciences, Tribhuvan University, Kathmandu, Nepal

Gerald Humphris PhD MClinPsychol CPsychol FRCP Edin

Professor, Medical School, University of St Andrews, St Andrews, UK

Honorary Consultant Clinical Psychologist, Edinburgh Cancer Centre, NHS Lothian, Western General Hospital, Edinburgh, UK

Foreword by
Catherine Calderwood MA Cantab FRCOG FRCP Edin FRCP Glas FRCS (Ed)

Hon Colonel 205 (Scottish) Field Hospital

Chief Medical Officer for Scotland

Obstetrician

ELSEVIER   EDINBURGH   LONDON   NEW YORK   OXFORD   PHILADELPHIA   ST LOUIS   SYDNEY   2019

ELSEVIER

© 2019, Elsevier Limited. All rights reserved.

First edition 1999
Second edition 2004
Third edition 2009
    Reprinted 2010, 2013, 2014 (twice)

Notices
Practitioners and researchers must always rely on their own experience and knowledge in evaluating and using any information, methods, compounds or experiments described herein. Because of rapid advances in the medical sciences, in particular, independent verification of diagnoses and drug dosages should be made. To the fullest extent of the law, no responsibility is assumed by Elsevier, authors, editors or contributors for any injury and/or damage to persons or property as a matter of products liability, negligence or otherwise, or from any use or operation of any methods, products, instructions, or ideas contained in the material herein.

ISBN: 978-0-7020-6298-8
[eBook: 978-0-7020-6299-5]
[Inkling: 978-0-7020-6474-6]

ELSEVIER your source for books, journals and multimedia in the health sciences
www.elsevierhealth.com

Working together to grow libraries in developing countries

www.elsevier.com • www.bookaid.org

The publisher's policy is to use paper manufactured from sustainable forests

Printed in China
Last digit is the print number: 9   8   7   6   5   4   3   2   1

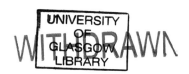

Content Strategist: Pauline Graham
Content Development Specialist: Kirsty Guest
Project Manager: Julie Taylor
Design: Renee Duenow
Illustration Manager: Amy Faith Heyden

Contents

Section 8: How do health services work? 148

Section 9: How do you fit into all this? 160

Foreword

Why would the Chief Medical Officer for Scotland be asked to write the foreword for this book?

You will be aware by now that these are challenging times for healthcare. The population is ageing, in the UK and across the world. A growing number of people live with multiple, complex and frequently changing health conditions. Our current models of care do not always suit our patients or their carers or the aspirations of our workforce. The demand on our services feels greater than ever.

In response, we need to change the culture of how we think about and practise healthcare. In 2016, I used my first annual report as Chief Medical Officer for Scotland to encourage the practice of Realistic Medicine. To put the person receiving health and care at the centre of decision-making and to adopt a personalised approach to care. To reduce the harm and waste caused by over-treatment and over-provision. To innovate and improve. These are bold ambitions but ones we can achieve. Already, Realistic Medicine has been embraced by healthcare professionals in Scotland and across the world, by policy-makers and, importantly, by the public.

Psychology is the science of behaviour and mind, including conscious and unconscious phenomena, as well as feeling and thought. Sociology is the scientific study of society, patterns of social relationships, social interaction and culture of everyday life. How important, therefore, that our future doctors have a grounding in and understanding of these subjects as they are fundamental to providing Realistic Medicine for our patients and to improving our healthcare for the future.

It therefore gives me great pleasure to introduce this textbook to such an audience. First published in 1999 and now in its 4th Edition, *Psychology and Sociology Applied to Medicine* has an established history of providing medical students and healthcare professionals with a rich understanding of the psychological and sociological processes crucial to delivering personalised care. Over the years, as with healthcare, the book has had to adapt to incorporate new evidence and reflect emerging health priorities. This 4th edition is no different and includes a new chapter on Obesity and updated material throughout pre-existing chapters. I am glad, though, that the original format of the book has been retained with time. It is rare for a resource to convey fundamental concepts as clearly and concisely as found here. And it is rarer still for these concepts to capture the key values that we require in our workforce.

So I conclude this foreword with optimism. These may be challenging times but future success depends on our most valuable asset – our workforce. Not just the doctors of today but also the doctors of tomorrow. You hold the values of Realistic Medicine. You are the drivers of change. The future of healthcare is in your hands.

Dr Catherine Calderwood
Chief Medical Officer for Scotland
October 2018

Preface to the fourth edition

In a world of fake news, increased social complexities, global warming uncertainties, rapid technological changes and social inequalities, one constant is the need for dedicated people to train in medicine to become our future generation of doctors.

Our expert social and behavioural scientists have created this textbook as a guide for medical students. Since the third edition, chapters have been updated and where necessary rewritten. However we kept the original straightforward structure of the book. We have also introduced a new chapter on obesity, which is currently one of the main public health issues in most high-income countries, as well as in a growing number of low-and-middle income countries.

We would like to thank the original editors for laying the excellent foundation for this fourth edition. Two of the original editors of the first three editions, Beth Alder and Charles Abraham, have stepped down and Mike Porter has unfortunately passed away. Mike Porter was a sociologist who taught at the Medical School at the University of Edinburgh for 40 years. He was killed by a 'freak' accident in 2013 while exercising his dog.

We would like to thank all those who have helped us in preparing this fourth edition, colleagues, friends, students and family.

EvT & GH

Contributors

Charles Abraham BA DPhil CPsychol FBPsS
Professor of Psychology Applied to Health, University of Exeter Medical School, Exeter, UK
1 *The bio-psycho-social model*
9 *Personality and health*
10 *Understanding learning*
15 *Intelligence*
35 *Health beliefs, motivation and behaviour*
36 *Changing cognitions and behaviour*
37 *Helping people to act on their intentions*
46 *Adherence*
63 *What is stress?*

Anna-Lynne Ruth Adlam BSc PhD DClinPsy
Senior Lecturer in Psychology, University of Exeter, Exeter, UK
13 *Memory problems*

Vanessa Allom PhD BPsych (Hons)
Research Associate, School of Psychology and Speech Pathology, Curtin University, Perth, Western Australia, Australia
20 *Changing patterns of health and illness*
32 *What are disease prevention and health promotion?*

Amanda Amos BA MSc PhD HonFFPH
Professor of Health Promotion, University of Edinburgh, Edinburgh, UK
41 *Smoking, tobacco control and doctors*

Niall C Anderson CPsychol MSc BSc (Hons)
Health Psychologist, Hywel Dda University Health Board, Carmarthen, UK
36 *Changing cognitions and behaviour*

Lindsay D. Apps CPsychol MSc BSc (Hons) AFBPsS
Lecturer in Psychology, Practitioner Health Psychologist, DeMontfort University, Leicester, UK
64 *Asthma and chronic obstructive pulmonary disease*

Susan Ayers PhD CPsychol
Professor of Maternal and Child Health, School of Health Sciences, City University London, London, UK
03 *Reproductive issues*

Thomas Bartlett BM BSc (Hons) MRCP
Specialist Registrar in Geriatrics and General Internal Medicine, Dorset, UK
81 *Life as a trainee doctor*

Timothy Battcock MB ChB FRCP
Consultant Physician, Poole Hospital, Dorset, UK
81 *Life as a trainee doctor*

Jill Bradshaw BSc PhD CertMRCSLT
Senior Lecturer in Intellectual and Developmental Disabilities, University of Kent, Canterbury, UK
60 *Learning disability*

Katie Brittain BSc (Hons) MA PhD
Associate Professor of Ageing and Health, Northumbria University, Newcastle upon Tyne, UK
70 *Coping with illness and disability*

Lucie M T Byrne-Davis PhD MSc BSc(Hons) CPsychol PFHEA
Senior Lecturer in Assessment and Psychometrics, Division of Medical Education, University of Manchester, Manchester, UK
10 *Understanding learning*

Kim M. Caudwell PhD BPsych (Hons)
Sessional Academic, School of Psychology, Curtin University, Western Australia, Australia
20 *Changing patterns of health and illness*
32 *What are disease prevention and health promotion?*

Jennifer A. Cleland BSc (Hons) MSc PhD DClinPsychol AFBPsS
Professor of Medical Education Research, Centre for Healthcare Research and Innovation (CHERI), University of Aberdeen, Aberdeen, UK
47 *Clinical communication skills*

Tracey Collett B.Ed(Hons)
Associate Professor (Senior Lecturer) in The Sociology of Health and Illness, University of Plymouth, Devon, UK
18 *Concepts of health, illness and disease*

Richard J Cooper PhD MA LLB BSC
Senior Lecturer in Public Health, ScHARR, University of Sheffield, Sheffield, UK
19 *Measuring health and illness*

Sarah Cunningham-Burley BSocSc PhD FAcSS FRSE MFPH
Professor of Medical and Family Sociology, The Usher Institute, University of Edinburgh, Edinburgh, UK
34 *The social implications of the new genetics*

Diane Dixon PhD BA(Hons) BSc(Hons)
Reader Health Psychology, University of Strathclyde, Glasgow, UK
33 *Health screening*
51 *Psychological preparation for surgery*
55 *Cancer*
59 *Physical disability*

Morag L. Donaldson MA PhD CPsychol
Senior Lecturer in Psychology, University of Edinburgh, Edinburgh, UK
16 *Development of thinking*

Flora Douglas PhD MPH PGDip Health Promotion BN RGN
Reader in the School of Nursing and Midwifery, Robert Gordon University, Aberdeen, UK
38 *The social context of behavioural change*

Frank Doyle BA(Hons) MLitt PhD C Health Psychol PsSI
Senior Lecturer, Royal College of Surgeons in Ireland, Dublin, Ireland
52 *Heart disease*

Andrew Eagle BA MA DClinPsy CPsychol
Consultant Clinical Psychologist, CNWL NHS Foundation Trust, London, UK
69 *Cognitive–behavioural therapy*

Winifred Oluchukwu Eboh PhD BSc (Hons) SFHEA RM RN
Lecturer in Adult Nursing, University of Essex, Essex, UK
24 *Ethnicity and health*

Helen Eborall BSc MSc PhD
Lecturer in Social Science Applied to Health, University of Leicester, Leicester, UK
31 *Perceptions of risk and risk-taking behaviours*

Catherine Exley BSc (Hons) MA PhD
Professor of Qualitative Health Research and Faculty Associate Pro-Vice Chancellor Research & innovation, Northumbria University, Newcastle, UK
70 *Coping with illness and disability*

R. Guy Fielding BSc PhD
Oxford, UK
17 *Understanding groups*

Arnstein Finset PhD
Professor Emeritus, Behavioral Sciences in Medicine, Faculty of Medicine, University of Oslo, Oslo, Norway;
Editor-in-Chief, Patient Education and Counselling, Elsevier
12 *Emotions*

Elizabeth Ford MA DPhil
Lecturer in Medical Research Methodology, Brighton and Sussex Medical School, Brighton, UK
03 *Reproductive issues*

Tamsin Ford FRCPsych PhD
Professor of Child and Adolescent Psychiatry, University of Exeter Medical School, Exeter, UK
05 *Childhood and child health*

Ruth Freeman BDS PhD MSc (DPH) MMedSci (Psychotherapy) DDPH.RCS (Eng) FFPH.RCPH (UK)
Professor of Dental Public Health Research, University of Dundee, Dundee, UK
66 *Counselling*

Alan Garnham MA(Oxon) DPhil CPsychol FBPsS
Professor of Experimental Psychology, University of Sussex, Brighton, UK
15 *Intelligence*

Ruth Garside BA (Hons) MA PhD
Senior Lecturer in Evidence Synthesis,
University of Exeter, Truro, Cornwall, UK
67 Urban nature, health and well-being

Colin J Greaves PhD C Psychol
Professor of Psychology Applied to
Health, University of Birmingham,
Birmingham, UK
62 Diabetes mellitus

Richard Hammersley MA PhD
Professor of Health Psychology,
Psychology, University of Hull, Hull, UK
06 Adolescence
39 Illegal drug use
40 Alcohol use

Gerald Humphris PhD MClinPsychol
  CPsychol FRCP Edin
Professor, Medical School, University of
St Andrews, St Andrews, UK
Honorary Consultant Clinical
Psychologist, Edinburgh Cancer Centre,
NHS Lothian, Western General Hospital,
Edinburgh, UK
Visiting Professor, Central South
University, Changsha, China
50 The patient experience

Adaeze Ifezulike Certified Lifestyle
  Medicine Physician MBBS MRCGP
  DFRSH
Aberdeen, UK
24 Ethnicity and health

Gail Johnston BSocSc PhD RGN DipDN
  CertMedEd
Programme Manager, HSC R&D Division,
Public Health Agency, Belfast, Northern
Ireland
08 Bereavement
48 Breaking bad news
65 Death and dying
71 Palliative care

Marie Johnston PhD FMed Sci FRSE
  FRCPE FAcSS FEHPS FBPS FSBM
Emeritus Professor of Health Psychology,
University of Aberdeen, Aberdeen, UK
33 Health screening
51 Psychological preparation for surgery
55 Cancer
59 Physical disability

Adam Jowett BSc PhD AFBPsS
Senior Lecturer in Psychology, Coventry
University, Coventry, UK
23 LGBT health

Steve Keen PhD MA BA(Hons) FHEA
Separated Child Seeking Asylum Manager,
International Care Network,
Bournemouth, UK
49 Self-care
77 Community care

Karen Forrest Keenan MA Hons MLitt
  PhD
Research Fellow, Health Services Research
Unit, University of Aberdeen,
Aberdeen, UK
*34 The social implications of the new
  genetics*

Michael P. Kelly BA (Hons) MPhil. PhD
  FFPH FRCP (Hon) FRCP Edinburgh
Senior Visiting Fellow, Primary Care Unit,
Department of Public Health and Primary
Care, Cambridge Institute of Public
Health, University of Cambridge, UK
30 Labelling and stigma
58 Inflammatory bowel disease
68 Coping and adaptation

Jennifer Kettle BA MA PhD
Research Associate, University of
Sheffield, Sheffield, UK
73 The management of pain

Jenny Kitzinger BA MA PhD
Professor of Communications Research,
School of Journalism, Media & Culture,
Cardiff University, Cardiff, UK
26 Media and health

Anita Laidlaw PhD
Senior Lecturer (Education Focused),
School of Medicine, University of St
Andrews, St Andrews, UK
46 Adherence

Susan Llewelyn BA MSc PhD FBPsS
Emeritus Professor and Fellow, Harris
Manchester College, Oxford University,
Oxford, UK
11 Perception
17 Understanding groups

Linda Long BSc (Hons) MSc PhD
Research Fellow, Evidence Synthesis &
Modelling for Health Improvement
(ESMI), University of Exeter Medical
School, Exeter, UK
72 Complementary therapies

Karen Mattick PhD
Professor of Medical Education,
University of Exeter, Exeter, UK
80 Medical students' experience

Suzanne McDonald PhD CPsychol
  AFBPsS
Research Methodologist, Newcastle
University, Newcastle upon Tyne, UK
35 Health beliefs, motivation and behaviour
37 Helping people to act on their intentions

Jenny McNeill BSc MSc PhD
Research Associate, University of York and
University of Sheffield, Sheffield, UK
27 Housing, homelessness and health

Karen Morgan PhD CHealth PsSI
Associate Professor Psychology &
Behavioural Sciences, Perdana University-
Royal College of Surgeons in Ireland
School of Medicine, Selangor, Malaysia
52 Heart disease

Kenneth Mullen MA MLitt PhD
Honorary Senior Research Fellow, School
of Medicine, Dentistry and Nursing,
University of Glasgow, Glasgow, UK
21 Social class and health
28 Work and health
29 Unemployment and health

Tamsin Newlove-Delgado MBChB (Hons)
  MRCPsych MPH MFPH PhD
Clinical Lecturer in Public Health
Medicine, University of Exeter, Exeter, UK
05 Childhood and child health

Diane O'Carroll LLB MBChB
Emergency Medicine Doctor, NHS Greater
Glasgow and Clyde, UK
57 Depression
61 Post-traumatic stress disorder

Ronan E. O'Carroll BSc (Hons) MPhil PhD
  FRSE FAcSS FEHPS
Professor of Psychology, University of
Stirling, Stirling, UK
57 Depression
61 Post-traumatic stress disorder

Daryl B. O'Connor PhD
Professor of Psychology, School of
Psychology, University of Leeds,
Leeds, UK
09 Personality and health

Sheina Orbell BSc PhD
Professor of Psychology, University of
Essex, Colchester, UK
20 Changing patterns of health and illness
*32 What are disease prevention and health
  promotion?*

Gozde Ozakinci PhD CPsychol
Senior Lecturer in Health Psychology,
School of Medicine, University of St
Andrews, St Andrews, UK
63 What is stress?

Elizabeth Peel BA PhD CPsychol FBPsS
Professor of Communication and Social
Interaction, Loughborough University,
Loughborough, UK
23 LGBT health

Emma Pitchforth PhD BSc (Hons)
Senior Lecturer and Senior Research
Fellow in Primary Care, University of
Exeter, Exeter, UK
79 Health: a rural perspective

Rachael Powell PhD MSc BSc (Hons)
Lecturer, Manchester Centre for Health
Psychology, School of Health Sciences,
University of Manchester, Manchester, UK
33 Health screening
51 Psychological preparation for surgery
55 Cancer
59 Physical disability

Rebecca Ellen Riddell MB ChB MSc
FRCGP
Former Head of General Practice and
Community Medical Education, Institute
of Education for Medical and Dental
Sciences, University of Aberdeen,
Aberdeen, UK
47 Clinical communication skills

Brian Rogers MA PhD
Emeritus Professor of Experimental
Psychology, University of Oxford,
Oxford, UK
11 Perception

Padam Simkhada MSc PhD
Professor of International Public Health
at Public Health Institute, Liverpool John
Moores University, UK
78 Health: a global perspective

Suzanne Skevington BSc PhD CPsychol
FBPsS
Project Diamond Chair in Health
Psychology, University of Manchester,
Manchester, UK
25 Quality of life

James Smith PhD MSc BSc (Hons)
Doctor, University of Oxford, Oxford, UK
20 Changing patterns of health and illness
32 What are disease prevention and health
  promotion?

Jane Rebecca Smith BSc (Hons) PGDip
PGCert PhD
Senior Lecturer in Primary Care,
University of Exeter Medical School,
Exeter, UK
62 Diabetes mellitus

Falko F Sniehotta PhD
Professor of Behavioural Medicine and
Health Psychology, Newcastle University,
Newcastle, UK
35 Health beliefs, motivation and behaviour
37 Helping people to act on their intentions

Edwin Roland van Teijlingen MA MEd
PhD
Professor, Bournemouth University,
Bournemouth, UK
Honorary Professor, School of Health
Sciences, University of Nottingham, UK
Visiting Professor, Nobel College, Pokhara
University, Kathmandu, Nepal
Visiting Professor, Manmohan Memorial
Institute of Health Sciences, Tribhuvan
University, Kathmandu, Nepal
01 The biopsychosocial model
02 Pregnancy and childbirth
07 Social aspects of ageing
14 How does sexuality develop?
22 Gender and health
43 Deciding to consult
44 Seeing the doctor
53 Malnutrition and obesity
54 HIV/AIDS
74 Organizing and funding health care
75 Assessing needs
76 Setting priorities and rationing
78 Health: a global perspective
79 Health: a rural perspective
82 The profession of medicine

Evelyn Watson BSc (Hons) PhD
Associate Lecturer (Education Focused)
School of Medicine, University of St
Andrews, St Andrews, UK
56 Anxiety

Mathew P. White PhD
Senior Lecturer in Environmental
Psychology, European Centre for
Environment & Human Health, Royal
Cornwall Hospital Treliske, Truro, UK
67 Urban nature, health and well-being

Brian Williams BSc PhD
Professor, School of Health & Social Care,
Edinburgh Napier University,
Edinburgh, UK
45 Placebo and nocebo effects

Martin R. Yeomans BSc PhD CPsychol
Professor of Experimental Psychology,
University of Sussex, Brighton, UK
42 Eating, body shape and health

Siyang Yuan BDS MPH PhD
Research Fellow, University of Dundee,
Dundee, UK
04 Development in early infancy

Acknowledgements

The editors would like to acknowledge and offer grateful thanks for the input of all previous editions' contributors, without whom this new edition would not have been possible.

Dedication

GH would like to dedicate this book to his 99-year-old father, Ken.

Mike Porter, one of the founding authors of this textbook, who died too young at the age of 66 in 2013. Mike taught medical students at the University of Edinburgh for over four decades before retiring in 2011.

1 | The biopsychosocial model

As doctors, you will be working face to face with patients – making sense of complex signs and symptoms, requesting and interpreting diagnostic tests, deciding on diagnoses, discussing their implications with patients and agreeing on treatment and longer-term management for those who have chronic diseases that cannot be cured. You may also find yourselves involved in trying to prevent, or at least delay, the onset of disease through screening programmes, opportunistic screening and secondary prevention (see pp. 64–65 and 66–67).

The World Health Organization (http://www.who.int/about/mission/en/) defined health as 'a state of complete physical, mental and social well-being and not merely the absence of disease or infirmity'. This definition emphasizes psychological and social aspects of health (see pp. 36–37). Any comprehensive framework for understanding health and health care services must embrace both psychological and sociological aspects of well-being and their interactions with biological processes (see pp. 36–37). Health depends on our perceptions, beliefs and behaviours and how these interact with physical systems such as the endocrine, immunological and cardiovascular systems. At the same time our perceptions and behaviours are shaped by our social context. Understanding how social, psychological and biological processes interact to create differences in health is what is meant by adopting a *biopsychosocial* perspective (Schwartz, 1980), as illustrated in the case study.

Bartholomew et al. (2006: 9) advocated a 'social ecological' model of health and health behaviours, which includes individual and social determinants of perception and behaviour (Fig. 1.1). For example, in the UK, where the wealthiest 10% of the population own more than half of all wealth, the difference in life expectancy between the poorest and the richest areas is about 10 years (Shaw et al., 2005). Thus just knowing where someone is

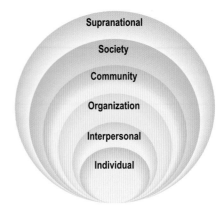

Fig. 1.1 Influences on health. *(From Bartholomew et al., 2006, with permission).*

born (e.g. part of the country or even which part of a city) allows us to make predictions about how long they will live, illustrating how our societal context shapes our well-being and health. Interestingly, in more equal societies such as those in Scandinavia there is less of a gap in life expectancy between the richest and the poorest 10%.

The health of a population generally is also significantly affected by public policy and legislation. For example, evaluating the law banning smoking in public places, Sargent et al. (2004) found that myocardial infarction admissions to a hospital fell significantly over 6 months during a smoking ban in public places, whereas surrounding areas (without a ban) experienced non-significant increases. Thus political action can sometimes be more effective in changing people's health behaviour than individual-level intervention.

Case study

Mr Brown is being interviewed by some third-year medical students and telling them about his experience of heart disease (see pp. 104–105). He is 65 years old and married with two children and two grandchildren. He was born in a relatively poor family and was one of four children living with their parents in a two-bedroom third-floor flat (see pp. 54–55). They ate what they regarded as good food: 'the best: eggs, butter, meat' as their mother worked as a cook for a local wealthy family. All six of them smoked (see pp. 82–83). He left school at 16 years old and became a bus driver, and his ability led him to be promoted to operations manager – 'quite a demanding and stressful job' (see pp. 56–57).

His first episodes of mild chest pain began in his early 40s, and when he went to see his doctor, he was strongly advised to stop smoking. However, he did not stop because, as he saw it, he wasn't *that* ill (see pp. 70–71, 76–77, 88–89). He had his first heart attack when he was 45 years of age, describing it as 'crushing pain; as if a ton of bricks had landed on my chest'. In hospital, he had a second heart attack (see pp. 100–101), and he needed coronary bypass surgery, which was successful (see pp. 104–105). He was discharged but has developed angina that has got worse over the years. Further surgery was not possible.

He finds it difficult to collect his newspaper from the local shop and takes tablets to help him cope with the pain and breathlessness. When he takes them first thing in the morning to help him get up, they give him a headache, and he has to take it easy until the side effect wears off. He tells the students that he has taken two to get to the interview – one to get him to the doctor's practice and another to get up the stairs to the room itself. He's got pain now as he's a bit nervous and stressed (see pp. 146–147).

Mr Brown explains he has changed a lot since his heart attack and become a lot more patient and relaxed, less irritable, adding by way of illustration, 'I used to shoo the pigeons off the windowsill, now I feed them' (see pp. 18–19). He is also concerned about his wife because she's a fairly anxious person at the best of times and she worries about him. He feels he can't give up living but is all too aware that this exacerbates her anxiety (see pp. 112–113). The best example he gives of how he manages his life is when, in answer to a question about how he's been recently, he describes a day the previous week when he showed his grandchildren a local historical tourist attraction. They were going to catch a bus, but his son-in-law decided that it was such a nice day so they would walk. So Mr Brown, who has a great love of history and doesn't want to disappoint his grandchildren or make a fuss, walks with them, mostly uphill, but taking frequent strategic breaks to describe other local historical and interesting sites while he gets his breath back and the angina subsides. He manages the outing this way but then has to spend the next three days, exhausted, in his bed (see pp. 50–51, 136–137). This interview today is his first day out since that outing. When the students presented this case study, a member of staff was overheard to comment: 'stupid patient'.

Apart from the psychosocial issues relating directly to Mr Brown and his disease, the case illustrates the importance of understanding how lifestyle and material disadvantage (see pp. 42–43), often experienced early in life, are important life-course risk factors for disease in later life (Davey Smith et al., 1997).

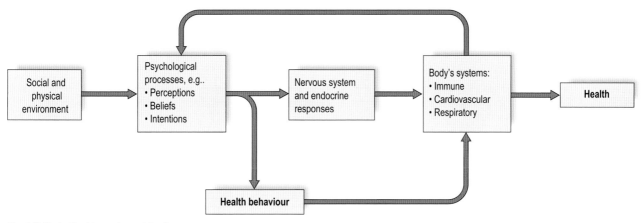

Fig. 1.2 Illustrative biopsychosocial pathways.

At a more local level, community culture and resources may shape health-related behaviour and health. For example, the North Karelia project (Finland) included education on smoking, diet and hypertension by using widely distributed leaflets, radio and television slots (see pp. 52–53) and education in local organizations. Voluntary-sector organizations, schools and health and social services were involved, and staff training was provided. The intervention included educating school pupils about the health risks of smoking and the social influences which lead young people to begin smoking as well as training them how to resist such social influences. This comprehensive intervention was found to be effective: 15 years later, smoking prevalence was 11% lower amongst intervention participants compared with controls (Vartiainen et al., 1998).

There are many examples of how insights from psychological research can help health care professionals with specific patient groups. For example, while adolescents have near-adult intellectual abilities and soon acquire adult physical abilities, neurological development continues into young adulthood, and it has been suggested that adolescents' cognitions and hence behaviours tend to be more impulsive and less risk-averse than those of adults because of this delay in brain development (Steinberg, 2007). Thus, compared with adults, adolescents tend to have poorer impulse regulation and heightened motivational drive in relation to rewards. Consequently, adolescents with chronic conditions are as likely as healthy adolescents to engage in risky health behaviour. This can have serious implications (e.g. adolescents suffering from asthma or cystic fibrosis who smoke are at increased risk of pulmonary deterioration). Smoking also accelerates the development of cardiovascular disease in individuals with diabetes and lupus. Yet health care professionals report less confidence and competence in dealing with adolescents than with other age groups (Sawyer et al., 2007). This strongly indicates a need to improve training for health care professionals in relation to care of, and health promotion for, adolescents, particularly those with chronic conditions.

Educational interventions by health care professionals have been found to enhance health impact. For example, a randomized controlled trial of an education programme for general practitioners focusing on social and physical activity promotion as well as prescribing and vaccination practices for elderly patients showed that patients in the intervention group increased walking by an average of 88 minutes every 2 weeks, spent more time on pleasurable activities and had better self-rated health than those in the control group (Kerse et al., 1999). Similarly, understanding how people plan actions and remember them can increase adherence amongst older patients. People who form 'if–then' plans are more likely to act on an intention in a specified context (Gollwitzer, 1999) (see pp. 74–75). Findings such as these demonstrate that educational interventions by family doctors and other health care professionals can have substantial effects on public health targets.

Understanding people's interpersonal context can also help health care professionals to offer more effective care. For example, stressful relationships have an impact on people's immune functioning and health (Fig. 1.2). Indeed, stress has been found to have multiple effects on health (see pp. 126–127), including slower wound healing (Kiecolt-Glaser et al., 1995), which is vital to the recovery process. Consequently, helping patients cope with stressful relationships for example, through referral to counselling or therapy (see pp. 132–133) and by helping them access social support (see pp. 154–155) including self-help groups (pp. 98–99), could enhance the effectiveness and cost-effectiveness of health care systems. Social support can also play an important role in recovery, including recovery from surgery: those who feel more supported need less medication and are discharged earlier (Krohne and Slangen, 2005). Those with more social support are more likely to take care of their health and so require less professional health care. Social support may be especially important to women's health.

Complementary therapies (see pp. 144–145) are increasingly popular because patients believe the health benefits are worth paying for. Because the effectiveness of some treatments (e.g. homeopathy) cannot be explained by evidence- or research-based theory, they are often regarded as capitalizing on placebo effects. Placebo effects (see pp. 90–91) demonstrate that apparently inert substances affect physiological processes. These generate positive health-related outcomes such as bronchodilation or pain relief (Stewart-Williams, 2004). Moreover, we know that adherence to placebo treatments generates greater health benefit (Epstein, 1984) indicating that adherence itself (apart from the effects of medication) has health benefits. Findings such as these indicate that people's perceptions and expectations about their health, symptoms and treatments strongly affect their health and well-being (Di Blasi et al., 2000).

The biopsychosocial model

- People's social context and interpersonal relationships and their perceptions, beliefs and expectations are important factors in the maintenance of health, the development of illness, help-seeking behaviour and responses to treatment.

- The model encourages doctors/health care professionals to be aware of these factors and to practise more sensitively and effectively at the individual, family, community and national levels.

2 | Pregnancy and childbirth

This textbook appropriately starts at the beginning of life, at birth. It is also appropriate to use one of the most 'natural' life events as an introduction to the behavioural sciences. The birth of humans differs from births in other mammals in our social construction of the event. Social behaviour is guided by institutions and customs, not merely by instinctual needs; and perhaps nothing illustrates this basic sociological principle better than the sheer diversity of human practices at the time of pregnancy and childbirth. In other words, where, how and in whose presence a woman gives birth differs from one social setting to another. Human societies everywhere prescribe certain rituals and restrictions to pregnant and labouring women. For example, the place of delivery is often prescribed, be it a special village hut or a specialist obstetric hospital.

Pregnancy and childbirth are important life events that are often influenced by doctors. Every medical student is required to attend a certain number of deliveries. Doctors may be involved directly by providing antenatal or postnatal care or attending the birth, more indirectly through the provision of infertility treatment or birth control methods, or as backup for midwives in case something unexpected happens during a normal delivery.

The nature of pregnancy and childbirth

There are two major contrasting views on the nature of pregnancy and childbirth (Table 2.1). The first argues that both pregnancy and birth are normal events in most women's life cycle. This is often referred to as the *psychosocial model*. It is estimated that some 85% of all babies will be born without any problems and without the presence of a special birth attendant. Many of the risks in childbirth can be predicted, and, consequently, pregnant women most at risk can be selected for a hospital delivery in a specialist obstetric hospital. The remainder of pregnant women can opt for a less specialist setting such as a delivery in a community hospital or a home delivery. A proponent of this view is Tew (1990), who discovered, to her own surprise whilst preparing epidemiological exercises for medical students in Nottingham, that routine statistics did not support the widely accepted view that increased hospitalization for birth had caused a decline in the mortality of mothers and their babies.

The second and most commonly held view in nearly all Western societies is that pregnancy and particularly labour are risky events, where a number of things could go wrong. This is referred to as the *biomedical model*. Childbirth is, therefore, potentially pathological. Because we do not know what will happen to an individual pregnant woman, each one is best advised to deliver her baby in the safest possible environment. The specialist obstetric hospital with its high-technology screening equipment and supervision by obstetricians is regarded as the safest place to give birth. In short, pregnancy and childbirth are only safe in retrospect. Consequently, the majority of deliveries occurs (singular) in hospital. Fig. 2.1 contrasts the percentage of home births in the Netherlands with England and Wales, with the latter reflecting the trend in most industrialized countries.

Place of delivery

Maternity services in the UK have changed significantly over the past four decades, and one of the key changes has been that the woman has been put more centrally in the doctor–patient relationship (see pp. 88–89). More emphasis has been given to the woman's own involvement in her maternity care. More recently we have also seen a move towards more midwife-led care, and a small but growing interest in home birth. Until the late 20th century the trend has been towards more hospital deliveries. For example, an official report in 1970 recommended 100% hospital deliveries on the grounds of safety. Political opinion changed in the late 1980s towards more choice for women and consequently more deliveries outside obstetric units. The Winterton Report (1992) moved away from total hospitalization: 'The policy of encouraging all women to give birth in hospital cannot be justified on grounds of safety'. More recently, the Birthplace study, the largest study of its kind worldwide, came to the following conclusion: 'Women planning birth in a midwifery unit and multiparous women planning birth at home experience fewer interventions than those planning birth in an obstetric unit with no impact on perinatal outcomes' (Birthplace in England Collaborative Group, 2011).

Birth attendant

The two views of childbirth also differ with regard to who the desired attendant at birth is. If one holds the view that pregnancy and childbirth are only safe in retrospect, then the only acceptable birth attendant is the obstetrician, a specialist, just in case something goes wrong. If one holds the view that childbirth is a normal part in the life cycle of most women, then the most desirable birth attendant is the expert in normal deliveries, the midwife or the general practitioner (GP). Throughout history midwives have been, and continue to be, key health care attendants at birth. Over the past three centuries in most industrialized countries female midwives have slowly lost their control over childbirth to male doctors.

Pregnancy is often a time of great expectations and excitement relating to the birth of the child and the start of parenthood.

Table 2.1 **Models of childbirth**		
Model	**Psychosocial**	**Biomedical**
	'Childbirth normal/natural until pathology occurs'	'Childbirth only normal in retrospect'
Emphasis	Normality	Risk
	Woman centred	Doctor centred
	Social support	Risk reduction
	Woman = active	Woman = passive
	Health	Illness
	Individual	Statistical

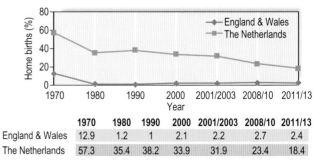

	1970	1980	1990	2000	2001/2003	2008/10	2011/13
England & Wales	12.9	1.2	1	2.1	2.2	2.7	2.4
The Netherlands	57.3	35.4	38.2	33.9	31.9	23.4	18.4

Fig. 2.1 Percentage of births out of hospital in England and Wales and the Netherlands. *(Sources: Office for National Statistics (England & Wales); Central Bureau voor de Statistiek (the Netherlands)).*

Women in modern Western societies have, on average, only two babies in their lifetime. At the same time, because obstetricians and/or midwives may attend deliveries many times a week or even a day, their expectations are considerably different from those of the expecting mother, and not only because the baby is not their own. Their priorities can be guided by medical requirements, hospital policies, or availability of resources (see Setting priorities and rationing, pp. 152–153). Such differences can easily lead to misunderstanding and dissatisfaction in the new parents (especially if the parties have not been able to get to know each other). Considering the role and status of health care professionals (see pp. 164–165) it is more likely that the mother would be disappointed than the birth attendant.

(see Setting priorities and rationing, pp. 152–153)

Case study

The Dutch example

The Netherlands is the only industrialized country where the proportion of all deliveries taking place out of specialist hospitals is substantial. At the moment approximately one-fifth of all deliveries take place in Dutch homes. The UK and the Netherlands are neighbouring countries with fairly similar levels of health care provision and a similar quality of specialist obstetric care; perinatal mortality rates do not differ substantially between the two countries. (*Perinatal mortality rate* refers to the number of stillbirths (after 28 weeks' gestation) plus the number of deaths occurring in the first 7 days after the delivery, divided by all live births and stillbirths.) Other outcome indicators suggest that the Dutch programme is good.

A number of factors have been suggested for this difference in the organization of maternity care:

- Pregnant women in the Netherlands are not regarded as patients, unless something goes wrong or the delivery is expected to be difficult for previously assessed reasons.
- Practical help is provided in the form of maternity home care assistants, who look after the mother and newborn baby at home for up to 8 days after the birth. They wash the baby, give advice on feeding, look after other children in the household, walk the dog, and so on.
- In case of low-risk pregnancies, the fee for a GP will be reimbursed only if there is no practising midwife in the area, and only in instances of high-risk pregnancies will the fee of an obstetrician be reimbursed.
- Midwives are trained to be independent and autonomous practitioners. They are not trained as nurses first but attend a separate 4-year midwifery course. The importance of independent training is, firstly, that nurses are trained to deal with illness and disease, whilst midwives are trained to deal with normal childbirth; and, secondly, that the hierarchical relationship between nurses and doctors tends to play a part in the medical decision-making process.
- Most midwives practise as independent practitioners in the community, similar to most dentists in the UK. As private entrepreneurs they have to be more consumer-friendly to attract customers.
- All major Dutch political parties agree that the midwife is the obvious person to provide maternity care and that birth should preferably take place at home.

One could, of course, argue that the UK and the Netherlands are different countries and therefore not comparable. However, the populations in these two neighbouring countries are not too different in terms of national income, the physiology of the average woman, life expectancy and many other socio-economic indicators. Although the funding for health care is different in these two countries, the organization of service provision and the quality of medical care are fairly similar. For example, the majority of all deliveries in the UK and the Netherlands are attended by midwives. In fact, one can turn the question of comparability round and ask, for example: Why is the proportion of home births equally low in the UK, Germany and the USA, whereas their organization of health care in general and of maternity care in particular is so different?

Stop and think

Pregnancy can be regarded as a 'normal state of health' in that it occurs without serious problems to most women in their lifetime. Pregnancy can also be seen as an 'illness' in that many women, for example, have morning sickness, experience a slowing down in physical functioning, seek medical care and/or deliver in hospital. How do you regard pregnancy and childbirth, and why?

Breast-feeding

Pregnancy is a time when many parents are particularly interested in health matters, and this offers an opportunity to promote health information. Breast-feeding has many health benefits (physical and psychological) and the World Health Organization (WHO, 2009) recommends that wherever possible infants should be fed exclusively on breast milk from birth until the first six months. Initiation rates are low (about 74% in England in 2014) and are closely related to educational levels. This contrasts with breast-feeding rates of about 98% in Scandinavia. Young mothers in low-income groups and who have fewer years of education are least likely to initiate and to continue breast-feeding. Health care professionals and peers can effectively support breast-feeding mothers to continue to breast-feed (Sikorski et al., 2003).

Stop and think

What does being pregnant and giving birth mean for:

- a midwife?
- an obstetrician?
- a medical student?
- a pregnant woman?
- her partner/husband?

Pregnancy and childbirth

- Biological events are never purely biological but always partly socially constructed.
- Where, how and in whose presence a woman gives birth differs from one culture to another.
- There are two different perspectives: (a) pregnancy is a normal event in most women's lives; and (b) childbirth is a risky event and only normal in retrospect.
- Pregnant women and health care professionals are likely to see the birth differently.
- Different ways of organizing health care can have profound effects on professionals and health care service users.

3 | Reproductive issues

Reproductive events include the onset of menstruation, conception, abortion, pregnancy, miscarriage, childbirth and menopause. Although mainly focussed on women, these events will involve men in areas such as sexual dysfunction, infertility and becoming a parent. Reproduction also encompasses a range of illnesses and processes such as testicular cancer, endometriosis, sexually transmitted infections, pelvic pain and premenstrual syndrome (PMS). These disorders and their treatments can have implications for fertility and reproduction. For example, endometriosis is associated with reduced fertility in women. Common procedures and treatments associated with reproduction include contraception, cervical smears and hormone replacement therapy (HRT). Reproductive issues raise strong ethical dilemmas such as at what point terminating a pregnancy is still morally defensible; the rights of donor parents and children of donors; and 'designer babies'.

Reproductive health can be viewed from different perspectives; for example, a biomedical perspective would see PMS as caused by fluctuations and imbalances in hormones associated with the menstrual cycle and requiring pharmacological treatment. A psychological perspective might examine how women's patterns of stress and behaviour contribute to worsening mood around menstruation, such as noticing particular triggers and maladaptive responses and finding coping strategies to help women respond in a more adaptive way. A social perspective might examine women's sociodemographic circumstances and levels of support or cultural expectations and narratives about PMS. This might lead to treatment providing practical or emotional support during critical times.

Often none of these perspectives on its own offers adequate explanation and hence a *biopsychosocial approach* (spread 1, see pp. 2–3) offers a more informed and holistic approach to treatment.

Menstruation

Intriguingly the menstrual cycle does not affect as many behavioural factors as is commonly believed. For example, research suggests that it does not affect food preferences. Chocolate cravings differ strongly across cultures, with 40% of American women craving chocolate during menstruation, compared with 4% of Spanish women (Zellner et al., 2004). This suggests that food preferences are culturally defined rather than physiological.

The menstrual cycle is also associated with physical and psychological symptoms just before menstruation (PMS), such as irritability, depression, labile mood, abdominal bloating and weight gain. PMS is most common in women aged between 25 and 35 years and is reported by up to 30% of women. In up to 8% of women these symptoms are very severe and affect their relationships, work and social functioning. This is referred to as *premenstrual dysphoric disorder* (PMDD). Women with a history of depression are more likely to suffer from PMDD, which is associated with poor overall health (Johnson, 2004). This makes it important to examine whether PMDD symptoms are being caused by the menstrual cycle or whether existing psychological problems are being made worse by it.

Transition to parenthood and mental health

Pregnancy and birth are a time of great physical and psychosocial transition (spread 2, pp. 4–5). Psychosocial factors such as stress in pregnancy are also associated with poor outcomes such as preterm birth, low birth weight and delayed development (see Case study).

The transition to parenthood is a time of great adjustment and change. In new parents this can exacerbate existing mental health problems or provoke new conditions. It has been estimated that up to 20% of women develop some form of mental health problem during pregnancy or after birth and that this costs the UK some £8 billion per year.

Potential mental health problems include 'baby blues', anxiety, depression, post-traumatic stress disorder (PTSD), puerperal psychosis and bonding disorders. 'Baby blues' is very common and comprises a brief period of emotional lability in the first week after birth. It is usually mild and resolves quickly without treatment. It can be linked to the large fluctuations in hormones in the first week after birth. Depression and anxiety are common and occur during pregnancy or after birth in approximately 10% to 15% of women. In addition, 3% of women develop PTSD after a traumatic birth. PTSD is particularly interesting because presumably a proportion of this could be prevented through providing appropriate support and care during birth. PTSD is associated with a negative subjective experience during birth, poor support, operative delivery and women dissociating. Puerperal psychosis is a rare but severe disorder that occurs in 0.1% of women. Women and their babies are at high risk of harm, including infanticide and suicide, so this requires immediate hospitalization. Women with a personal or family history of psychosis or bipolar disorder are more likely to develop puerperal psychosis. Some women develop severe mental health disorders, but many more develop moderate symptoms. These moderate symptoms can still be distressing and can have severe consequences, as shown in Fig. 3.1, which presents some results from a survey of 1,500 women.

A number of risk factors make it more likely women will develop perinatal mental health problems. Some of these risk factors are remarkably consistent across different disorders and cultures. For example, mental health problems are more likely to occur if women live in social adversity (e.g. deprivation, low socio-economic status, domestic violence), have a history of

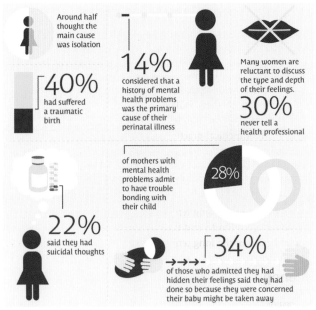

Fig. 3.1 Perinatal mental health survey of women with moderate distress.

psychological problems or childhood adversity and poor support available to them. In addition, if women are anxious or depressed during pregnancy, this is likely to continue or worsen postpartum.

Mental health problems during and after pregnancy are important because of the negative impact they have on women and their families. Women's mental health during pregnancy affects the developing foetus through neuro-biological foetal programming, which can have a long-term effect on the child's development and health. Infants of mothers who are stressed and anxious in pregnancy show more fearful behaviour and increased physiological stress responses. Longer-term anxiety and depression in pregnancy are associated with poor emotional and behavioural development, which can persist into adolescence (see Case study).

After birth, mental health problems have a negative impact on the relationship between the mother and the baby and between the woman and her partner. Women with mental health problems are less sensitive to their babies' emotional state and display less optimal parenting, such as being withdrawn and unavailable to the baby or over-intrusive. It is therefore not surprising that postnatal mental health problems are associated with children developing an insecure or disorganized attachment style, which, in turn, is associated with poor mental health in childhood and later in adulthood. Similarly, poor mental health in parents is one of many factors associated with child maltreatment. These are some of the mechanisms through which mental health problems and social adversity can be transmitted inter-generationally.

Treatment and interventions at this time are therefore important to prevent the transmission of social adversity and mental health problems between generations. Progress in this regard is patchy, with a recent report showing very few areas in the UK have adequate perinatal psychology services (www.everyonesbusiness.co.uk). More advances have been made in providing parenting interventions, some of which have been shown to be effective at improving parenting and secure attachment in infants (www.CANparent.org.uk).

High-risk pregnancies and birth

Pregnancy loss can be particularly difficult and includes miscarriage, termination of pregnancy and stillbirth. Approximately one in five pregnancies ends in miscarriage. Although often thought of as a lesser event than stillbirth, miscarriage can be distressing for women and result in depression or PTSD with between 10% and 50% of women reporting symptoms of depression (Lok and Neugebauer, 2007) and around 11% reporting symptoms of PTSD (Daugirdaite, van den Akker and Purewal, 2015).

Worldwide every year 2.64 million babies are stillborn after 24 weeks of pregnancy and in most cases the reason for death is unexplained. Studies unanimously find this is an intensely painful loss for parents, with reports of intense grief, marital difficulties, feelings of worthlessness, isolation, shame and guilt. Around a third of women report high levels of anxiety, depression and/or PTSD. Current medical practice offers parents a chance to see and hold their dead infants on the assumption that it will help them in their grieving process. However, the evidence for this is inconsistent, and some research suggests that although parents appreciate the opportunity to do this, they may have poorer mental health in the long term. Stigma and reduced chances to talk about the stillbirth and the baby appear to contribute to poor mental health in the long term (Crawley, Lomax and Ayers, 2013).

Menopause

Menopause is defined as the last menstrual period, which happens on average around 50 years of age (range 45–55 years). During menopause the majority of women in Western cultures experience symptoms such as hot flushes, night sweats, loss of libido, irritability, problems with skin or hair, vaginal dryness and headaches. In terms of mental health, there is no consistent evidence for poor psychological well-being during this period. A biomedical perspective would see menopause as caused by a hormonal deficiency. Treatment would therefore be using HRT to replace the missing hormone, oestrogen. In contrast, a socio-cultural perspective would view menopause as a natural process, where symptoms or experiences are culturally constructed. Thus any distress would result from negative stereotypes or attitudes about menopause and ageing and the coincidence of menopause with significant role changes in women's lives. In cultures where menopause increases prestige for women, such as the Indian and Native American cultures, much lower levels of symptoms are reported. However, when migrant populations move from such cultures to live in Western cultures, their menopausal symptoms increase. In Western cultures it has been found that concurrent stressful events are important predictors of women's well-being during menopause. Stress may also influence the production of hormones, having a physiological effect on women's experience, supporting the biopsychosocial approach mentioned previously.

Stop and think

A young woman who was sexually abused as a child is now accidentally pregnant. She is not in a committed relationship with the father of the baby. How might she feel about the pregnancy? What kind of issues might she be facing?

Case study

The foetal programming hypothesis suggests mental health problems during pregnancy can affect the neuro-biological development of the foetus and therefore the health of the child later in life. O'Donnell et al. (2014) used data on 7944 families to examine this hypothesis. Their results showed that anxiety in the mother during pregnancy predicted more behavioural and emotional problems for the child throughout childhood and adolescence. Children of mothers who were anxious or depressed in pregnancy were also up to two times more likely to have a mental health disorder. These associations remained after controlling statistically for potential confounding factors such as psychosocial and obstetric risks, mental health in mothers and fathers and parenting styles, illustrating the inter-generational transmission of mental health problems.

Reproductive issues

- Reproductive issues cover a wide variety of issues, events and illnesses that are relevant to both men and women.
- Reproductive issues exist in biomedical, psychological, social and cultural contexts, and thus a biopsychosocial approach needs to be taken.
- Becoming a parent is a time of transition and adjustment and is associated with relationship strains and mental health problems.
- Perinatal mental health problems have a severe and potentially long-lasting impact on mother and baby, so appropriate intervention is critical.
- Many symptoms associated with the menstrual cycle and menopause are associated with psychosocial and cultural factors.

4 | Development in early infancy

Early infancy is a crucial period for building the foundations of physical, cognitive and emotional development. What happens during the early years will have a profound effect on various dimensions, including physical and psychosocial well-being, educational attainment and socio-economic status in later life. This spread will discuss key issues relating to (1) the assessment of infant behaviour in the days and weeks after birth; (2) the early development of communication in the first year of life; (3) the emotional attachments between infants and their mothers (or other carers) and (4) the consequences of maternal mental health problems for infant development. Research on these topics shows us how important it is to see infants within the context of their relationships with their carers.

Neonatal assessment

Infants are born with reflexes and behaviours that enable them to respond to the world and develop rapidly. For example, in the first few days after birth, babies are able to imitate facial expressions, selectively respond to humans or human-like objects and rapidly develop a preference for characteristics associated with their carers.

A variety of physiological and observational methods have been developed to assess aspects of development and behaviour in the first few months after birth such as visual acuity, auditory assessments, stress immune responses, temperament, learning and attention. Advances in ultrasonography have also enabled researchers to examine prenatal foetal development as a precursor of neonatal development.

A widely used measure of early neonatal development is the Brazelton Neonatal Behavioral Assessment Scale, which measures behavioural and reflex responses and is used to assess 10 areas of sensory, motor, emotional and physical development at birth and during the first 2 months of life. After 1 month, development can be measured by the Bayley Scales of Infant and Toddler Development, which are appropriate for infants up to 42 months of age. These scales involve specific interactions with the infant through play to assess cognitive, motor and language development, as well as two parent questionnaires to

social–emotional development and adaptive behaviour.

The advantages of these kinds of measures of neonatal development are that they help us build a detailed profile of infants' functioning, identify developmental delays or difficulties and recommend appropriate interventions. They are also helpful for understanding how particular psychosocial circumstances such as drug use in pregnancy or maternal depression (see following section on maternal mental health) may be associated with delayed development.

Communication in the first year

Careful studies of infants' interactions with other people have revealed the extensive growth in communicative skills during the first year of life. Although it is not until around 12 months of age that infants produce their first words, they start cooing (vowel-like sounds such as 'oo') and babbling (consonant–vowel combinations such as 'bababa') much earlier. Furthermore, infants show they can understand some words from as young as 6 months (Tincoff and Jusczyk, 1999).

To understand the building blocks of language development in infancy, we need to look at more than the comprehension and production of spoken language. Infants' earliest experiences provide them with opportunities to learn about turn-taking and to use and respond to emotional expressions. For example, activities such as nappy-changing, breast-feeding and bathing often involve 'dialogues' where the baby and the carer respond to each other's sounds, gestures and facial expressions. Research has demonstrated that infants in the first year of life can interpret others' emotional expressions and use them to guide their own behaviour (see Case study). Moreover, babies can also give cues for carers to respond to their needs by crying, giggling and seeking eye contact (see section on Infant-carer attachment later).

A particularly important aspect of early communication is *joint attention*, a state where both the infant and the mother are focussing on the same object or event. Between 9 and 15 months, babies develop an increasingly refined ability to follow the gaze of an adult and also to initiate and direct joint attention by using gestures such as pointing (Carpenter et al., 1998;

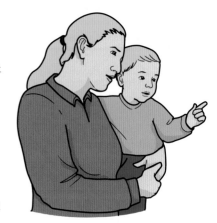

Fig. 4.1 Pointing.

Fig. 4.1). Psychologists have shown that infants can use gestures to direct carers' attention to an interesting sight or object (e.g. pointing to a dog) and to get carers to do something (e.g. pointing to ask for a toy). Carers often respond enthusiastically to these gestures, providing verbal labels (e.g. 'Oh yes, what a lovely doggy!') that contribute to the infants' language development.

Infant–carer attachment

The great strides made by infants in their communicative skills take place within emotionally intense relationships, or *attachments*, formed with their mothers (or other primary carers) during the first 2 years of life.

Previous behavioural theories indicated that attachment was the result of the feeding relationship between infants and the carers, but psychologists now view this as simplistic. Bowlby's (1969) attachment theory suggests that attachment has an evolutionary basis, involving inbuilt signals from the infant (crying, smiling, grasping, etc.) that elicit caregiving responses from the mother. The mother/primary carer's availability and responsiveness to the infant's needs will provide the child a secure base to explore the world and develop healthy trusting relationships with others in later life.

In the first few months of life, infants become increasingly able to differentiate between their mothers and unfamiliar individuals in terms of how they look, sound and smell. But it is not until around 6 to 8 months that infants begin to show the key features of attachment to their mothers or other primary carers. These include a desire to maintain physical closeness to the carers and distress upon separation from them. As babies begin to crawl and explore the world around them, the carer becomes an important secure base. The distress that infants display when separated from their carers tends to increase into the second year of life, but then starts to decline as the infants develop into more self-aware, independent toddlers.

Importantly, the nature of the attachment relationship can differ widely from one family to another. Ainsworth's (1978) pioneering work observing infants' interactions with their mothers demonstrated that whereas most attachments showed the qualities described earlier, others did not: some 12-month-olds seemed to have little interest in maintaining proximity to their mothers and were untroubled by separation, whereas others were extremely clingy with their mothers and were so distressed by separation that they could not even be comforted by their mothers upon reunion. Research has shown that these kinds of differences relate to features of the infant (e.g. temperamental characteristics such as irritability), as well as to qualities of the care received from the mother (e.g. the sensitivity and responsiveness shown towards the infant).

Case study

In one famous series of studies, Sorce et al. (1985) showed that 12-month-old infants clearly pay attention to their mothers' facial expressions in ambiguous situations. The studies made use of the so-called visual cliff apparatus – a Plexiglas table with a 'shallow' side created by placing a patterned material immediately beneath the table top and a 'deep' side created by placing the patterned material some distance beneath the table top. Infants were placed on the shallow side and were encouraged to approach an attractive toy placed on the deep side. As most infants approached the 'cliff' separating the shallow and deep sides, they looked to their mothers for guidance (Fig. 4.2). In one of these studies 14 out of 19 infants who saw their mothers posing a happy expression went on to cross the deep side. But out of the 17 infants whose mothers posed a fearful expression, not one ventured across the cliff, highlighting their sensitivity to carers' facial expressions as a source of information about the world.

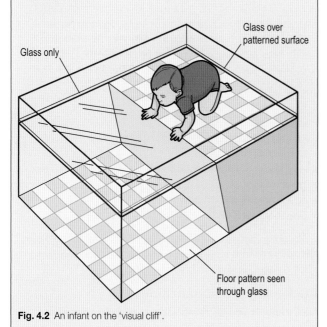

Glass only

Glass over patterned surface

Floor pattern seen through glass

Fig. 4.2 An infant on the 'visual cliff'.

Effects of maternal mental health problems

Maternal mental health has a variety of effects on infant and child development. A considerable amount of evidence shows that maternal depression is associated with poor cognitive and emotional development in the first 2 years of infant development (Murray and Cooper, 1997). This may be caused by the impact of postnatal depression on the quality of the interaction between the mother and infant. For example, one study found that impaired cognitive development in babies at 18 months was predicted by features such as mothers' insensitivity to their baby's experience and their failure to communicate actively with their baby (Murray et al., 1996). The effect of postnatal depression on later development of the child is less clear, although there is some evidence that children of depressed mothers, particularly boys, have more behavioural difficulties. Furthermore evidence shows that mothers from socially excluded groups (single mothers, immigrant mothers, etc.) are more susceptible to maternal depression during the postpartum period (Falah-Hassani et al., 2015).

An exciting and relatively new area of research examines the effects of stress and mental health during pregnancy as a precursor to early infant development. This research suggests that stress in pregnancy is associated with a range of adverse infant outcomes such as increased risk of hyperactivity, anxiety and delayed language and cognitive development (Talge et al., 2007). In line with this, Diego et al. (2005) found that babies of mothers who were depressed in pregnancy were more likely to cry, fuss and show signs of stress compared with babies of women who were not depressed during pregnancy or were only depressed after birth.

Finally, it is important to remember that infant development needs to be examined in the context of the whole family. For example, a recent study of over 10,000 children found that even after controlling for maternal depression, paternal depression was associated with poor emotional and behavioural outcomes in children aged $3\frac{1}{2}$ years (Ramchandani et al., 2005). However, other studies also showed that social support provided on the basis of the needs of families during the postpartum period will empower mothers who suffer from postpartum depression to bond with their babies (Yuan et al., 2011; Dennis and Dowswell, 2013; Reid and Taylor, 2015).

Stop and think

- Compare the reactions of a 2-month-old infant and a 12-month-old infant to separation from their mother (or other primary carer). How do they differ, and why?

- Observe a parent with a baby under the age of 1 year, and note how they communicate with each other. Pay attention not just to words and sounds but also to facial expressions, gestures and turn-taking.

Development in early infancy

- Neonatal behavioural assessment can be used to screen for early developmental problems.

- Infants learn to communicate with their carers through vocalizations, gestures and turn-taking before they produce their first word.

- Infants form intense emotional relationships with their primary carers during the first year of life, with significant increases in proximity-seeking and separation distress between 6 and 12 months of age.

- Mothers' mental health problems can have significant consequences for the early cognitive, social and emotional development of their infants.

5 | Childhood and child health

Childhood is a process of transition from vulnerability and high dependence towards autonomy. The risk of serious ill health interfering in this process has been significantly reduced in most affluent countries, but there remain considerable inequalities in health and life chances between the least and the most deprived children in the UK. There were dramatic reductions in children's mortality in the 20th century from infectious and environmental diseases, but congenital disorders and cancers are now relatively more predominant, and there are increasing numbers of children with chronic health problems and complex disabilities (Crowley et al., 2011).

Key topics

Child poverty and inequalities in health

Social and economic factors that affect child health and development include parental unemployment, parental depression, smoking during pregnancy, household overcrowding and financial stress. Evidence suggests that anxiety, aggression, confidence, emotional and cognitive development, concentration, and readiness for school at the end of reception year are all related to socio-economic status. Fig. 5.1 displays some key child public health indicators for 2012 to 2013 for England as a whole and for the 10% most deprived and least deprived areas. These inequalities in physical and psychological health can then persist throughout the life course, and consequently there is now increasing emphasis on the importance of early interventions and getting a good start in life. Schools have taken a greater role in both universal and targeted approaches to promote health and build resilience. Examples of such programmes include Healthy Schools and Place2Be (see Case study box: Place2Be).

Mortality

In 2012 over 5000 children under 19 years of age died in the UK. In data from 1980 to 2010, all-cause mortality continued to decline (RCPCH and UCL, 2013). The leading cause of child death after the first year of life was injury, followed by cancer and blood conditions. The most common causes of injury were transport accidents, drowning and self-harm. Whilst deaths from unintentional injuries decreased between 1980 and 2010, probably as a result of new

policies, there was no parallel decline in deaths resulting from self-harm, assault or other undetermined intentional injuries in 10 to 18-year-olds, and the UK's child mortality rate remains higher than comparable countries in Western Europe (Fig. 5.2).

Childhood obesity

Childhood obesity has been identified by the World Health Organization (WHO) as one of the top public health challenges for the 21st century. Obesity in childhood is associated with wide-ranging effects from low self-esteem to school absence, and an increased risk of overweight, ill health and premature mortality as an adult. Obese children are more likely to become obese mothers later in life, carrying health risks for mother and child. Prevalence of childhood overweight increased markedly between 1995 and 2004, and although this rise may now have tapered off, levels remain a concern (see pp. 106–107). Approximately a fifth of children aged 4 to 5 years and a third of those aged 10 to 11 years are overweight or obese, and unhealthy weight in children is twice as prevalent in the most deprived 10% of the population as in the least deprived 10%.

Mental health and well-being

One in ten children in the UK has a mental health disorder, with the most common being conduct and oppositional defiant disorders, anxiety disorders and attention deficit hyperactivity disorder. Despite evidence for the existence of effective interventions such as cognitive behavioural therapy (see pp. 138–139), only a minority is estimated to receive treatment.

Children experiencing mental health problems are at increased risk of a range of adverse outcomes, ranging from school exclusion and educational underachievement to relationship problems and poorer physical health. There is a high rate of continuity between child and adult mental health disorders – around half of adults with a psychiatric disorder aged 26 years first met diagnostic criteria between the ages of 11 and 15 years, and almost three-quarters had symptoms by the age of 18 years. Mental health and well-being in children is influenced by individual factors such as genetics but is also affected by the wider home and community environments. Whilst a secure home and supportive parenting build resilience, a number of factors represent risks to mental health. Such factors may be present even before the child is conceived or born, and include the following (WHO, 2012):

- Substance use in pregnancy
- Parental mental illness
- Insecure attachment
- Family violence or conflict
- Physical ill health
- Poor housing and overcrowding
- Trauma and abuse
- Adverse learning environment
- Neighbourhood violence and crime

Emerging concerns related to social media, new technology and mental health also include sleep disturbance from gadget use, 'selfie culture', 'sexting' and cyberbullying.

Adolescence and transitions

Adolescence is a time of rapid and extensive psychological and biological growth. It is also a crucial time for adult health, as five of the ten WHO main risk factors for adult disease may be initiated or established. These are tobacco use, physical inactivity, overweight, unsafe sex and alcohol use. Improvements have been made recently in some of these risk factors: there have been

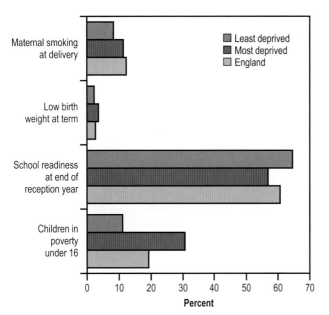

Fig. 5.1 Key Child Public Health Indicators for 2012–2013, for England and by deprivation decile *(from Department of Public Health, England, 2015).*

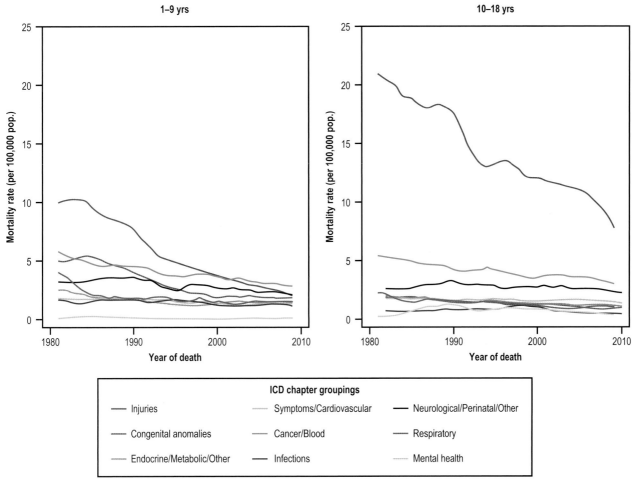

Fig. 5.2 Smoothed child mortality rates by age group, year and underlying cause (grouped), UK 1980–2010 *(from RCPCH and UCL, 2013).*

reductions in the prevalence of smoking, drinking and drug use amongst people aged 10 to 24 years, as well as in the numbers of teenage pregnancies (Public Health England, 2014). Young people are also learning to manage chronic conditions such as asthma and diabetes, meaning that help to initiate positive self-management in adolescence is crucial to longer-term health.

Late adolescence is full of transitions to be negotiated, in the spheres of education, employment and relationships. Historically in health services the transition from child to adult services has taken place at 16 or 18 years. This transition of care has been associated with adverse health outcomes such as poorer glycaemic control in diabetes as well as increased loss to follow-up from services for those who have been through cancer or cardiac surgery. There is now increasing recognition that the phase of late adolescent brain development continues into the mid-20s and that the under-25s are likely to have needs best met by youth-oriented services.

Stop and think

Did any changes in your adolescent years worry you at the time?

Childhood and child health

- All-cause child mortality has continued to decline since 1980; but the UK's child mortality rates are higher than comparable European countries.

- The leading cause of death in children over one year is injury.

- There remain considerable inequalities in health and life chances between the least and the most deprived children.

- Mental health disorders affect one in ten children in the UK, and such children are at increased risk of a range of adverse psychological, educational and social outcomes.

- The transition from adolescence to adulthood is a crucial period for health when many risk factors for disease are initiated or established. Young people with health problems are likely to require specialist services during this time.

Case study *Place2Be (http://www.place2be.org.uk/)*

Place2Be is a charity that is commissioned by schools nationally to provide emotional and therapeutic services, building children's resilience through talking, creative work and play. This charity currently works in over 200 schools. Place2Be also provides support for parents, teachers and other school staff to deal with issues such as depression, divorce and stress management.

Over four years of analysis, consistent improvements in well-being have been reported by teachers, parents and children. Of children identified as having problems that interfered with their classroom learning, 59% were more able to focus on their classroom learning after support from Place2Be. Children who fell into the 'abnormal' clinical category pre-intervention reported lessened difficulties after intervention according to self-reporting by teachers, parents and children. The programme estimated that for every £1 spent on the counselling support services, there is a cost saving of £6. This includes reduced costs associated with social services, welfare benefits and the criminal justice system.

6 | Adolescence

Adolescence describes a period of transition between childhood and full adult roles. In some cultures this follows rapidly after puberty and sometimes involves a formal initiation rite but, in Western societies such as the UK, many people in their mid-20s have still not taken on all adult responsibilities. For example, they may still not have left home, are unlikely to have children and may have several shorter-term relationships and jobs rather than a sole marriage or career. The ages at which different adult activities are permitted vary. Thus adolescents are expected to behave in some ways like adults and in other ways like children. Parents and children often disagree about which roles are appropriate at a given age. Since the 1950s there has also been increasing identification of 'youth' as a distinct and positively valued life phase, which has changed rapidly (Table 6.1).

The physical changes of puberty are important. However, the psychological changes are also vital to understand and are caused very often by the difficulties of adolescent roles. Adolescents have near-adult intellectual abilities (although not necessarily adult knowledge or experience) and soon acquire adult physical abilities. Neurological development continues into young adulthood, and it has been suggested that adolescents' cognitions and hence behaviours tend to be more impulsive and less risk-averse than those of adults because of this delay in brain development (Steinberg, 2007). Adolescents also have to cope with important emotional, sexual and moral development. Parents and children can often disagree about which behaviours are appropriate and at what age. The influential theorist Eric Erikson (1968) described adolescence as a time of forming adult identity.

Two sources of strain are:

1. Having to choose and adjust to adult roles. Many adolescents experiment with a variety of roles and behaviours before settling down with what suits them. This experimentation often includes activities that seem extreme to adults; for example, youth fashions often offend older sensibilities.
2. Disputes over rights and responsibilities. Adolescents often complain that adults expect them to have adult responsibilities without adult freedoms: to be responsible enough to baby-sit, but not responsible enough to choose when to have sex. Adults often feel the opposite, that adolescents expect adult freedoms without adult responsibilities: to be free to choose what time to come in, but not to be willing to help with housework.

Despite these strains, most adolescents have a fairly untroubled time and get on relatively well with their parents, and Table 6.2 shows how parenting styles can affect children. Most adolescents' interests and aspirations are similar to adults'. However, about 20% of adolescents experience personal problems (Coleman and Hendry, 1999). Many troubled adolescents abuse drugs or alcohol, engage in some criminal activities, may do poorly or drop out of school and are likely to be depressed or unhappy. They are also likely to engage in behaviours inappropriate for their age, although not considered a problem for older people. Both sexual intercourse and drinking alcohol are considered age-inappropriate for people under 14 years of age (note this is not just a legal definition, but a social norm). For most this is a temporary phase lasting a few years, but some troubled adolescents become adults with problems. Early intervention can help some adolescents, but there is also a risk of labelling someone as mentally ill, drug-addicted or delinquent, actually making problems worse (see pp. 60–61).

The two most common social psychological explanations of risk-taking in adolescents are that they have a sense of invulnerability and that they do not think in abstract ways about the future consequences of their own actions. More sociological explanations have suggested that risk-taking behaviour is a part of some youth subcultures that provide identity and meaning within a larger or dominant adult culture that is seen as irrelevant, unrewarding (or even punitive) and meaningless to their experience and life chances.

Table 6.1 Life for young people today has changed compared with 50 years ago

More	Less
Celebrating diversity	Marriage
Brands	Permanent jobs
Travel	Local community
Virtual and networked interactions	Social class
Social media	Left–right politics
Serial monogamy	Physical activity
Body decoration and body concerns	Perceived safely and security
Reality TV	
Recreational drug use	

Table 6.2 Effects of combined parenting styles on adolescent development

Two dimensions of parenting style	Hostile Cold, neglects or ignores child's needs, uses punishment to control behaviour	Loving Warm, accepts child's needs, attends to child, uses praise to control behaviour
Authoritarian Makes strict, rigid unrealistic demands on child's behaviour	Parent is consistently strict and punishing Some parents may be physically or sexually abusive Adolescent develops internalized anger: neuroses, depression or anxiety, suicide attempts	This extreme combination is unlikely because rigid demands require ignoring child's needs In less extreme form, the child may become an 'overachiever' in an unsuccessful effort to please the parent
Authoritative Has clear expectations for behaviour, but these are flexible, realistic and negotiable	This combination of styles is unlikely because hostility precludes clear flexible expectations	Parent provides good guidance The ideal combination, likely to lead to a well-adjusted adult
Uninvolved	Adolescent is withdrawn, has low self-esteem, performs more poorly academically and is mistrustful of others	How can a parent be 'loving' yet uninvolved?
Permissive Makes few demands on behaviour and provides few guidelines for child	Parent largely ignores child's behaviour and punishes inconsistently Some parents may be physically or sexually abusive Adolescent develops externalized anger: acting-out behaviour, delinquency, drug abuse	Parent treats child too much as an equal: child is 'spoiled' Major role conflicts, less extreme acting-out behaviour Child forced to 'be the parent'

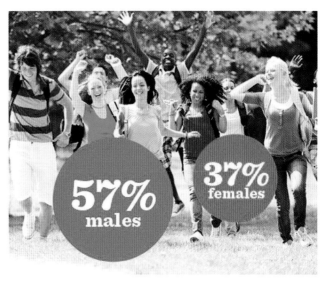

Fig. 6.1 Percentage of high school students who reported 60 minutes of physical activity on 5 or more days in the past week.

Youth is perceived as a time of resilience when a young body can cope with overindulgence: young people will take exercise more because of concerns about attractiveness than for health reasons. Even a simple review of the health statistics tends to support this. With the exception of accidents for boys, young people are generally much healthier than older people, so the class gradient in health is less steep for adolescents.

Health care needs of adolescents

Drug abuse, alcohol abuse (including accidents whilst intoxicated) and suicide are among the leading causes of death in adolescents, and there are also concerns about rising obesity levels in this age group as a result of sedentary lifestyles (caused by too much screen use, car use and overheated buildings) and overeating. Interventions to improve health and well-being nowadays tend to try and tackle lifestyle holistically and involve parents and entire communities; one example with evidence of success is the EPODE

international network (epode-international-network.com) (Fig. 6.1). Adolescents may also have special health concerns related to their rapid physical development, including concerns about their sexual development, acne, allergies, fatigue, headaches and concerns about body size, diet and exercise. Many adolescents are somewhat uncomfortable about their bodies, and they may be very self-conscious about aspects of health care.

The provision of health care to adolescents can be problematic because they do not fit easily into child or adult services.

7 | Social aspects of ageing

There is a widespread view that ageing is an inevitable process of physical and psychological decline produced by biological change. In this biomedical view (see pp. 2–3), ageing is seen rather mechanistically as a result of the increase in life expectancy. The solutions proposed to the 'problem of ageing' tend, therefore, to be medical. Ageing, however, is a lifelong process involving an interaction between biological, psychological and social factors. Therefore care for older people must involve these three dimensions.

Social scientists acknowledge biological ageing but highlight that the process must be understood in terms of the social environment. Thus ageing can be described as a *relational experience*: that is, changes taking place in the body alter our relationships with other people, the environment and the wider society. For example, a statutory retirement age changes people's status in personal and public spheres, but there is no biological reason for retirement at 60 or 65 years. Ageing into old age is a gradual process that varies individually. Hence there is no universal answer to the question: when does old age begin?

Ageism

Ageism, or prejudice and discrimination against people simply because they are old, is perhaps simply a reflection of our fears of growing old in a society that values youth. This fear is associated with the belief that chronological age inevitably results in mental and physical decline. Jerrome (1992) studied old people's clubs and concluded that old age should be defined as a state of feeling and behaving rather than a chronological state. She observed that older people work hard to cope with the ageing of their bodies and often turn physical ageing into a personal challenge. Involvement in club activities helps them explore the meaning of growing older and negotiate the point at which it is socially acceptable to acknowledge frailty or illness and withdraw from social activities. Talking about illness is not, therefore, a self-pitying preoccupation, but a social process through which older people come to understand changes in their roles and decide how they should behave: 'One cannot be ill by oneself and know that one is ill' (Jerrome, 1992 p. 101) – feelings and experiences have to be tested out with others.

The ageing body and the self

A better understanding of ageing as a personal experience grounded in social relationships requires more information about the relationships that older people experience in everyday life. Language, for example, has an important part to play. Coupland et al. (1991) showed how age identities are shaped in sequences of talk. References to ageing and old age by both younger and older women do not necessarily indicate the older women's experience of ageing but reflects assumptions that older people are preoccupied with old age. Aspects of age-related speech include the disclosure of chronological age, references to time passing, self-association with the past and recognition of social change over time. Age identity is a fluid process that varies according to time, place and the people involved.

Older people may retain an image of themselves as younger. This leads to a disjunction between how people experience themselves and how their bodies are, so the self may be experienced as a kind of 'ageless' or youthful prisoner inside an ageing body. The ageing body and face act as a kind of mask disguising the inner sense of personal selfhood or identity (Hepworth, 1995; Biggs, 1999). The relationship between the body and the self is, therefore, complicated by perceptions of the body and the value placed upon it. People who value their youth and beauty may be much unhappier with their bodies as they grow older compared with those who value the inner self more. The latter may find physical ageing less burdensome and an opportunity for personal development. It is, therefore, important to find out how people perceive their bodies as they grow older as well as looking for information about biological change.

Perhaps the reason why health care professionals think all old people are infirm and ill is that they encounter this group most frequently. However, acknowledging that older people may not think of themselves as 'older' may help understand their feelings and behaviours. It also cautions us against stereotyping older patients.

The ageing mind

It is commonly believed that older people are incapable of learning new things and are depressed and that intelligence declines with age. At one time there appeared to be a substantial body of evidence showing that intelligence declines with age (see pp. 30–31). However, longitudinal studies (Schaie, 1996) showed that when the same individuals were tested over time, there was very little change in intelligence scores (Fig. 7.1).

Does the ability to learn decline with age? It seems to take older people longer to search their memory stores to retrieve information. Therefore doctors should give older patients more time to 'find' the answers to questions. Filling the silence with other questions can lead to a breakdown in communication (see pp. 94–95).

Older and younger subjects differ in the ability to filter out irrelevant information, referred to as the 'cocktail party' effect. When young people go to a party they have little difficulty filtering out the irrelevant conversations around them. Older people find this difficult. Studies involve asking subjects to listen to headphones in which one message is played to the left ear and a different one to the right. The subject is asked to follow only one message (so-called dichotic listening experiments). As people age, more and more information from the 'wrong' ear appears in the test (Stuart-Hamilton, 1994).

These findings are relevant to the practice of medicine:

● When taking a history or explaining something to an older patient, ensure that there are as few distracting and irrelevant

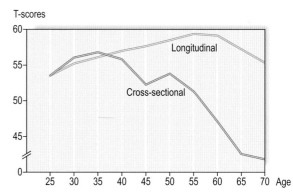

Fig. 7.1 Findings from cross-sectional and longitudinal studies of intelligence and age.

noises about as possible; patients find it stressful to have to struggle to listen to and concentrate on one particular conversation.

- It is not uncommon for middle-aged patients to ask GPs to have their hearing tested or for earwax to be removed. Testing often reveals no wax and little decrement in the acuity of the patient's hearing. The patient goes away frustrated and still convinced that he or she is going deaf. Explanation of this 'central processing' phenomenon usually provides reassurance.

Dementia and Alzheimer's disease

Alzheimer's disease has been described as the loss of self. Sabat and Harré (1992) divided the self into two parts: self i and selves ii. Self i is the personal singularity indicated by the use of expressions such as 'I', 'me' and 'mine', which is made possible by the structure of language. The 'I' is the sense of personal identity we all possess. Selves ii is the social aspect of identity, and this is made up of an ensemble of social selves that is displayed during our relationships with others. Selves ii require the collaboration of other people in recognizing our various social identities. These are the selves that are socially presented: public expressions of a type of character drawn from a 'local repertoire' (Sabat and Harré, 1992: 452). For example, we may present different identities as 'student', 'neighbour' and 'daughter'.

Sociological studies of dementia suggest that the process may be more than simple loss of capabilities caused by physical changes. Kitwood (1997: 31) developed a person-centred approach to understanding dementia, suggesting that the changes that are observable not only tend to result from biomedical factors but also are related to loss of resources, including social support for the self. Biomedical change is, therefore, aggravated by changes in the responses of other people to the sufferer when they withdraw the social support he or she needs to continue maintaining a social self. Thus social support and interaction are also factors in the development and manifestation of dementia. Kitwood (1997) argued that 'those who are well supported only very rarely suggest that their relative has acquired a different personality or "disappeared". Perhaps they have found ways of maintaining relationships and communication and can deal more accurately with their own feelings of loss and bewilderment'.

Ageing and social change

Comments on the increasing prevalence in dementia are often followed by a statement about our 'ageing society'. Increased life expectancy and decreases in the birth rate mean that people over 50 years will no longer be a minority group in industrialized countries. This change will not necessarily result in an increased burden of older people (Coleman et al., 1993) because evidence shows that many older people continue to make an active contribution to social life. As politicians recognize the votes to be won in the age group, it may affect policy proposals about health care facilities that favour older people. For example, the Netherlands saw the emergence of the 'old folks' party in politics. The role of grandparents as babysitters (and carers for others) and debates in many countries about increasing the retirement age are examples of active roles of older people.

Demographic change means that the traditional views of the roles of older people in society are less relevant. The experience of ageing is changing and becoming more diverse as societies become more complex, and new models and images of ageing have to be created (Fig. 7.2). Hence it is no longer acceptable to regard life after the age of 50 years as a period of decline into old

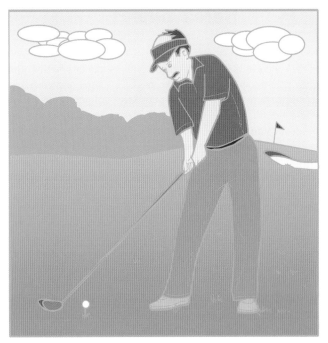

Fig. 7.2 The experience and image of ageing are changing.

age. Care provision is not just a matter of looking after the body but must, therefore, change to ensure the continuity of personal identity and individual independence in later life.

Case study

The writer Linda Grant (1998) provides a moving account of the effects of Alzheimer's disease on the 'self' of her mother Rose (who suffered from Alzheimer's disease) and on herself. She discusses in vivid detail Rose's gradually developing sense of confusion as a threat to her mother's sense of identity. Rose is sometimes aware of the changes taking place in her ability to control her presentation of self, on the occasions when she would show she was 'ashamed, embarrassed and afraid of [the] response [of other people]. She had cut herself off because she could no longer manage the skills she needed to be in company ... "I cringe inside when someone tells me I'm repeating myself," she said once, in a rare acknowledgment'.

The experience persuaded Grant that individuals do not have a fixed identity through their lives, but experience a range of selves throughout their lives.

Stop and think

- 'You're only as old as you feel!' How does this relate to the old people you know, perhaps your grandparents or older family friends?

Social aspects of ageing

- Biological ageing occurs in social environments.
- Ageing is a relational process.
- Physical and mental decline are not inevitable in later life.
- As people grow older, they work to maintain their own sense of personal identity.
- People may experience the self as 'younger' than the body.
- Dementia and Alzheimer's disease do not necessarily mean loss of self.
- New models of ageing and old age are emerging to replace traditional beliefs and attitudes.

8 | Bereavement

In the course of their careers, doctors will often have to care for people who are coming to terms with the loss of someone through death. The process occurring after the death, during which individuals learn to adjust to the loss, is known as *bereavement. Grief* can be described as the emotional response to that loss, whereas *mourning* refers to the expression of grief (Stroebe and Stroebe, 1987). The bereavement period can provide the opportunity for doctors to assess the needs of the surviving spouse or family and to intervene, where appropriate, with relevant back-up and services. This is important because studies show that bereaved people can have higher levels of morbidity and mortality compared with non-bereaved people, and the way they cope will determine the amount and type of support they need (Parkes, 2006; Relf et al., 2010).

Determinants of grief

Many factors can affect the way in which someone reacts to being bereaved. These may precede the bereavement, for example, a childhood experience, a previous life crisis such as divorce or mental illness or the nature of the relationship between the bereaved person and the deceased. The reaction may also be influenced by the bereaved person's present circumstances, for example, his or her age, sex, religion, type of personality or even cultural background. Reactions may also be determined by the circumstances of bereaved people after the death, for example, the amount of support they have and other stresses in their life such as having young children. Such determinants have been referred to as the antecedent (previous experience), concurrent (present circumstances) and subsequent determinants of grief (Parkes, 1996).

Cultural and religious beliefs may also affect how people display grief and feel they should behave during bereavement. In some cultures, strict rules govern the preparation of the body after death and the rituals associated with burial and mourning among different ethnic groups (Firth, 2001) (see pp. 130–131).

The mourning process

In the same way that the dying process has a series of stages (Kubler-Ross, 1970; see pp. 130–131), the process of mourning has similarly been defined as a series of phases that must be passed through before grief can be resolved. The initial phase of numbness gradually gives way to feelings of pining, yearning and searching, as the bereaved person seeks to recover what has been lost. When the intensity of this second phase diminishes, it is replaced by feelings of depression, disorganization and despair when it becomes apparent that the loss is irretrievable. Finally the bereaved person moves to a phase of recovery and reorganization when he or she begins to adjust to a new way of life without the deceased (Parkes, 1975; Bowlby, 1998). Worden (1991) defined the process as a series of tasks that must be worked through. He described these as accepting the reality of the loss, working through the pain, adjusting to an environment in which the deceased is missing and moving on with life. Although these stage and phase theories can be a useful way of beginning to understand the complexity of the grief process, they are not intended to be prescriptive. Individual reactions will vary and may not conform to a specific pattern.

The more recent Dual Process model suggests that bereaved people move between confronting grief (loss-oriented behaviour) and avoiding grief (restoration-oriented behaviour) (Stroebe and Schut, 1999). This and other newer models propose that the bereaved do not return to the way they were before the death as the stage models may have implied but adapt to a new way of living that incorporates a continuing bond with the dead person (Klass et al., 1996; Walter, 1999).

Normal grief

Normal grief reactions can include a range of different feelings, moods, symptoms and behaviours. The Dyer Model describes 6 dimensions of the normal grief process (Fig. 8.1).

Risk factors

Parkes (2006) identified four factors that affect the bereaved person:

- Personal vulnerability
- Relationship with the deceased person
- Events and circumstances leading up to the death
- Amount of social support

Atypical grief

Abnormal or complicated grief reactions occur when bereaved individuals are unable to express or work through their grief, which prevents their recovery from the loss and adaptation to life without the deceased. These reactions can be excessive and prolonged or absent and short-lived. They can be classified as delayed or absent, chronic, masked or exaggerated grief.

Delayed or absent grief

The bereaved person is unable to mourn the loss. This may be conscious, when the person's situation makes it difficult for him or her to grieve freely, e.g. in the case of a mother who carries on normally for the sake of her children. It can also be unconscious, when the bereaved person does not believe that the death has occurred, e.g. when there has been no definite confirmation, as in the case of soldiers missing during a war. This may be called *absent grief* (Faulkner, 1995). Delayed grief reactions are often triggered by other losses occurring a long time after the death, e.g. a later divorce or other unrelated loss (Worden, 1991).

Chronic grief

The bereaved person continues to experience the immediate pain of the loss months or even years later. That person is therefore unable to move on in the grieving process and adapt to life without the deceased. Usually chronic grief reactions occur in people who have had ambivalent or dependent relationships with the deceased (Parkes, 2006).

Masked grief

The grief reaction is masked by the development of physical or somatic symptoms that appear to the bereaved to be unassociated with the loss. Often these are physical symptoms that replicate those experienced by the deceased and these commonly appear on the anniversaries of the loss (Worden, 1991).

Exaggerated grief

The grief reaction is excessive and intense. In these cases the bereaved person's experience may develop into a serious psychiatric illness, e.g. clinical depression or acute anxiety (Worden, 1991).

Disenfranchised grief

Some people may react to other losses or illnesses in the same way as they would to bereavement through death, e.g. reaction to a cancer diagnosis (see pp. 96–97), amputation, miscarriage, stillbirth, physical dependence, divorce, unemployment or even relocation to a new town or city. With these losses the grief experienced and exhibited by the person may be as intense

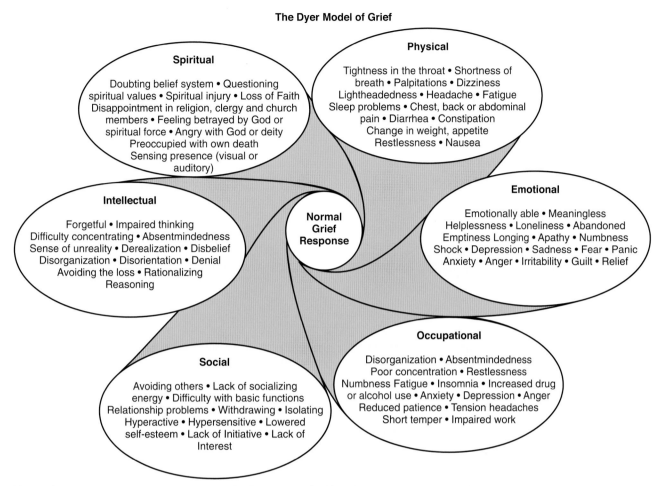

Fig. 8.1 Six dimensions of the normal grief response, The Dyer Model of Grief *(from Dyer, 2005, with permission).*

as grief expressed at a death. However, the grief may not be acknowledged by others, making it difficult for the bereaved to grieve openly or gain support (Doka, 2002). These types of reactions may also occur when a relationship with the deceased has had to be hidden. For these reasons health care professionals may miss or fail to appreciate the extent of a person's distress. This may mean that the person experiencing the loss is not offered the help needed to come to terms with it.

Bereavement care

The amount of support available for the bereaved varies greatly according to the setting where patients and their relatives are cared for. Tools now exist to help identify those people who may be at risk of an abnormal grief reaction and the type of support that would be most helpful (Relf et al, 2010; Parkes, 2006). Doctors working in general hospitals may not have the time or resources to follow up carers during bereavement. Often this is done by general practitioners or community nurses, who are able to visit the bereaved at home. Not every bereaved person will want or need professional support at this time. The majority of people rely on family and friends or find their own ways of coping.

In cases where the grief reaction is problematic, the doctor should recognize his or her limitations and summon the help of someone who is specially trained in bereavement counselling. In extreme cases, it may also be necessary to refer the person on to a clinical psychologist or psychiatrist (see pp. 132–133, 136–137).

Case study

Ethel was a 61-year-old woman whose husband Jack had died 6 months earlier after a sudden heart attack. At the same time her youngest daughter Ruth had left home to start university. Her two elder children were both married and living abroad. Ethel had been a lively woman, with many interests, and had shared most of these with her husband as they both enjoyed early retirement. Lately, however, Ethel had become withdrawn and morose and seemed to have lost all interest in anything. She preferred to spend her days looking at old family photos or going through her husband's belongings, with which she refused to part. She constantly phoned her daughter in tears and said she did not want to live without her husband. As a result Ruth felt guilty at leaving home and was at a loss to know what help to give her. Eventually Ruth asked the family doctor for help who suggested that Ruth phone a local voluntary bereavement counselling service. After a few visits from a trained counsellor, Ethel began to come to terms with her husband's death. Although she knew that her life would no longer be the same without her lifetime partner, she realized that she had to make a new beginning. Ruth was relieved that her mother was now able to resume some of the hobbies and her own life at university became happier.

Stop and think

• Which factors do you think might have influenced the way Ethel reacted to her husband's death?

• Think about how you would cope with Ethel if you were Ruth.

• Think about the counsellor's task in helping Ethel through her grief (see pp. 132–133).

Bereavement

• *Bereavement* is when someone who has experienced the loss of a loved one, and *grief* is the emotional response to the loss.

• Normal grief can be described as a series of stages individuals must work through until they adapt to life without the deceased.

• The way people react to a loss will depend on their past experiences and present circumstances.

9 | Personality and health

The term *personality* refers to enduring and distinctive features of individual behaviours across time, place and situation. The term *personality traits* refers to stable individual differences in thinking, feeling and behaving across a range of different situations. Research has found that particular dimensions of personality are associated with poor health and reduced longevity, whereas some others are linked to good health and increased length of life. The magnitude of these effects can be similar to those of known biological risk factors such as high cholesterol and blood pressure as well as other factors such as low socio-economic status (Hampson, 2012; Bogg and Roberts, 2013).

Big Five Taxonomy of personality

Personality is best understood in terms of five broad personality traits: openness to experience (or intellect), conscientiousness, extraversion, agreeableness and neuroticism (or emotional stability). This is often referred to as *the Big Five Taxonomy* or *the OCEAN* (Openness to Experience, Conscientiousness, Extraversion, Agreeableness and Neuroticism) *model of personality* (Fig. 9.1). An established body of research now relates traits from the Big Five Taxonomy to numerous health-promoting behaviours, health status and longevity. Moreover, a recent theoretical review by Ferguson (2013) highlighted that personality is a central concern in improving our understanding of health and illness processes in terms of diagnosis, treatment and prognosis. The Big Five model is based on the assumption that a range of more specific personality traits can be understood as blends of the different Big Five traits. Some of the best evidence for the impacts of personality on health outcomes arises from work looking at more specific personality traits such as optimism, type D personality or hostility. In terms of the Big Five model, however, there has been less research on how openness to experience and agreeableness link to health outcomes. Information from some of this research in relation to conscientiousness, neuroticism, extraversion, type D personality and dispositional optimism are presented in the following section.

Conscientiousness

Conscientiousness is characterized by a propensity to follow socially prescribed norms, control impulses, delay gratification, be planful and be both task directed and goal directed. It is well established that conscientiousness influences physical health and

longevity. The Terman Life Cycle Study showed that in any given year people high in conscientiousness have a significantly reduced risk of dying. A growing body of work has focussed on exploring potential explanatory mechanisms that may transmit these beneficial effects over the life course. Friedman et al. (1995) found that the protective influence of childhood conscientiousness on health status was accounted for, in part, by its impact on health-risking behaviours such as alcohol use and smoking. Similarly, high levels of conscientiousness has also been found to be associated with better health status, greater adherence to medication and lower obesity risk across populations. Recent work is emerging to suggest that conscientiousness may affect health and well-being through its influence on the stress process (e.g., O'Connor et al., 2009). For example, conscientiousness may be associated with the experience of less stress and may influence how individuals appraise stress that might be protective for health over time.

Neuroticism

Neuroticism refers to the tendency to frequently experience negative emotions such as distress, anxiety, fear, anger and guilt. Those high in neuroticism (also sometimes known as *negative affect*) and worry about the future, dwell on failures and shortcomings, and have less favourable views of themselves and others. A large number of studies have shown that individuals high in neuroticism are at greater risk of poorer physical and psychological health. Goodwin and Friedman (2006), in a large nationally representative sample in the United States, found that neuroticism was associated with numerous common mental and physical disorders, including major depression, stroke, asthma/bronchitis, persistent skin problems, ulcers and alcohol/substance use disorder. Another study by Shipley et al. (2007) reported the impact of neuroticism on mortality in a sample of over 5000 UK adults over a period of 21 years. High neuroticism was associated with mortality from all causes and with mortality from cardiovascular diseases.

Extraversion

Individuals high on extraversion tend to be outgoing, social and self-confident, seek stimulation and show high levels of energy. Extraverts also tend to enjoy new challenges, but they get bored easily. In contrast introverts tend to be more cautious and serious and avoid over-stimulating environments and activities. Unsurprisingly extraversion has been found to be associated with a myriad of positive physical, mental and behavioural health outcomes. Early research showed that extraverts reported lower rates of coronary heart disease, ulcers, asthma and arthritis. More recently Goodwin and Friedman (2006) found that high levels of extraversion were associated with the absence of common disorders such as major depression, generalized anxiety disorder, high blood pressure, stroke and sciatica/lumbago. In addition to exploring the effects of neuroticism, higher levels of extraversion are associated with reduced risk of respiratory disease at 21-years' follow-up.

Type D personality

Type D, or distressed, personality is a relatively new trait, not part of the Big Five Taxonomy, but is, instead, a blend of traits. It describes individuals who experience high levels of negative emotions (negative affectivity) and inhibit the expression of these negative emotions in social interactions (social inhibition). Denollet et al. (1996) showed that type D personality is a risk

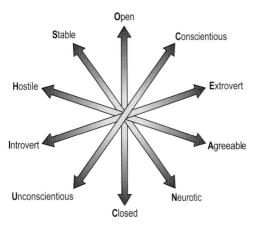

Fig. 9.1 OCEAN (Openness to Experience, Conscientiousness, Extraversion, Agreeableness and Neuroticism) dimensions of personality *(from McCrae and Costa, 1987, with permission).*

Chapter 9 Personality and health • 19

factor for adverse health outcomes in cardiac patients. Patients with type D personality were more likely to have died eight years earlier compared with patients with non–Type D personality. A majority of the deaths were caused by heart disease or stroke. These effects have been replicated in several studies, but the relationship between type D personality and risk of death is not entirely clear. Those with type D personality appear to have more highly activated immune systems and more inflammation (perhaps indicating more damage to blood vessels in the heart and throughout the body). They also show greater increases in blood pressure reactivity to stress. Recent research has suggested that individuals with type D personality engage in fewer health-promoting behaviours and experience lower levels of social support and that these effects remain after controlling for neuroticism (Williams et al., 2008).

Stop and think

- Personality is associated with longevity. Which personality traits are likely to be most important in the ageing process?
- Do you think personality can be changed? If the answer is yes, which personality trait would you try to alter?

Dispositional optimism

Dispositional optimism refers to the expectation that in the future good things will happen to you and bad things will not. Although we all may be optimistic in some areas of our lives and pessimistic in others, optimism taps the extent to which an individual is optimistic in general across a range of domains and across time. The outcomes of optimism include:

- increased psychological well-being,
- better physical health, and
- greater longevity (Carver and Scheier, 2014)

Recently it has been argued that physical health effects associated with optimism are likely to occur through differences in both health-promoting behaviours and physiological concomitants of coping with stress.

How does personality influence health outcomes?

Numerous explanations have been suggested through which personality traits may influence health outcomes (Table 9.1). An important one may be that personality traits can be damaging to health through changing physiological mechanisms. For example, type D personality might cause damage to arteries that, in turn, leads to a greater likelihood of heart disease. A second explanation considers the notion that particular personality traits may be associated with approaching certain risky situations. Friedman (2000) referred to this idea as *tropisms*. For example, individuals low in conscientiousness and who have less self-control may be more likely to be drawn to risky situations and to engage in riskier behaviours (e.g. substance abuse) that may be potentially damaging to their health. A third explanation is that personality

Table 9.1 **Explanations of the relationship between personality traits and health outcomes**

Physiological changes	The personality trait causes physiological changes that, in turn, influence health outcomes.
Tropisms	The personality trait has the effect of making the individual more likely to be exposed to risky situations.
Health behaviours	The personality trait has the effect of making the individual more likely to engage in health-risking behaviours and less likely to engage in health-promoting behaviours.
Stress processes	The personality trait has the effect of making the individual more likely to experience stress and/or less likely to be protected from the effects of stress through coping mechanisms or social support.

traits may lead to negative health outcomes through influencing the engagement in health-related behaviours. For example, again, conscientious individuals appear to be less likely to engage in health-risking behaviours such as smoking and more likely to engage in health-promoting behaviours such as exercise. In addition, personality traits such as conscientiousness might make individuals more likely to engage in health-promoting behaviours such as exercise by influencing how they think and plan about such behaviours.

A final set of explanations for the relationship between personality traits and health outcomes relates to the stress process and the variables that protect against the negative effects of stress. Personality traits may directly influence the number of stressors an individual experiences, thereby increasing or reducing any direct effects of stressors on various bodily systems over time. For example, individuals high in neuroticism may perceive themselves as experiencing more stress, and as a result their body will be exposed more to excessive wear and tear. Moreover, personality traits may influence how people respond to stress. For example, an individual high in conscientiousness might be more likely to engage in exercise on days when they encounter stress compared with their low-conscientiousness counterparts.

Personality and health

- Some personality traits are associated with poor health and reduced longevity, whereas others are linked to good health and increased length of life.
- The Big Five model is based on the assumption that a range of more specific personality traits can be understood as blends of the different Big Five traits.
- Individuals high in conscientiousness have been found to live longer than individuals low in conscientiousness.
- Type D personality has been found to be a risk factor for adverse health outcomes in cardiac patients.
- Extraversion and dispositional optimism have been found to be associated with better health outcomes.
- Personality traits may influence health through physiological changes, tropisms, health behaviours and stress processes.

10 | Understanding learning

Learning is not just about acquiring facts or knowledge. Skills, beliefs, values, attitudes, emotions and behaviours can also be learned (Fig. 10.1). Understanding how people learn equips us to do many important things. We may be able to change our own behaviours or help other people change theirs. We may be able to learn how to study more effectively to pass examinations or do our jobs more effectively and efficiently. Understanding learning has been of central concern to psychologists and the source of much debate (Eysenck, 1996).

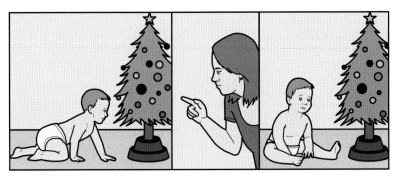

Fig. 10.1 If an infant approaches the Christmas tree decorations, he or she will be restrained: this will decrease the frequency of approach. In practice, however, punishment is a very poor way of changing behaviour and often arouses emotional responses. What does the baby do when he or she is not allowed to touch the tree (or approach medical equipment)?

Learning can be defined as a relatively permanent change in behaviour. Behaviourist theories of learning assume that there are laws of learning that are fundamental to all animals and that humans are no different in this respect. Behaviourism suggests that learning results from stimulus–response associations. A stimulus can be any change such as the sight of food or a moving ball. A response is a reflex action such as salivation or a muscular response such as catching the ball. Once learned, behaviour is hard to change. This explains why people can be very motivated to change their lifestyle but find it hard or impossible to do. Of course, much learning is cognitive – such as the acquisition of knowledge and concepts that is taking place as you read this book. Research into adult learning has informed medical teaching, and the way in which you are taught is likely to differ from the experience of senior medical staff. It is recognized that adults learn in different ways from children, so you may find a very different approach to learning from your school experience.

Operant conditioning

A kind of learning, known as *operant conditioning*, was described by Skinner, an American psychologist. In operant conditioning, the likelihood of a response occurring again is increased if the behaviour is followed by reinforcement. Thus the behaviour is controlled by its consequences. The principles of operant conditioning have been established through experimentation on animals such as rats and pigeons as well as on humans (Table 10.1).

For example, sucess in walking after an amputation would be rewarded internally by feelings of mastery and enhanced self-efficacy and externally by the approval of others. Praise (especially from medical staff) can be a very powerful reinforcer.

Classical conditioning

Operant conditioning is contrasted with classical conditioning described by Pavlov, a physiologist. In classical conditioning an initially neutral stimulus becomes associated with an involuntary response by its association with a previously conditioned stimulus. Pavlov worked with dogs because they naturally salivate at the sight of food. After a bell was paired with the food, the dogs learned to salivate at the sound of the bell alone. These principles were later tested on human emotional responses.

Watson and Raynor (1920) used classical conditioning to produce a phobia in a 9-month-old child known as Little Albert. Before the experiment, the child had no fear of white rats but was

Table 10.1 **Principles of operant conditioning**			
Principle	**Definition**	**Effect on behaviour**	**Example**
Positive reinforcement	Provides positive, pleasant consequences	Increases probability that response will occur again	Verbal praise in rehabilitation
Negative reinforcement	Removes unpleasant conditions	Increases probability that response will occur again	Adjusting gait to avoid pain in walking
Punishment	Removes a positive reinforcer or applies an aversive stimulus	Decreases the probability that response will occur again	Prescribing disulfiram (antabuse) to make someone feel sick after drinking alcohol.
Extinction	Removes positive reinforcer	Decreases the probability that response will occur again	Ignoring tantrums in waiting room
Shaping	Reinforces successive approximations to the one required	Gradually increases approximation to desired behaviour	Teaching a medical student how to take blood

frightened by loud noises. In the experiment the loud noise was paired with the presence of a white rat. After six pairings Albert showed a fear response in the presence of the white rat alone. Fear had now become a response conditioned to the previously neutral stimulus of the white rat. Moreover the fear became generalized to other furry animals. White rats and loud noises are not an everyday occurrence, but nurses may be associated with painful injections.

Some patients may develop conditioned responses to the sight or smell of hospitals. If hospital treatment has been associated with nausea, for example, in the case of chemotherapy for cancer, the mere sight or smell of a hospital can induce nausea or even vomiting (Fig. 10.2). Both operant conditioning and classical conditioning probably occur together in many learning situations. Food elicits salivation but also acts as a reinforcer.

Observational learning

This model suggests that behaviour patterns can be learned by watching other people's behaviours and being part of a group (Wenger, 1998). Many clinical skills and professional skills are learned through modelling and socialization. Both voluntary and

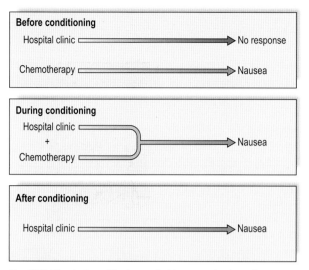

Fig. 10.2 Classical conditioning applied to nausea in chemotherapy.

involuntary responses can be learned through modelling. Sometimes we are not aware that learning is happening, but we adopt the practices of those around us. This is called *implicit learning*.

Children who were going to be admitted to hospital were shown a film about an unstressed child going into hospital, undergoing surgery and going home. Compared with others who were shown an unrelated film, these children showed less anxiety both before and after the operation (Saile et al., 1988). The closer in age and sex the model was to themselves, the more imitation took place. Interestingly the films may have reduced the anxiety of the parents as much as that of the children so that the child had a very powerful model of a relaxed parent to imitate as well! In the same way anxiety or embarrassment shown by a doctor will be quickly picked up and learned by a patient. Doctors and medical staff are powerful models.

Systematic desensitization

Systematic desensitization or graded exposure would treat a phobia (e.g. Little Albert's learned fear of furry animals) by gradually exposing the person to the feared object while replacing the anxiety with a relaxed condition. This can be achieved by reassurance or relaxation training. In a diabetes outpatient clinic, someone with a needle phobia might be treated by such methods so that he or she can tolerate injections. Initially this might be done by imagination alone, by visualizing the object, and once this is achieved without fear, the syringe could be introduced in the form of a picture. Later it might be shown in vivo, firstly at a distance and then gradually brought nearer (see pp. 112–113).

Cognitive behavioural therapy tries to alter behaviour by undoing the learning of maladaptive behaviours and by learning new behaviour patterns (see pp. 138–139). Principles of learning such as rational emotive behaviour theory and biofeedback have also been used in theories that enhance coping with stress.

E-learning

Learning by using modern information technology gives learners control over the content, learning sequence, pace of learning, time and a choice of media. Research has shown that this is at least as effective as traditional instructor-led lectures (Ruiz et al., 2006). Faculty may become facilitators of learning and assessors of competency rather than imparters of information. This will mean a radical role change (see pp. 162–163). Having constant access to information through mobile devices will increasingly change the way doctors learn. The theory of transactive memory (Wegner, 1987) proposed that we deliberately do not learn information if someone else in our team knows it because we can access it through our colleague. If we have constant access to information through the internet, this might influence how much information a modern doctor needs to learn or chooses to learn.

Learning factual material

Medical students find that they have to learn and recall difficult material (see pp. 26–27). Various strategies have been proposed to help this. Mnemonics can be associations of two words or letters, or a word and a visual image. Rehearsal can establish words in long-term memory, and this is most effective if they are organized. Many students make lists or mind maps of a topic. Spaced learning, which is learning the same content across multiple sessions with breaks in between, has been shown to improve recall of information. A recent report detailed common learning techniques and the evidence for the efficacy of each one (Dunlosky et al., 2013).

You will find that much of your course uses self-directed learning, and this is thought to promote learning skills and team-working as well as factual knowledge. Problem-based learning has also been adopted by many medical schools.

11 | Perception

What is perception? Is perception separate from cognition? Isn't all perception just physiology? What are illusions? How do we perceive what we do? Typically, we think about perception in conscious, subjective terms – a beautiful sunset, the sound of our favourite music or an annoying toothache. But the patterns of stimulation reaching our senses constantly control or influence our behaviour, without any awareness on our part (think of riding a bicycle), and the study of perception is concerned with both subjective experiences and the sensory control of behaviour. Of course, there are brain mechanisms underlying all those perceptual processes, and these are worthy of investigation, but the study of perception is about the *relationship* between sensory information and our behaviour/subjective experiences. To study perception, psychologists use both phenomenology (what things look like) and psychophysical techniques (e.g. signal detection) to separate off the influences of bias from an individual's awareness/sensitivity to sensory information.

The main emphasis in this spread will be on visual perception, but many of the ideas and general principles also apply to other aspects of perception such as audition, olfaction and proprioception.

How should we think about perception?

Many scientists consider perception to be an active (rather than passive) process that creates and enriches our subjective experiences, from rather limited or impoverished sensory data. In the 19th century, Hermann von Helmholtz suggested that our perceptions are 'unconscious inferences' – guesses or hypotheses, based as much on learning, knowledge and experience as on sensory input. When only part of an object is visible, for example, the top half of a person sitting behind a desk, we perceive this as a 'whole' person, not just half a person despite the absence of sensory information. However, if our perceptions are only guesses or hypotheses, then it is not surprising that our perceptions can be fooled. The study of illusions provides some dramatic examples.

In contrast, the American psychologist James Gibson claimed that perception is better thought of as the direct 'pick-up' of information rather than an inferential process. In particular, he showed that

patterns of motion reaching the retina when we move – optic flow – provide rich information about both the three-dimensional structure of the surrounding world and also about our movements within it. This idea of a direct pick-up of information is particularly relevant when we consider the perceptual systems of animals lower down on the phylogenetic scale – it seems unlikely that flies make inferences!

What these theories share is the idea that perception is all about extracting *meaning* from the patterns of sensory stimulation, rather than creating 'pictures' in our heads. A smile or frown tells us something about the emotional state of another person. The discomfort we feel when peering from the top of high buildings is not just about the perception of distance, it is about the potential danger the situation offers.

What are illusions, and what are their causes?

Illusions are typically defined as 'departures from reality' – situations where what we perceive does not correspond to what is actually there. In the Müller–Lyer illusion (Fig. 11.1), the horizontal lines are physically the same length but the line with the outgoing fins is typically perceived

(a) Ponzo

(b) Müller–Lyer

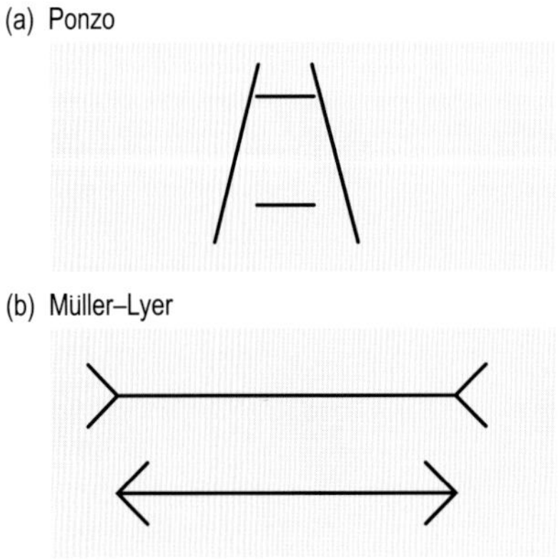

Fig. 11.1 Müller–Lyer illusion.

as longer. In the Ebbinghaus illusion (Fig. 11.2), the circles are the same physical size but the circle surrounded by the small circles is typically perceived as larger. Although physically stationary, the moon appears to move in the opposite direction to the clouds passing over it.

We are fooled by these illusions not because we are unintelligent but rather because of the particular ways in which our perceptual systems work. Most often information about the *relative* characteristics of objects in the surrounding world is more important than their *absolute* values and this is what our perceptual systems are able to do accurately and reliably. Hence we are good at perceiving the relative movement between the moon and the clouds but poor at perceiving their absolute motions. Our ability to discriminate subtle colour differences between surfaces is much better than our ability to identify a particular shade. From the psychologist's point of view, illusions are interesting not because they represent failures of the perceptual system but because they reveal how our perceptual systems work.

Learning, past experience and context

Learning is crucial for our perceptions. Young children do not perceive the solid-looking surface of an ice-covered pond as potentially dangerous, and the subtle signs of a cancerous tumour in a CT or MRI scan will not be obvious to newly trained medics. However, note that there is a subtle but important difference between learning and knowledge. Past experience and learning can affect our perceptions and behaviour, but the resultant changes in our perceptual abilities may or may not be available as conscious knowledge. Few of us have any idea of how we manage to balance and ride a bicycle, but we can still

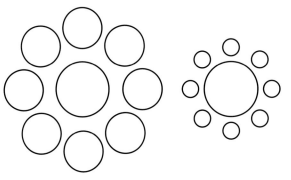

Fig. 11.2 Ebbinghaus illusion.

learn to do so. Moreover, conscious knowledge, by itself, does not typically affect our perceptions. We might know that the moon is about a quarter of a million miles away but this does not affect our perception of its apparent distance – as being like that of the passing clouds.

At a conscious level, we are likely to be influenced by our previous experience when making a diagnosis (see Case study). Perceptions may also be influenced by past experiences. For example, we tend to be more positive towards physically attractive people even though we are unaware of this. In studies of social perception, people were asked to choose the company with whom they would prefer to watch television. Most chose people who were not physically disabled. In many cases this may have simply resulted from lack of experience with disabled people. Patients with congenital deformities may at first seem distressing to observe, but as you become familiar with such patients, you will find that their deformity becomes less distressing and less pertinent. In a sense, you no longer 'see' the deformity. Instead you are able to see past it to the person within.

Context is also vital for understanding perceptual processes. What surrounds a particular object or event, in space or time, affects what we perceive. Traditionally these influences have been divided into those resulting from automatic, 'bottom-up' processes and those resulting from 'top-down' processing. Our perceptions would therefore be based on an initial analysis of low-level 'features', which then have to be assembled to form our perceptions. But in the 1920s, the Gestalt psychologists rejected this, arguing that the 'wholes' (Gestalten) are 'more than the sum of the parts'. In other words, the distinction between a 'stimulus' and its 'context' is probably artificial.

Perception and attention

It is tempting to consider perception as a process in which we cast a spotlight and 'pay attention' to aspects of the 'picture' that has been created by lower-level perceptual processes. However, if we consider perception as a process of extracting information (rather than creating 'pictures'), then it is clear that the selective aspect of our perception (attention) is not an 'add-on' but is essential and integral. Our perceptions may be:

- Selective. We attend to stimuli that are changing, repeated, intense and personally meaningful. Certain words catch our attention, for example, our names, words connected with significant events or important concerns such as the word 'sex'.
- Divided or focussed. Our ability to divide our attention is limited, although it can be improved with practice. It is easier to divide attention if different types of stimuli or different sensory modalities are involved. For example, you can probably look at pictures and listen to music simultaneously, but not both to read and listen to speech.
- Negatively affected by stress and fatigue. When tired, or when more demands are placed upon us than there are resources to meet those demands, our ability to attend may decrease. This can have disastrous results. Tired doctors are likely to make more errors because they are no longer able to pay full attention to all the details of a particular set of diagnostic signs.

Perception and cognition

What is the role of cognitive processes in perception? According to traditional understanding, there are lower-level processes that create representations that are subsequently subject to cognitive or 'thinking-like' processes. These then determine the meaning of those representations. We are typically unaware of these, but what we expect to see, or want to see, can affect our perception. For example, the doctor learns from a patient that she has been in contact with someone suffering from rubella. This creates an expectation, and a perceptual 'set' when examining the patient's rash. When expectations are strong, this can lead to misdiagnoses.

Our impression of people depends on how we perceive and think about them (constructs). This includes our perception of their sociability, likability and intelligence, and this perception depends partly on context. When forming impressions of people you meet at a party, your cognitive constructs differ from those you use when seeing patients in an outpatient clinic. Sometimes we make errors in assuming that the behaviour of a patient results from his or her personality rather than the situation of being ill in a hospital. Alternatively you may also wrongly attribute a patient's behaviour to having a particular disease, rather than the fact that he or she behaves in that manner always.

Relevance of psychology of perception to medicine

All of the processes we call *perception* occur in the brain. Consequently, brain damage will result in perceptual distortions and errors and hence may be an early indicator of organic damage. The study of neuropsychology is very important in this respect.

There is no such thing as a 'correct' way to perceive something: our perceptions vary because the perceptual process is a creative one. Usually we do not notice this, but sometimes the differences are critical. A pathologist may carry out a postmortem examination, with an assumption about the cause of death. This may lead her to seek, identify and report an incomplete finding. A second pathologist may discover another, highly significant sign that can change the course of a police enquiry completely.

We are all prone to see what the context indicates we should see. Given ambiguous cues, we 'recognise' things according to our expectations and experience.

Attention can be divided with practice. When you start to acquire a skill (e.g. taking blood), it is almost impossible to do anything else at the same time such as talking reassuringly to the patient. In time, however, the skill of attending to both aspects of the patient encounter simultaneously can be learned.

Stop and think

- Consider whether you have recently experienced an illusion that you believe has influenced your perception. What relevance might this experience have to your work, for example, working with patients, or your involvement in treatments such as surgery?

Perception

- Perception is an active process.
- Illusions teach us how the perceptual system works.
- Cognitive 'sets' or representations influence our perception.

12 | Emotions

Emotions are transient, internal experiences involving sensations, feelings and changes in bodily arousal. They also have a strong cognitive component, connecting us to thoughts and images and influence how we react to and communicate with others. It is, however, difficult to define emotions. The specific quality of a feeling, the feeling of being emotionally moved, is difficult to explain without going in circles, and define it by another word that, in turn, requires definition, such as affect or sentiment. Whilst emotions are transient experiences, moods are more stable conditions, not as reactive as emotions (Gross, 1998). *Affect* is a more general term, covering both the short-term emotions and the longer-lasting moods.

A common way to classify emotions is to make a distinction between the *valence* (positive or negative) and *intensity* of emotional experience. However, not all emotions are easy to classify. Even if all would agree that fear is an emotion, most often there is also a significant cognitive component in the sense that we are afraid of something. Moreover there are many nuances in our experiences of emotion, reflected in the language. The feeling of awe, for instance, may be said to be a combination of fear and the cognitive component respect.

The perception of basic emotions in others' faces may be biologically determined, rather than learned. This was first suggested by Darwin in 1872 but only systematically studied later. Ekman (1993) proposed that six primary emotions could be recognized from the same facial expressions across cultures: (1) fear, (2) anger, (3) disgust, (4) sadness, (5) enjoyment or happiness and (6) surprise. Evidence supports the universality of the first five.

Emotion as social communication

Even subtle emotions influence social expectations and our relationships, informing others about our responses to them (Fig. 12.1). In this way, emotions play an important role in all social interactions. Different cultures have different display rules (i.e. what is socially acceptable in terms of the expression of emotion).

Processing of emotions in the brain

To understand how emotions function, it is helpful to know how they are processed in the brain. Somewhat simplified, we may say that there are three stages in the processing of emotion in the brain:

- Autonomic activation
- Perceptual and cognitive processing
- Integration and regulation of emotions.

Autonomic activation

Emotions are elicited by stimuli. You see or you hear things that somehow are emotionally evocative. Sometimes emotions are evoked by thoughts without an apparent external stimulus, as when you suddenly remember that you forgot your mother's birthday.

Let us say that you are confronted by a dangerous animal, which immediately scares you (Fig. 12.2). The sensory input from your eyes reaches the thalamus, an important relay station centrally placed in the brain in the posterior part of diencephalon. The thalamus makes the first rudimentary evaluation of the stimulus (the dangerous animal) and immediately sends signals to the amygdala, an almond-shaped structure deep in the temporal lobes (see the blue arrow in Fig. 12.2). The amygdala immediately defines the animal as a dangerous stimulus and, in a matter of milliseconds, sends down a stream of signals to the hypothalamus, which, in turn, activates the sympathetic part of the autonomic nervous system. You feel physiologically aroused (increased heartbeat, sweat in your hands, etc.) and react by running away from the animal (a fight-or-flight response). These bodily reactions are then fed back to the brain and will represent important input in further emotional processing.

Perceptual and cognitive processing

From the thalamus, signals also go to the posterior parts of cerebral cortex, which are specialized in analyzing sensory input. These areas of the cortex that make a more detailed interpretation of the stimulus (indicated by the red arrow from the thalamus in Fig. 12.2). How dangerous is this animal really? This interpretation is fed back to the amygdala, and we may see a subsequent increase or decrease of activation of the autonomic system.

Controversy – what comes first: arousal, perception or identification of emotion?

The sequence in this chain of events (stimulus – sensation – physiological arousal – interpretation of the stimulus – experience of fear) has been a matter of controversy in psychology. In the late 19th century, James (1884) and Lange independently proposed that we experience emotion (e.g. fear) after perceptual events (e.g. I see the animal in Fig. 12.2) and subsequent physiological changes (e.g. heightened sympathetic arousal, reinforced by running away from the animal). James would say 'We are afraid because we run', instead of the conventional 'We run because we are afraid'. However, the James–Lange theory could

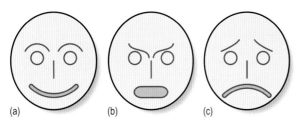

Fig. 12.1 Universally recognized facial expressions of emotion – (a) happy, (b) angry, (c) sad.

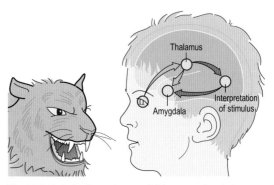

Fig. 12.2 Both the faster 'low road' *(blue arrows)* and slower, cortical-mediated 'high road' *(red arrows)* by which emotion-related information can affect behaviour.

not explain emotions reported by people with spinal injuries blocking physiological feedback to the brain. Two physiologists, Cannon (1931) and subsequently Bard argued that heart-pounding corresponds to fear, but one does not cause the other: they represent two outcomes of the same (or parallel) processes. Later, Le Doux (2000) found evidence for the two parallel pathways in the processing of the emotional stimuli, described previously. The fast pathway from the thalamus to the amygdala is called the 'low road', and the somewhat slower connection from the thalamus to the posterior cortex is called the 'high road'. So both classical theories have some merit. There are parallel processes (Cannon–Bard), but the full emotional response appears subsequent to the physiological arousal (James–Lange).

Emotional integration and regulation

Immediately after the autonomic activation and the perceptual and cognitive processing of stimuli, the processing sequence continues with an integration and regulation of emotions before expression and action, described as a perception – valuation – action sequence (Etkin, Büchel and Gross, 2015). Signals from the body indicating physiological arousal are fed back to the insula, a medial structure of the temporal lobes that plays an important role in the processing of these interoceptive signals. Pathways from the insula and other areas of the brain involved in early processing of emotional stimuli converge in the medial areas of the prefrontal cortices. Here the valence (positive versus negative) of the input is evaluated, guiding our actions towards or away from the stimuli.

Prefrontal cortex is also important in the regulation of emotions. Gyurak, Gross and Etkin (2011) made a distinction between explicit and implicit emotion regulation. An example of explicit emotion regulation would be preparing an anxious child for a scary medical procedure by explaining it beforehand and giving the child an opportunity to control the situation, for instance by giving a signal to indicate pain. Emotion regulation may also be implicit, without conscious awareness. For instance, the mere labelling of emotions may be associated with activation of the right ventrolateral prefrontal cortex and downregulation of the amygdala. Thus by putting feelings into words, the individual may be better able to control his or her emotions (Lieberman et al., 2007). These findings have implications for how doctors should handle emotional reactions in their patients.

Emotions and disease – negative and positive emotions

Emotional dysregulation (both overregulation and underregulation) is implicated in many examples of psychopathology, including mood and anxiety disorders and addictive disorders (Williams et al., 1997), as well as somatic disorders such as irritable bowel syndrome, fibromyalgia, chronic pain syndrome (Montoya et al., 2005).

Disconnecting from emotional experiencing may be harmful. If a person consciously or unconsciously tried to limit his or her awareness of difficult emotions, over time the arousal associated with the 'blocked' emotions can contribute to physical symptoms as well as chronic states of depression or anxiety.

Positive emotions are important to promote health and counteract the harmful effects of negative emotions. People can experience positive emotion even when they are upset or stressed. This may be important to effective coping.

Health care professional–patient communications

Many medical consultations have an emotional dimension. Patients may be afraid of what their medical condition is and what the consequences may be; they may be sad and distressed because of lost functions caused by their physical disability; or they may be angry at doctors who they feel have not provided optimal and timely treatment. Yet patients tend not to express their worries and concerns explicitly. More often they express their concerns by cues and hints to their emotional states and reactions (Zimmermann, Del Piccolo and Finset, 2007). It is important for the doctor to be sensitive to these hints to respond adequately to patients' emotions and to provide empathic acknowledgement of patients' emotions.

Adequate responses to patients' emotions are important to secure patient satisfaction, bolster patients' adherence to medical regimes and ultimately to promote recovery and health. Recent studies have shown how empathic physician–patient communication may have impact on the clinical outcome on a number of diseases such as diabetes, irritable bowel syndrome and pain (Finset, 2013).

Stop and think

- Imagine you are told you need to be admitted to hospital for major surgery. List some of the emotions you might experience. Think about how you might respond to these emotional experiences. What kind of support would be helpful to you? How would you like your doctor to handle your emotions? How could you regulate your emotional reactions?

Case study

George is recovering from a myocardial infarction in hospital. A nurse notices he is upset and talks to him. He begins to explain some of his worries and the nurse says: 'Don't worry about those things now – you just relax and get well'. He talks to a doctor, who says, 'There's no need for you to be worried. Everything will be fine'. Although both clinicians want to help, George feels somewhat rejected and isolated because he has no one to talk to about his feelings. This may affect his decision to enter into a rehabilitation programme and his recovery. A more helpful response from the clinicians would be to acknowledge George's upset and allow him to talk through his worries.

Emotions

- Emotions involve physiological arousal and cognitive interpretation. They often evoke fast responses to something unexpected, or highly positively or negatively valued.
- Facial expressions of certain basic emotions are recognized across many cultures, but cultures also have their own 'display rules'.
- Emotional processing in the brain includes autonomic activation (amygdala, hypothalamus), perceptual and cognitive processing (posterior cortices) and emotional integration and regulation (insula and prefrontal cortex).

  Emotion regulation may occur by a conscious effort (explicit) or implicitly, for instance when putting words to emotion may downregulate negative emotions.

  Disconnecting from emotional experiencing is disconnecting from important information, and can contribute to the development of symptoms of psychological distress or physical illness.

- People can experience positive emotion even when they are upset or stressed. This may be important to effective coping.
- Sensitivity to patients' subtle hints and empathic emotional management of consultations is crucial to patients' responses to doctors and, therefore, to the effectiveness of consultations.

13 | Memory problems

We are all familiar with lapses of memory – not being able to put a name to a face; forgetting to keep an appointment; and poor recall during an exam. Psychologists have learned a great deal about the process of memory in the past 100 years both through laboratory-based experiments and by studying individuals with brain damage resulting in unique forms of memory loss. Although it presents a very simplified view, Fig. 13.1 is a useful summary of a widely held basic model of memory. Items are initially held in a short-term store and whether they become permanently represented in a long-term memory (LTM) store will depend on a host of factors such as how important and interesting they are and whether we engage in active rehearsal strategies to encode items into permanent memory or LTM. There are also many different divisions of LTM, in particular a distinction between *declarative* and *non-declarative* (including *procedural*) memory (i.e. between memory for facts *(semantic)* and autobiographical events *(episodic)*, and memory for skills and other cognitive operations that do not require conscious awareness).

Stop and think

- What were you doing on 15 March last year?

Stages of memory

If we listen to a list of unrelated words read out to us and then are required to recall the words immediately, items presented either first or last are better remembered than those in the middle. This better recall for the more recent items *(recency effect)* is because we are retrieving them directly from the short-term memory (STM) store. If we were to delay recall of the word list by 30 seconds, then this recency effect disappears (Fig. 13.2).

Even items that do successfully enter into LTM may not be recalled when we need them but much later are recalled. This illustrates the problem of *retrieval*, rather like a book that has been stored in a library: if we lose the catalogue slip, then the book is very difficult to find. This problem of memory loss is clearly very different to being unable to locate the book because it was never stored correctly in the first place. A good practical illustration of this distinction is the difference between testing your knowledge about anatomy by *recall* ('describe the structure of the brain') and

recognition ('which of the following is part of the limbic system?'). Multiple-choice exam questions have already carried out the retrieval part of remembering, leaving only the recognition component to be necessary.

When we consider the problems of forgetting and the poor memory associated with clinical conditions such as brain injury, dementia, mood disorder, or typical ageing, and we are trying to devise methods to aid recall, we first need to have clear ideas about the stage at which the process is disturbed. Is it the initial *encoding* of the information that is impaired, a difficulty accessing the relevant information *(retrieval)*, or do those with poor memories simply forget more quickly *(storage)*?

How much can we remember?

Realising that we have seen a film previously, but only about 10 minutes before its end, or revisiting a childhood home and having a flood of forgotten memories are powerful experiences, which may tempt us into thinking that we do, indeed, store all events and, given the right conditions, can retrieve such memories. Although there are well-documented cases of people with exceptional memories (one fascinating account, *The Mind of a Mnemonist*, is provided by the Russian neuropsychologist Luria (1969)), there is no scientific evidence to support this 'videotape' view of memory. To acquire permanent representation in memory we need to organize the new material and establish connections with the existing LTM store. Hence the use of mnemonic techniques, which rely on devices such as learning a list of items in relation to an easily remembered rhyme, or first-letter mnemonics such as Richard Of York Gave Battle In Vain for the colours of the visible spectrum. Memory tricks like this should not be scoffed at and have proved useful in helping elderly patients remember people's names.

Helping people to remember better

When individuals have been asked to recall what they have been told during a clinical consultation, they have been found to forget almost half. Memory for medical advice as opposed to diagnostic information can be particularly poor, especially in the case of individuals experiencing high anxiety or older adults. Statements

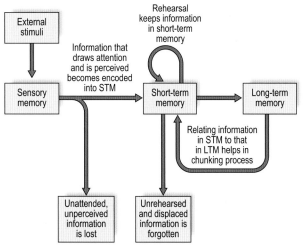

Fig. 13.1 Memory: short-term and long-term storage. STM, short-term memory; LTM, long-term memory.

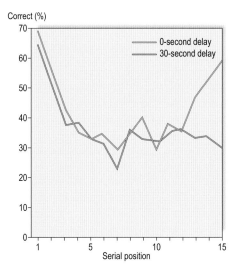

Fig. 13.2 The recency effect and short-term storage.

made early in the consultation are more likely to enter LTM (the *primacy effect*) and those at the end are remembered better initially but then tend to be forgotten (the recency effect). General or abstract statements are more difficult to remember than more specific concrete suggestions. Researchers have concluded that recall is aided by following some simple rules:

- Give the most important information early in any set of instructions.
- Stress the importance of relevant items (e.g. by repetition).
- Use explicit categorisation under simple headings (e.g. I will tell you what is wrong … what treatment you will need … what you can do to help yourself).
- Make advice specific, detailed and concrete rather than general and abstract.
- Summarize the relevant and important information into smaller 'chunks'.

Memory after traumatic brain injury

Memory problems often follow accidental trauma to brain (traumatic brain injury; TBI). Individuals with the most dramatic form of TBI may be unable to recall not only the events leading up to the accident but also those that occurred many years prior to that time. This memory loss extending backwards in time is known as *retrograde amnesia*, as distinct from the inability to form new memories, which is known as *anterograde amnesia*. Individuals with TBI may well report themselves as 10 years younger than they are and be unable to recall all the events of those 10 years, such as marriage, birth of children and employment. At the same time, they will repeatedly need to be told why they are in hospital and the names of the nurses and doctors caring for them. Eventually these years of memory loss will be recovered, indicating that the problem was difficulty of retrieval, but they may be left with enduring deficits of memory, which may be secondary to attentional or concentration difficulties. The exact nature of the deficit will require extensive assessment by a neuropsychologist. A collection of essays dealing with the effects of brain damage is Oliver Sacks' book *The Man who Mistook his Wife for a Hat* (1986).

Stop and think

- How would you set about establishing the extent of retrograde amnesia in someone for whom you have no autobiographical information?

Organic amnesia

Permanent memory loss is a serious problem necessitating continuous care of such individuals. These instances of organic amnesia may be caused by long-term alcohol abuse and development of Korsakoff's syndrome; to the brain damage resulting from viral encephalitis; or to some surgical interventions. In cases where the memory loss is primary and not secondary to other cognitive deficits, individuals are likely to have suffered damage to components of the limbic system and the related neural network, with the hippocampus being a key structure (see Case study).

Brain imaging

Brain imaging techniques such as magnetic resonance imaging allow researchers to directly examine the parts of the brain and related networks associated with cognitive processes. In the last 20

years there have been several important discoveries that are relevant to understanding memory mechanisms and which also demonstrate the considerable plasticity of the brain with respect to function. Animal studies have long implicated the hippocampus as playing a particular role in spatial memory (Professor John O'Keefe, University College London, won a Nobel Prize in Physiology or Medicine in 2014 for his work on place cells in the brain), and this has also been shown to apply to humans in a particularly interesting study of London taxi drivers performed by Maguire et al. (1998). The researchers studied taxi drivers qualified in the 'knowledge' – a two-year acquisition of street locations and one-way systems in London. In comparing taxi drivers and a control group of casual drivers, they found differences in the cellular density of the left and right hippocampus, with the posterior hippocampus having a larger volume on both sides in the taxi drivers, whereas in the control group the anterior hippocampus was larger. The researchers found a positive correlation between years of experience in the job and volume of the right posterior hippocampus and a negative correlation for the anterior hippocampus. This strongly suggests the changes are acquired as a result of the experience of taxi driving and the spatial maps formed as a result. There are clear implications here for rehabilitation, suggesting that a similar environment-related plasticity is possible in other regions of the brain.

Stop and think

- Can you recall the moment you first encountered a younger sibling? Your first day at school? Why do such memories endure?

Case study

HM is an engineering worker who, in 1953, in his late 20s was operated upon in an experimental procedure intended to relieve his epileptic seizures. The operation involved a radical bilateral medial temporal lobe resection, destroying the anterior two-thirds of the hippocampus, as well as the uncus and the amygdala. The operation was successful in alleviating the epileptic symptoms but left HM with profound memory impairment. Although he can remember events and facts he acquired up to 2 years before his operation, he can remember essentially nothing that has occurred since. He does not know what he had for lunch an hour ago, how he came to be where he is now, where he has left objects used recently or that he has used them. He reads the same magazines over and over again. He has learned neither the names of doctors and psychologists who have worked with him for decades nor the route to the house he moved to a few years after his surgery. Yet despite such difficulties he is not intellectually impaired. His language comprehension and production and conversational skills are normal, he can reason competently and do mental arithmetic. His IQ measured in 1962 was an above-average 117 – higher than the 104 measured presurgery in 1953. This neurological dissociation supports the idea that the temporary retention of information in working memory and the permanent storage of new information depend on different brain mechanisms (for a lengthier account of HM's problems, see Hilts, 1995).

Memory problems

- There is clear distinction amongst the encoding, storage, recall and recognition processes in memory.
- Different kinds of memory mechanisms underlie STM and LTM, as shown by the serial position effect and the nature of the amnesic syndrome in individuals with brain damage.
- Improving memory recall by means of mnemonic aids is especially useful for unconnected items and events.

14 | How does sexuality develop?

Sexual identity and behaviour are fundamental to the development of a person, and the relevant influences are diverse and complex. The nature of sexuality is such that it has an important effect on health and well-being, and sexuality, in turn, is strongly influenced by these factors.

Gender identity

Biological influences

Gender identity (whether you feel male or female, see Gender and health, pp. 44–45) usually coincides with sexual identity indicated by chromosomes, hormones and sexual organs, but not always. Biological indices can occasionally be different so that gender may be ambiguous or contradictory. Also some women and men feel they are in the wrong biological body (transsexual) and may decide to undergo a sex change operation, which can be very stressful both psychologically, because it affects the notion of identity (who we are), and socially, because it upsets our common-sense and legal notions of gender/sex as a fixed entity. We as a society are slowly beginning to understand the complexity and fluidity in taken-for-granted notions of sex and gender.

The sex chromosomes determined at conception and the subsequent hormonal activity in the foetus set the pattern for development of the internal and external sex organs and the sexual differentiation of the brain. There are exceptions. For example, abnormal chromosomes may give rise to a definite gender identity but altered sexual organs and atypical social and sexual behaviour; or a foetus with normal chromosomes may be exposed to unusual levels of hormones in utero. Some mothers who were given progestogens to prevent abortion had daughters who developed genital abnormalities and atypical sexual and social behaviours.

Social and cultural influences

During puberty, gender identity becomes linked to sexual activity. There is often a period of sexual experimentation before individuals feel confident of their orientation. In the development of homosexual orientation, there is some evidence for a genetic factor: monozygotic twins show higher concordance than dizygotic twins, but cultural factors and individual learning experiences will also determine attraction to a partner.

Psychological influences on gender start at birth; in the UK traditionally we dress baby boys in blue and girls in pink. Also our interactions are determined by the perceived sex of the baby, which we often only notice when babies are dressed non-gender-specifically (Fig. 14.1). We have certain expectations of boys and girls from a very young age, which may lead to playing more 'rough and tumble' games with boys and more talking and cuddling with girls. This process quickly extends to peers, school and the media. It is thought that a core gender identity is fixed by about the age of 4 years.

Cultural pressures may delay the acceptance of sexual identity because in many societies variations from the norm are not accepted. It may take a long period of adjustment and considerable courage to 'come out', accepting one's own sexuality and letting others know. Fear of one's sexuality being discovered may lead to secretive or reclusive lifestyles and can be the source of enormous distress. Social norms are changing: witness the changes in the media's (see pp. 52–53) portrayal of sex and sexuality in, for example, documentaries, soap operas and discussion shows over the past decades.

The development of sexual activity

Although some sexual behaviour (genital play and stimulation) is seen in infants, the level of activity rises before puberty, and this takes the form of sexual play with other children or solitary genital stimulation (masturbation). Peers are often a key source of knowledge about sexual behaviour.

Although a young person's interest in a sexual relationship is also influenced by hormones, the age at which sexual intercourse first takes place varies from culture to culture, also across time and according to social class. A UK study in the early 1990s indicated that average age of first intercourse has fallen in the last 40 years from 21 to 17 (Table 14.1). More recently, it is reported that an increasing proportion of young people have sexual intercourse before they are 16 years old (Wight et al., 2000), and studies have found that sexual intercourse before the age of 16 years is often regretted. In the 1960s surveys in Europe showed that sexual activity, including intercourse, took place at an earlier age in working-class males and females than amongst the middle classes. By the 1970s these differences had disappeared.

The most common pattern of long-term sexual partnership is heterosexual monogamy. Although in many societies polygamy is part of religious and cultural structures, in practice many men do not take more than one wife at a time, through lack of availability or resources. Worldwide the pattern of human attachment is often serial monogamy (one partner after another) rather than lifelong monogamy. The high rates of divorce in the industrialized world are one example of this.

Sexual activity continues through adulthood into old age (see pp. 14–15). Although the sexual behaviours of young adults and those in middle age are often discussed and form the subject of films and plays, the sexual needs of older people are seldom portrayed. Sexual interest continues in the older age group, although functioning changes; for example, in postmenopausal women, reduced oestrogen may cause thinning and dryness in the vagina, making intercourse more painful. In men, ageing is associated with increased time to achieve an erection, longer refractory periods and increased need for tactile rather than psychic stimuli. For men these changes are most marked after the age of 70 years. It may be difficult for older people to discuss sexual problems with a doctor because their interest in sex is sometimes seen as inappropriate.

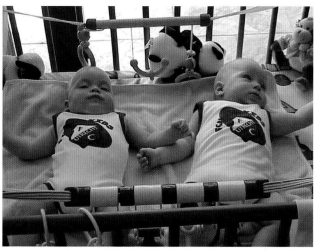

Fig. 14.1 Girls or boys? Two babies in gender-neutral outfits.

Table 14.1 **Age at first sexual intercourse by age at interview**				
	Women		Men	
Age at interview (years)	Median age at first intercourse (years)	% (No.) reporting first intercourse before age 16 years	Median age at first intercourse (years)	% (No.) reporting first intercourse before age 16 years
16–19	17	18.7 (182/971)	17	27.6 (228/827)
20–24	17	14.7 (184/251)	17	23.8 (271/1137)
25–29	18	10.0 (152/1519)	17	23.8 (268/1126)
30–34	18	8.6 (116/1349)	17	23.2 (235/1012)
35–39	18	5.8 (73/1261)	18	18.4 (181/982)
40–44	19	4.3 (55/1277)	18	14.5 (150/1042)
45–49	20	3.4 (37/1071)	18	13.9 (115/827)
50–54	20	1.4 (13/933)	18	8.9 (61/684)
55–59	21	0.8 (6/716)	20	5.8 (35/603)

Analysis was based on weighted data.

Data from Wellings et al. (1995).

Case study

Karen, a 29-year-old woman came to see her family doctor because of infertility. Karen stopped the contraceptive pill 2 years ago but had not conceived. She was well and reported no relationship difficulties. Her 34-year-old husband Chris was a manager on a short-term contract.

Before referral to the infertility clinic, the doctor asked to see each partner separately. Both said that the frequency of sexual intercourse was low. Karen assumed that this was because of her husband's tiredness through overwork and did not want to put pressure on him. Chris acknowledged that he was very anxious about work, had resumed heavier drinking again, resulting in a recurrence of gastritis, and was experiencing erectile difficulties. Afraid of impotence, he did not initiate sex but wished that Karen would do so sometimes. He was too embarrassed to say this to her.

Instead of referral for infertility, the couple was sent to a sexual problems clinic. There was a ban on intercourse at first to take the pressure off both. With the therapist acting as intermediary, the couple began to communicate honestly about their own worries and expectations of sex. Chris was given advice on anxiety management and drinking less. For their homework non-threatening goals were set for increasing sexual activity, which included Karen taking the initiative sometimes. By the fourth session, Chris was drinking less, and the frequency of intercourse had increased to two or three times per week. Karen conceived 7 months later.

Sexual problems

Sexual difficulties can arise through problems in functioning (e.g. erectile difficulties in the male or failure to achieve orgasm in the female); incompatibility (differences in appetite for or style of sexual activity); problems of fertility (inability to conceive or fear of conception); psychosocial problems arising through sexual behaviour (e.g. problems of sexual identity or problems with the law); and sexually transmitted infections (see pp. 108–109). A number of medical conditions give rise to sexual problems. Most common amongst these are multiple sclerosis, cardiovascular disease, diabetes, epilepsy and renal disease (see Heart disease, pp. 104–105 and Diabetes mellitus, pp. 124–125). A person who is dependent on alcohol (see pp. 80–81) is also likely to

experience sexual problems, and some prescribed drugs have as side-effects loss of interest in sex or problems in sexual functioning. For example, drugs given to reduce blood pressure may cause erectile and ejaculatory difficulties in men. Psychological factors, especially anxiety and depression, frequently affect sexual interest and performance (see pp. 112–113 and pp. 114–115).

Sexual problems arising from medical treatments may be overlooked by doctors through their own embarrassment or that of their patients. Yet many sexual problems can be effectively treated by a combination of approaches: medical intervention (e.g. changing a drug (e.g. Viagra), the use of hormones), surgical interventions (e.g. vascular surgery) or counselling (see pp. 132–133).

Stop and think

- Transvestism (most commonly males dressing in female clothing) has always existed in many societies, either as entertainment for others or in secret. Many cross-dressers have no wish to change their sexual identity but get pleasure from cross-dressing. Sexual excitement is sometimes involved, but cross-dressing is also done in private by the individual for comfort and to relieve stress. What does this say about society's sex role stereotypes and expectations of men?

How does sexuality develop?

- Sexual development is influenced by biological, social and cultural factors.
- Difficulties can arise in sexual functioning, compatibility, fertility and psychosocial functioning, or as a result of sexually transmitted disease.
- Medical and psychological disorders can interfere with sexual functioning.
- Sexual problems can be effectively treated by medical or surgical interventions or by counselling (e.g. behavioural psychotherapy).

15 | Intelligence

Intelligence has been described as the ability to learn from everyday experience; think rationally; solve problems; act purposively and engage in abstract reasoning. Assumptions about intelligence may affect how we treat others, and, for very few people, intelligence limits their capacity for self-care.

'Intelligence' is a value-laden term. No one wants to be categorized as unintelligent, and stereotyping patients or students as 'intelligent' or 'unintelligent' has consequences for how they are treated. When someone is perceived to be unintelligent, people may think it is not worth explaining things to them, resulting in communication breakdown, loss of confidence and uninformed decision-making. This can be especially problematic when we want to encourage self-management and adherence amongst patients (see pp. 92–93). Thus health care professionals should be cautious about making inferences about their patients' intelligence.

What do intelligence tests measure?

Intelligence tests assess how well a person learns or acquires skills and depends, to some extent, on prior experience and learning. Intelligence tests identify individual differences in general reasoning abilities, whereas aptitude tests such as tests of musical ability focus on particular abilities.

Psychologists distinguish *crystallized* and *fluid* intelligence. Crystallized intelligence is based on skills and knowledge learnt within particular cultures. Fluid intelligence is the capacity to reason and solve problems, which enables us to learn from experience. Tests that measure abstraction and generalization primarily assess fluid intelligence. For example, the Raven Progressive Matrices test involves a series of pattern-matching problems. The test measures the ability to infer abstract relationships and patterns from data and assesses the capacity to decompose problems into subtasks and hold multiple subtasks in mind.

Tests that assess vocabulary, general knowledge and scholastic attainment provide information about crystallized intelligence. For example, the Wechsler Adult Intelligence Scale (WAIS) has 11 subscales. Six of these generate a *verbal intelligence* score: (1) information, (2) comprehension, (3) arithmetic, (4) similarities, (5) digit span and (6) vocabulary. The other five offer a *performance* score: (1) digit symbol, (2) picture completion, (3) block design, (4) picture arrangement and (5) object assembly. Tests of this nature draw on culture-specific learning, assessing crystallized as well as fluid intelligence by using questions such as 'What is the capital of Spain?' (comprehension) and 'How are a comb and a brush alike?' (similarities). A children's version (the Wechsler Intelligence Scale for Children; WISC) is used to assess performance and progress at school.

Intelligence tests are scored so that the average (or mean) score is 100 and the standard deviation is 15. So that 68% of the population have scores, or intelligence quotients (IQs), between 85 and 115, and 95% score between 70 and 130. A score of 148 is required to join MENSA, a society for those with an exceptionally high IQ, and people scoring less than 70 (two standard deviations below the mean) may have learning disabilities and need special help in school and with everyday living.

Scores on intelligence tests are stable. Successive test scores correlate highly and children's scores (e.g. at age 6 years) predict adult scores (e.g. at 18 years ($r = 0.8$)). Children's scores also predict performance at school and the number of years they stay

at school ($r = 0.5$–0.55). However, other determinants are also important. IQ scores can predict measures of job performance such as supervisor ratings but other characteristics such as interpersonal skills, particular knowledge and aspects of personality are probably of equal or greater importance to job performance.

Thurstone (1938) proposed that intelligence consists of seven distinct mental abilities. Guilford (1967) considered 120 separate mental abilities, and Gardner (2001) has suggested that as well as linguistic, logical/mathematical and spatial intelligence (measured in tests such as the WAIS), we should also consider musical, body-kinetic, interpersonal and intrapersonal intelligence. Thus, rather than thinking of intelligence as a single dimension, we may be better able to understand differences in people's abilities by investigating a range of distinct intelligences. An alternative view (Sternberg, 1996) is that intelligence has three crucial components: analytic, creative and practical.

Is intelligence genetically determined?

Performance on intelligence tests is affected by many factors. Closer genetic relationships lead to more similar scores. The correlation between the IQ scores of monozygotic (MZ) twins brought up in the same family is 0.9 whereas the correlation for MZ reared apart is 0.7 to 0.8. In contrast, the correlation between genetically unrelated children reared together in adoptive families ranges from 0.0 to 0.2. These facts do not mean that performance on intelligence tests cannot be changed. One of the mechanisms by which genetic make-up affects performance is through the selection of environments that enhance particular skills. If the environment and available learning experiences change, so will performance, including on intelligence tests (see Neisser et al., 1996). Interestingly children's IQ scores correlate better at age 18 years than at age 6 years with their parents' IQs, suggesting a role for shared learning experiences.

Group differences on intelligence scores

Most intelligence tests have been standardized for sex; items with different scores for men and women have been eliminated. Consequently, men and women tend to have equal intelligence scores. Differences have been found between other groups such as black and white Americans, with the white mean being about 10 points higher. A range of explanations has been proposed for this difference. Most controversially, that there may be differences in the black and white gene pools that confer a different range of intellectual abilities. This explanation is problematic if other factors differ between the two groups. By analogy, imagine two plants with the same genetic make-up planted in soil that is either rich or poor in nutrients. The plants will grow to different heights even though height is genetically determined. If environments relevant to intelligence test performance differ, on average, for black and white Americans, then group performance might differ, even if the two populations share the same intelligence-relevant genes. A larger proportion of black Americans live in poverty, which is associated with poor nutrition, less adequate parenting and a lack of intellectual resources and stimulation. In addition, not long ago, black Americans did not have equal civil rights (in relation to voting, schooling, etc.) and they continue to suffer discrimination (Neisser et al., 1996). Another explanation for group differences is that intelligence tests draw on particular cultural experiences so that people brought up in a different culture are disadvantaged.

Health and intelligence

In 1997 Whalley and Deary (2001) traced more than 2,000 children born in Aberdeen in 1921. Mental ability scores based on childhood tests converted into IQ scores were positively related to survival to age 76 years in both women and men. Overcrowding in the school catchment area, estimated from the 1931 UK census, was weakly related to survival. Such data suggests that intelligence scores are related to mortality. However, intelligence scores and socio-economic status (SES) are also correlated. For example, the correlation between parents' SES and one's own IQ is about 0.33. Mortality and morbidity rates are inversely related to SES.

Environmental factors can affect intelligence and health, for example, malnutrition, exposure to lead and antenatal exposure to alcohol are all associated with lower IQ scores. Associations between lower IQ and antenatal exposure to aspirin and antibiotics have also been reported (Zigler and Valentine, 1979).

Are we getting more intelligent?

Yes! The Flynn (1987) effect. Average scores on intelligence tests have increased over time. Interestingly, the largest gains are on tests of fluid intelligence. For example, Raven's Matrices IQ scores in the Netherlands increased by 21 points between 1952 and 1982. So, if we transported a person with an average IQ today back 70 years, that person would be regarded as exceptionally intelligent (e.g. scoring up to 149). By comparison, US WAIS scores, which reflect crystallized as well as fluid intelligence, have risen by about three points per decade. Similar effects have been observed in other countries, and these effects are typically larger than IQ differences between groups. The Flynn effect may be attributed to better schooling and a more visually sophisticated and information-rich culture; it might also be related to improved nutrition. For example, increases in the IQ scores of Spanish children over time primarily resulted from improvements at the lower end of the distribution. More recently it has been suggested that the Flynn effect has halted or even been reversed in certain European countries (Dutton, van der Linden and Lynn, 2016).

Does intelligence decline with age?

Yes and no. Fluid intelligence declines with age, but as we get older, we also get wiser. On many tests of intelligence, especially those of crystallized intelligence, IQ increases with age, peaking around the mid-50s. Older people, including those in their 80s,

can draw upon knowledge built up over their lives. Younger people may outperform older people on tests focussing on fluid intelligence, especially when these are timed tests. The best predictor of an older person's IQ is likely to be his or her IQ when younger.

Can we boost intelligence?

During Project Head Start, a series of preschool schemes run in the USA in the 1960s, children were provided with extra teaching and play opportunities designed to enhance the intellectual content of their environment. Children participating in such schemes had higher intelligence test scores compared with similar children not participating in the schemes. However, once the schemes ended, these differences tended to disappear by age 11 to 12 years. However, children taking part were less likely to be: assigned to special education, held back in school and leave school than matched children not in the schemes (Neisser et al., 1996).

Intelligence

- Intelligence can be defined as the ability to learn from everyday experience and to think rationally.
- Psychologists distinguish between fluid and crystallized intelligence.
- About 68% of the population has IQs between 85 and 115.
- People with closer genetic relationships tend to have similar IQs.
- Average group differences in IQ are not helpful in predicting an individual's intelligence.
- IQ is associated with mortality, but both are associated with socioeconomic status.
- Average scores on intelligence tests have increased over time (the Flynn effect).
- Older people do better than younger people on test of intelligence that draw on their experience.

Stop and think

Traditional intelligence tests (e.g. WAIS) assess individual problem-solving ability by using a limited set of problem types that have clearly defined answers. Howard Gardner includes intrapersonal and interpersonal intelligence among his types of intelligence – the abilities to understand oneself and other people. Other psychologists have suggested that we have a (related) type of intelligence called *emotional intelligence*, or EI.

The items in EI tests, similar to personality tests, do not have right or wrong answers, how might we say that IQ and EI are two subtypes of a single characteristic – intelligence?

Case study *High IQ: Grigori Perelman*

Having, or being estimated to have, an exceedingly high IQ indicates a particular set of analytic skills but may not correspond to a lay notion of extreme intelligence. In particular, high IQ does not guarantee worldly success, which is why authors such as Robert Sternberg (1996) have suggested a largely unrelated type of intelligence – practical intelligence. People estimated to have very high IQs (160+) include successful business people, for example, Paul Allen, co-founder of Microsoft, as well as chess players (Judit Polgar, Gary Kasparov) and mathematicians (Andrew Wiles, who proved Fermat's Last Theorem; Grigori Perelman). Perelman is an interesting case. He has had difficult relationships both with other mathematicians and with the world at large. Perelman's IQ is unknown. Indeed, there is no satisfactory way to measure very high IQs because they are too rare to occur in the samples on which IQ tests are standardized. A case could be made for describing Perelman as the world's top mathematician. In 2000 seven unsolved mathematical problems were identified as 'Millennium Prize' problems, and a private institution, the Clay Mathematics Institute, offered a US $1 million prize for a solution to any of the problems. Only one has been solved, the Poincare Conjecture (a problem in topology), by Perelman. Perelman has refused both the Millennium Prize itself and the Fields Medal (the nearest thing to a Nobel Prize in Mathematics), partly because he did not want the fame and publicity (or the money) and partly because he thought other mathematicians on whose work he had built (particularly that of Richard S. Hamilton) was not being recognised. Perelman left his job in academia and may have abandoned mathematics altogether. He went to live with his mother in St Petersburg, Russia, and avoided all contact with the media.

16 | Development of thinking

Do children simply know less than adults do, or do children and adults think in qualitatively different ways? For example, are children just as capable as adults of understanding why they are ill or why they should take their medication, if they are presented with the relevant information? Or do children under a certain age lack the necessary concepts to make sense of such explanations? Questions such as these are addressed by psychological research into cognitive development, which investigates age-related changes in thinking and other intellectual abilities. This chapter will focus on evidence from research into children's understanding of illness, both because this illustrates some general issues regarding the nature of cognitive development and because it has important implications for health care and health education.

Does understanding of illness develop through distinct age-related stages?

Early research on children's understanding of illness was heavily influenced by the work of Jean Piaget (1896–1980). Piaget revolutionized the study of cognitive development by arguing that young children not only know less than older children and adults do but also view the world in radically different ways. For example, Piaget argued that until the age of about 7 years children are not able to reason logically and lack an understanding of fundamental concepts such as causality. He proposed that children's cognitive abilities develop through a series of stages that differ qualitatively from each other and that apply to children's understanding across all domains (e.g. mathematics, causality, morality).

Findings from pioneering studies of children's understanding of illness were interpreted as reflecting Piaget's stages of cognitive development (Bibace and Walsh, 1980; Kister and Patterson, 1980). For example, it was argued that 4- to 7-year-olds typically view illness either as being a punishment for their misbehaviour or as being caused by proximity to ill people or to particular objects – that is, they have a very basic concept of contagion without any understanding of an underlying causal mechanism. In contrast, 7- to 11-year-olds are able to give explanations based on a concept of contamination in that they see illness as caused by physical contact with an ill person or by germs. From the age of about 11 years, children have a more sophisticated understanding of illness, including a concept of internalization processes (e.g. swallowing, inhaling) through which external causes influence internal bodily processes.

However, more recent research suggests that these stages present an over-simplified picture that may under-estimate both the complexity of children's understanding of illness and the extent to which it is influenced by knowledge about specific illnesses (e.g. Myant and Williams, 2005). Also since young children do not usually receive explicit tuition about the causes of illness, the typical stages may partly reflect what they have had the opportunity to learn, rather than representing the limits of children's ability to understand explanations of illness.

How do children understand different types of illness?

Myant and Williams (2005) explored this issue by asking 4- to 12-year-old children questions about cartoon characters that had

various types of ailment (injuries, contagious and non-contagious illnesses). Children of all ages understood injuries (bruise and broken leg) better than illnesses and showed a good understanding of how injuries are caused and could be prevented. This may be because children tend to have more experience of injuries than of illnesses and because the causes of injuries are usually more observable and more directly linked to the child's behaviour (e.g. *Sally got a bruise because she fell off her bike*). However, greater familiarity did not always result in more sophisticated understanding. Although colds are familiar illnesses, misconceptions about them being caused by cold weather rather than by contagion were evident even in older children. Myant and Williams suggested that this may be because similar misconceptions are often evident in what adults say to children (e.g. 'you'll catch a cold if you go out in the snow without your scarf').

Within the category of contagious illnesses, children gave more accurate causal explanations of chickenpox than colds. Even the 4- to 5-year-olds showed a basic ability to explain chickenpox in terms of the biological factor of contagion (e.g. catching chickenpox by 'germs' being passed on from a friend who has chickenpox), although a more detailed understanding of the biological mechanisms involved in contagion takes time to develop.

Within the category of non-contagious illnesses, children gave more accurate explanations of toothache than of asthma. Children's explanations of toothache showed a similar level of understanding to their explanations of injuries, perhaps because some of the causal factors that contribute to toothache relate to directly observable physical behaviours such as eating sugary foods and not brushing teeth. Also these factors have typically been emphasized in dental health education. (Our current knowledge concerning tooth brushing, however, is that it is the fluoride additive that confers the protection to the tooth enamel and not the thoroughness of the tooth brushing itself.) Even 4- to 5-year-olds were able to explain toothache in terms of these behavioural causes, whereas older children were more likely to refer also to underlying biological mechanisms of toothache such as tooth decay processes. Children of all ages understood asthma less well than toothache. Again younger children's explanations tended to focus on physical factors – from about the age of 7 years, children showed a basic understanding of physical triggers of asthma symptoms (e.g. exercise or allergens). Older children were more likely to refer also to biological causes (e.g. genetic inheritance).

Although some earlier research found that young children tend to over-extend the concept of contagion by explaining non-contagious illnesses as if they were contagious, even the youngest children in Myant and Williams' study did not show this type of misunderstanding when explaining toothache.

Stop and think

- What would you do or say to help a 4-year-old child in hospital who was worried about catching appendicitis from the child in the next bed?

Does personal experience of illness influence children's understanding of illness?

Case study *Children's understanding of their blood*

When a 3-year-old girl with leukaemia joined a playgroup, the staff members were concerned about how to explain her illness to the other children, and a group of researchers decided to investigate this topic (Eiser, Havermans and Casas, 1993). They interviewed healthy 3- and 4-year-old children about their knowledge and experiences of blood and then gave the children an explanation of the functions of different types of blood cells, illustrating their explanation with drawings. Although on the whole the children had difficulty understanding the explanation, the children who showed most understanding were those who had mentioned a personal experience involving blood.

The researchers also interviewed the 3-year-old girl with leukaemia. In the course of her treatment, she had received more extensive and more frequently repeated explanations about blood than the healthy children had, and these explanations obviously had clear personal relevance to her. Her knowledge of the structure and function of blood was found to be much more advanced than that of the healthy children: 'she knew that blood... is full of red cells which make new blood, white cells which fight infection, and platelets which stop bleeding'. 'Sometimes the platelets don't come and then you keep bleeding.' About the leukaemia, she said that she was 'full of bad cells – they just come' (Eiser et al., 1993, p. 535).

Although this explanation includes some misunderstandings and some of the phrases may be simple repetitions of adults' speech without full understanding, and although we do not know how typical the explanation is of other 3-year-olds who are receiving treatment, the explanation is, nevertheless, extremely impressive for such a young child, and it suggests that young children's ability to understand explanations of illness may be much greater than has often been supposed.

How can children's understanding of illness be enhanced?

Children's understanding of illness can be enhanced by providing them with explicit tuition. For example, when children under the age of about 14 years produce spontaneous explanations that refer to germs, these typically relate to mechanical mechanisms (e.g. the movement or path of germs), rather than to biological mechanisms (e.g. germ reproduction). However, when 8- to 9-year-olds were taught about AIDS and other infectious diseases in an intervention study, they learned to give explanations based on biological mechanisms. Similarly when adolescents participated in interventions regarding HIV/AIDS prevention, their learning was more effective if the intervention encouraged them to learn about biological mechanisms of disease transmission (e.g. the role of micro-organisms in AIDS) than if it involved memorizing factual information about risk factors (Zamora, Romo and Au, 2006). The central role of explanations in enhancing children's understanding of illness is highlighted further by a study in which 7- and 11-year-olds were taught about contagious illnesses (e.g. colds, chickenpox). There were three types of intervention that involved presenting factual information: (1) in an illustrated story with explanations, (2) in a formal scientific style with explanations or (3) in a story without explanations. The children who received an intervention that included explanations showed more improvement in their understanding of contagious illnesses compared with those who received an intervention without explanations. The two groups of children who received interventions involving explanations showed comparable levels of improvement, irrespective of whether the factual information was presented as a story or in a formal scientific style (Myant and Williams, 2008).

The case study suggests that children's understanding of illness may be influenced by their personal experience. Further evidence in support of this conclusion comes from a study by Crisp, Ungerer and Goodnow (1996), which found that 7- to 10-year-olds with cancer showed a more advanced understanding of illness than those who had experienced only more minor or acute illnesses. However, the extent of children's medical experience (duration of illness, frequency of hospitalization) does not affect their understanding of the causes of illness. Similarly, Crisp et al. noted that various factors, including the nature of the specific chronic illness that children experience, may influence whether their understanding is enhanced. Therefore to communicate effectively with children about illness, health care professionals should be careful to neither over-estimate the knowledge of children with prior experience of illness nor underestimate the extent to which children's understanding could potentially be enhanced by presenting explanations geared to their individual cognitive levels.

Development of thinking

- The development of children's thinking about illness, like other aspects of the development of thinking, involves a complex interplay between learning factual information and developing conceptual understanding.

- Although children's understanding of illness becomes more accurate, detailed and sophisticated as they get older, it is not as constrained by specific stages of development as earlier research suggested.

- The way children think about illness depends not only on their age but also on:
  - The type of illness (e.g. contagious illness, non-contagious illness, injury) and the specific illness within these types
  - Their personal experience of illness or specific illnesses
  - The nature and extent of explicit tuition they receive about illness

- Children's understanding of illness is more likely to be enhanced by explicit tuition that provides explanations and emphasizes causal mechanisms, rather than that which simply encourages memorization of factual information.

17 | Understanding groups

The effectiveness of medical staff depends on team work. No doctor works completely alone. So if they are to be effective, doctors must know how to work with and in groups. Research shows that groups can produce more effective solutions than the sum of individuals working on their own. Groups can also have negative effects, which can, if understood, be avoided or minimized: e.g. we may behave in ways we would not if we were on our own. Finally groups are central to our social and personal identity. Joining the medical profession after university involves becoming part of a different group, becoming a different person with different identification, interests and loyalties (see spread 82, pp. 164–165). Becoming aware of the power of groups is an important part of professional training.

What are groups?

Groups are essential and pervasive. Each of us belongs to many groups of different kinds. It has been estimated that typically we have membership of about 100 groups, ranging from our family, professional and friendship groups, to neighbourhood or sports teams, to our country or religion.

A group can be defined as consisting of three or more people who have shared goals, interact with and have relationships with each other, have mutually agreed ways of doing things and share an identity.

Features of groups

Conformity

In groups we tend to conform. We 'go along with' the group despite private reservations. Conformity can be problematic: for example, going along with poor decisions because of actual or imagined pressures. Not surprisingly as a medical student you will tend to conform to decisions made by more senior colleagues even if you disagree privately. The more we want to belong to a group or are tied in to the group, the more we conform. Also the lower our status in the group, the more we conform. But conformity is also valuable and important; groups and teams depend on doing things 'the group way' to work together efficiently and effectively.

There are three underlying dynamics of conformity:

1. Normative pressures – be like others to get rewards or avoid punishment.
2. Informational pressures – the group provides information, but restricts access to alternative sources.
3. Intergroup pressures – we may support our group versus other groups because we may perceive them as threatening to our group.

These pressures are especially strong when the situation is new or unclear; we look to other people for clues about what to do.

Obedience

Most people obey authority. In one well-known series of experiments, participants were asked by an experimenter to administer electric shocks to other volunteer participants. The prediction was that only 1/1,000 would obey. Two-thirds, in fact, did as requested. (The shocks were not, in fact, real!)

Factors that influence the likelihood of obedience are similar to those affecting conformity but also include the perceived benefit

of obeying the person in authority. Many human systems depend upon obedience to authority (e.g. the armed services). To some extent hospital medicine also relies on obedience to authority to ensure that there is a clear and appropriate understanding of responsibility towards patients. If consultants are ultimately responsible for patient care, they must be able to trust that junior medical staff will carry out instructions. Automatic obedience, however, is not wise. Occasionally senior staff make errors, and young doctors need to think critically as they work and be courageous enough to question a wrong decision.

Deviance

Groups do not easily tolerate people who do not conform (dissenters). Dissenters:

- Are normally unpopular because they threaten the cohesiveness and "self-esteem" of the group.
- If they persist, are likely to be rejected and excluded.
- If won over, are usually seen as particularly valuable.
- But can offer alternative and better solutions, which may be vital for the group's long-term survival.
- Can challenge the group to review, explore, elaborate and justify its position.
- Are more effective if there is at least one other dissenting voice, even if the dissenters do not agree with each other.

It is not comfortable being a dissenter, but dissenters are often important over time and may therefore need protection and support.

Structure

Groups consisting of people who are very similar to each other are called *homogeneous*. These groups often get on well together and can quickly establish their working practices. They may, however, be poor at dealing with difficult problems and at innovating and adapting in the long run. Groups with different kinds of people are known as *heterogeneous*. These take more time to settle down and may experience more conflict within the group as they do so, but they are able to generate better solutions in the long run.

There is a natural development of virtually all new groups. This has been described elegantly by Tuckman (1965) and involves four stages, namely: Forming, Storming, Norming and Performing. A final stage, known as Adjourning, which reflects the phase when the group disperses after the tasks are completed, has been added.

Groups have both social and task aspects: that is, there is a social, interpersonal aspect to the group as well as its formal, stated objective or task. A group that only focusses on tasks may seem efficient, but it engenders little loyalty and does not survive long (Fig. 17.1). Paying attention to people's social and emotional needs as well as the task is therefore important for the long-term effectiveness of the group.

Intergroup competition and conflict

Sometimes groups conflict with one another. Intergroup conflict is very common and occurs between rival sport clubs, schools, religions, nations and health care professions. Although competition can be healthy, if it escalates, conflict can lead to serious disputes, even war, and eventually genocide. Conflict can be triggered by simply labelling people as members of different groups. The need for the 'in-group' to generate a positive group identity is achieved by competing with and being better than the

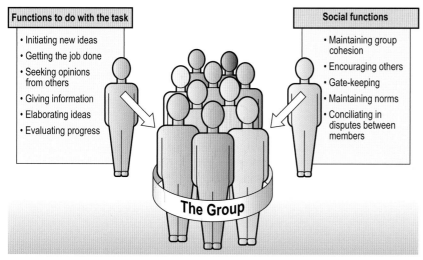

Functions to do with the task	Social functions
• Initiating new ideas • Getting the job done • Seeking opinions from others • Giving information • Elaborating ideas • Evaluating progress	• Maintaining group cohesion • Encouraging others • Gate-keeping • Maintaining norms • Conciliating in disputes between members

Fig. 17.1 Typical roles in a group.

'out-group'. Conflict often results from competition for the same resources or goals. In these cases identifying super-ordinate goals (both groups want, but also need each other to achieve them) can drive co-operation.

One notable feature of intergroup conflict is stereotyping whereby members of the 'out-group' are lumped together and seen as bad, weak or aggressive or as possessing admired but feared characteristics such as intelligence, cunning or sexuality. Individual differences between people are minimized and differences between in- and out-group members are exaggerated: for example, all working class people are seen as racist, all women are gossips, all football supporters as hooligans and so on.

Effective groups

Research by Michael West (2004) demonstrated clearly that a number of highly significant health outcomes in both acute-care and community settings are affected by group or team structure and processes. These include the quality of health care provided, patient morbidity and mortality rates, accidents and error rates, staff satisfaction and staff turnover. Teams are the vehicles by which staff deliver health care to patients. It, therefore, makes good sense for health care services to pay close attention to exactly how staff teams work together. Effective teams provide a much better standard of care compared with less effective teams and are characterized by having the following:

- A clear, shared purpose or vision (people knowing exactly what their team uniquely is trying to achieve)
- Agreed goals spelling out how to achieve that purpose
- Job clarity: everyone in the team knowing what is expected of them (since lack of job clarity is a prime cause of job dissatisfaction)
- Clear communication processes and agreed methods for decision-making
- Participation by all, and making effective use of diversity (since having a range of professional groups and a range of cultural perspectives enhances decisions)
- Regular team reviews to check the team is on track
- Having clear leadership (although this can be shared)

Teams that regularly take time out to look at how they are performing as a unit are much safer places than teams that do not. Doctors are in a good position to ask questions about how the team is working and when the team last checked on its own health as a performing unit.

Case study *Intergroup conflict*

The staff of a large inner-city general practice decided to establish an asthma clinic in response to increasing patient numbers. Part of the strategy was to include assessment of patients at home, carried out by practice community staff. The medical staff announced the plan to the community staff, without consulting them about the feasibility of the procedures. Some tried to carry out the assessments as requested, whereas others declared the whole strategy unworkable, given other time constraints. One of the nurses who was eager to implement the strategy was criticized heavily by the others and soon left the job. Some medical staff felt some sympathy for the nurses and suggested that the plan had been implemented too hastily but were accused by others of being behind the times. Each group of staff considered the other group to be thoughtless, unprofessional, selfish and lazy. The atmosphere in the practice became unpleasant and hostile, and even the patients began to notice this. Only the appointment of a practice manager (an outsider), who agreed to review the whole issue, allowed the situation to calm down and return to normal.

Understanding groups

- Groups can reach better outcomes than the sum of individuals working alone.
- Groups give us a sense of belonging but also create conformity pressures.
- Groups may punish non-conformers by making them feel odd, unwanted and excluded.
- Groups can be a force for good, providing support, allowing team work and fostering engagement and loyalty.
- Effective teams provide safe, higher-quality care.
- Group identity can lead to in-group/out-group conflict.

Stop and think

- Consider groups you have been in such as a tutorial or work group.
- Most groups or teams tend to show the previously mentioned features, especially if the team has worked together for a long time. You may have noticed that group members tend to do different things to keep the team functioning (Fig. 17.1). Also although people tend to behave fairly consistently in one group, they may behave differently, playing a different role in another group.
- Why might a person's role change depending on the particular group he or she is in?

18 | Concepts of health, illness and disease

Ideas matter. Beliefs matter. They influence how we see and what we expect of ourselves, and how we see and what we expect of others.

Medical concepts

The implicit assumption of the biomedical model (Fig. 18.1) is that to be healthy is to be 'without disease': to have no identifiable signs of physical abnormality. However, this model does not align with the reality of medical work or acknowledge the tensions that biomedicine can give rise to. Many patients seek medical assistance for conditions that are not classified as disease (e.g. psychological illness, pain, fatigue and post-viral syndromes). In addition, we can suffer from diseases that have not been identified or fully understood (e.g. in the past, multiple sclerosis, swine flu or toxic shock syndrome). Potentially irresolvable conflict between biomedically minded doctors and ourselves as patients can occur when we experience a form of suffering yet feel that this is rejected. Even where disease is clearly identifiable, doctors relying on a biomedical perspective alone, frequently understand things differently from their patients. Doctors can be puzzled if we claim to be healthy when we are diseased or if we do not seek or follow conventional medical advice.

To practise medicine effectively doctors need to acknowledge that patient or 'lay' perspectives of health and illness co-exist alongside the medical perspective and will have a profound effect on medical care. Once this is understood, communication can be learned for doctors and patients to work more collaboratively.

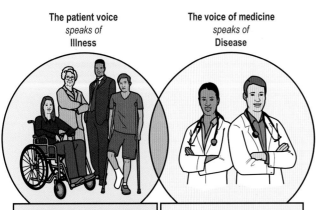

The patient voice *speaks of* **Illness**

The voice of medicine *speaks of* **Disease**

Illness is often <u>subjective</u>. Being ill may incorporate medical ideas of disease but it will also be influenced by individual circumstance and affected by culture, psychology and social factors such as age, gender, marital status and economic status.

Illness/health means different things to each of us

Disease is <u>objective</u>. It can be discovered or 'ruled out' using scientific measures such as blood tests, x rays, ultrasound.

Typically health is simply the absence of disease
(You are either diseased or you are not)

Doctors need to know that both conceptual worlds exist and to be skilled in taking patients' ideas about illness into account. This understanding forms the basis of communication skills teaching, where students are given a framework for exploring illness and disease during the consultation. This model is also useful for understanding the value of shared decision making and resource allocation.

Fig. 18.1 A model for concepts of health, illness and disease.

Lay (or non-specialist) concepts

How we as patients interpret our bodily experiences may have no direct relationship to the presence of medically defined disease. Rather our knowledge is drawn from our immediate culture (families and communities) and from broader societal views, via the (social) media, or other healers that operate alongside the biomedical system (e.g. Indian Ayurvedic, homeopathic, herbal or Chinese medicine). For example, many health care professionals believe that poor knowledge and fatalistic attitudes are the main barriers to healthy lifestyle choices amongst British Bangladeshis with type 1 diabetes. However, studies have shown that interventions (designed for a white population), have little impact because Islam has more significance than medicine in terms of Bangladeshi food choices. The solution to the treatment and prevention of diabetes therefore lies in recognising that the norms and expectations of Islam offer opportunities for supporting patients.

Over the past 40 years there has been extensive research into how we think of health and illness. Listed below are three common conceptualizations of health that exist in modern Western societies today and one important point about illness.

Health as absence of disease

This view of health is passive and fatalistic because it assumes that if there is nothing overtly wrong, then you 'just carry on'. From this point of view, few measures are taken to prevent illness. Persisting in the most deprived, least empowered populations, this perspective has been found traditionally to be held by men who are more likely to adopt health-damaging behaviours (see pp. 44–45 on gender).

Large-scale surveys and in-depth studies have found that individuals can often consider themselves to be healthy *despite* experiencing symptoms. For example, a study of women (average age 51 years) with few material resources in northeast Scotland found that they had low expectations of good health. As such 'you keep going until your number's up' (Blaxter and Paterson, 1982). The idea that illness is something 'that you don't lie down to' was also reported by Cornwell (1984) in her classic study of (working class) Bethnal Green. Evidence suggests that these attitudes have persisted over time:

I believe in God. Like I told you, he has his Big Book. Your expiration date is written in there somewhere. When that day comes, that's it … when the product is past its due date, it's not good anymore. (Max, 44, former tow truck driver, in Savage et al., 2013, p. 1218).

Although health interventions have been aimed predominantly at changing individual behaviours, attitudes towards health are influenced significantly by our social environments and the psychosocial stressors and lack of control that they can engender. Paradoxically indulging in unhealthy behaviours may act as a short-term buffer to poor circumstances. For example, among both men and women, drinking and smoking or drug abuse can be part and parcel of social activities that temporarily alleviate stress and strengthen kinship and belonging within many communities. (It is also important to note that not all individuals in deprived circumstances take a fatalistic approach to health.)

Health as functionality and being able to cope

This is a more proactive view of health taking into account not only 'being able to function physically' but also 'being able to manage things well'. In this sense well-being is also an indicator of health. Here health is described as 'having lots of energy', 'feeling good' and 'not being bothered by anything'. Having a positive attitude towards life counts as does taking active measures to prevent ill health.

Traditionally women have been found to be more proactive than men. Not least because of reproduction, women at all ages are more 'used' to medical intervention. They are also more likely to be informal care givers within the family, and therefore more knowledgeable about health issues. Several recent studies have shown that men (shown in earlier work as privileging physical fitness over wellbeing) are increasingly interested in health issues.

Doctors need to be aware that ideas about functionality and health can change with age. Thus, we tend to relate potential symptoms to signs of ageing or to symptoms of pre-diagnosed conditions. Significantly a sense of wellbeing can *override* physical functioning (and potential help seeking). The sentiment here is that 'there is no point in moaning about trivial aches and pains, because overall, life is good'.

Health as positive fitness and well-being

Here health is 'an aim in life', with individuals working actively to maintain 'equilibrium' or, as D'houtard and Field (1984) suggested, achieve 'a life without constraints'. This perspective recognises overtly that disease can be a product of chance but more so, illness is dependent on events in life and the stressors of modern society. As wellness is central to this perspective, it is possible to define oneself as healthy and having a good life despite also being diagnosed as ill.

Taken to an extreme, this form of proactivity towards health is sometimes described as a form of health consumerism known as 'healthism'. Characterized by high health awareness and expectations, healthism can be problematic for medics, who are increasingly finding their diagnoses and explanations contested. The growing phenomenon of self-diagnosis has been influenced by the availability of medical information on the internet; lay social movements; the rise in the 'well-being market'; commercial forces keen to exploit the growing interest in self-diagnosis (e.g. private laboratories that test blood) and encouragement from

health services for patients to be experts (Jutel and Dew, 2014). Doctors are not immune from labelling patients, and a key concern is that as demands on health care professionals increase, an individual who is, indeed, 'ill' may be passed off as 'worried well'.

The moral dimension of health and illness

Any consideration of lay concepts of health and illness must take into account the moral dimension of illness. Society emphasises personal responsibility for health. In Cornwell's study (1984), a more stoical stance towards health was associated with a commitment to a strong work ethic and fear of being seen as being work shy, letting people down or becoming dependent. Reminiscent of an age before biomedicine where illness and religion were more closely linked, a theme in Blaxter and Paterson's study (1982) of

working class women was that illness was seen as a state of spiritual or moral (rather than physical) malaise associated with personality and a lack of fibre. Illness was seen as 'God's punishment', striking the wicked or the lazy.

Crucially the moral dimension of illness can be seen in our everyday fears of being thought of, by our families, friends and medics, as morally deviant: as 'abnormal', 'weak', 'stupid', 'a problem' or 'disgusting'. Moral judgement can make us feel stigmatized about: obesity, our sexuality, being in an abusive relationship, smoking, drinking or drug-related conditions and more. This stops us seeking help, leaving much illness undiagnosed and untreated (Fig. 43.1). An example here is health amongst the transgender community, who have frequently reported not attending appointments for fear of negative bias and who as a group experience higher rates of morbidity and worse life chances.

Concepts of health, illness and disease

- How we as patients *think* about health, illness and disease is not just a matter of philosophical debate; it is a matter of life and death.
- Different groups within society and different cultures will have varied concepts of health and disease.
- Concepts of health, illness and disease are inherently social and it is important to recognise this in medical practice.
- Doctors and patients may have different views about health, and patients may not reveal their subjective experiences in the belief that

these are not important or valid.
- If medicine is to deal with patients in the context of their family and social relationships, then listening to and understanding the patient's perspective is the prerequisite for good practice.

Stop and think

- What does being healthy mean to you? What do you think it may mean to someone who is 75 years old? How about other people that you know?
- What impact might define something as a disease have on a patient?
- Why is it important to understand the patient's own beliefs?

Case study *Health as absence of disease/fatalistic approach*

Michael Brady has lived almost all his 65 years in a traditionally working class part of Manchester. Michael made his living as a builder and, like many men he worked with, enjoyed a drink and a smoke. A few years ago he developed chronic obstructive pulmonary disease (COPD). Last Tuesday, Michael was also diagnosed with lung cancer. 'It's a very small one, about as big as a pea,' Michael said, describing the tumour. 'If it had gone on any longer, it possibly wouldn't have been curable … I'm just carrying on as normal. I've had quite a few friends that have had cancer and died through it.'

Manchester has the highest number of premature deaths because of lung cancer in England. Lung cancer is often hard to detect until it is too late. In more deprived communities, this occurs because those at greatest risk of lung cancer already have other health conditions. These can mask the symptoms of the cancer, leading to a later diagnosis.

Note: A solution to the problem of non-detected cancer in this population has been to set up mobile screening units in shopping centre car parks, thus targeting members of the population who would not ordinarily seek cancer screening.
Source: BBC News, 14 November, 2016. <http://www.bbc.co.uk/news/health-37923708/>

19 | Measuring health and illness

The measurement of health and illness has become increasingly important as health care professionals, governments and researchers try to assess the effectiveness of treatments, the performance of health services and the consequences of inequality. Important sources of routine and other data are available in many countries globally, although measuring health and illness can be problematic. All births and deaths in developed countries and in many developing countries are legally required to be registered so that, together with census data, accurate counts can be made of birth and death (mortality) rates and of population (demographic) change.

Mortality

Mortality rates, particularly infant and maternal mortality rates, are often used as proxy measures of a country's health and development (see pp. 156–157). Life expectancy also provides a summary measure of health in an area or country, and Fig. 19.1 summarizes overall life expectancy and healthy life expectancy (Box 19.1) for selected countries.

Crude death rates are calculated by dividing the total number of deaths by the number of people in the population. However, because older people and men are more likely to die over a given time period compared with younger people and women, allowance is normally made for the age and sex of the population when making comparisons amongst areas/countries.

Cause-specific death rates are also useful. Cause of death is entered on death certificates and then coded using the International Statistical Classification of Diseases and Health-Related Problems (ICD-10). Table 19.1 gives details of a selection of death rates for selected countries.

Care is required in the interpretation of data because of many factors such as differences in how deaths are categorized and reported and even simple coding errors, which can lead to apparent differences.

Standardized mortality ratios (SMRs) (Box 19.2) are commonly used to compare deaths for specific subgroups in a population. An SMR of 100 indicates that observed deaths equals the expected number of deaths (average mortality). An SMR >100 indicates that observed deaths exceed expected deaths, and an SMR <100 indicates that observed deaths are lower than expected deaths. SMRs are useful summary indicators of mortality in a subpopulation or specific social group, and social scientists have used SMRs particularly to investigate social inequalities in health (see pp. 42–43).

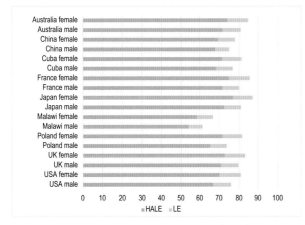

Fig. 19.1 Life expectancy (LE) healthy life expectancy (HALE) for selected countries 2016 *(Global Health Observatory Data Repository WHO 2018 http://www.w.who.int/gho/en/).*

Box 19.1 **Definition**

Healthy life expectancy: the average number of years that a person can expect to live in 'full health', taking into account 'years lived in less than full health due to disease and/or injury'. For details and methods of estimation, see http://www.un.org/esa/sustdev/natlinfo/indicators/methodology_sheets/health/health_life_expectancy.pdf.

Box 19.2 **Standardized mortality ratio (SMR)**

$$SMR = \frac{\text{number of observed deaths} \times 100}{\text{number of expected deaths*}}$$

*which would have occurred if the study population had experienced the same mortality as the reference population, allowing for age and sex differences.

Table 19.1 **Mortality for selected Sustainable Development Goal (SDG) indicators**

	Maternal mortality ratio (2015)	Under 5 mortality rate (2016)	Suicide mortality rate (2016)	Road traffic mortality rate (2013)	Pollution mortality rate (2016)
Australia	6	3.7	13.2	5.4	8.4
China	27	9.9	9.7	18.8	112.7
Cuba	39	5.5	13.9	7.5	49.5
France	8	3.9	17.7	5.1	9.7
Japan	5	2.7	18.5	4.7	11.9
Malawi	634	55.1	3.7	35.0	115.0
Poland	3	4.7	16.2	10.3	37.9
UK	9	4.3	8.9	2.9	13.8
USA	14	6.5	15.3	10.6	13.3

Under 5 mortality rate (per 1000 live births), Road Traffic Mortality Rate and Suicide Mortality Rate (both per 100,000 population), Maternal Mortality Ratio (per 100,000 live births), mortality rate attributed to household and ambient air pollution (age standardised per 100,000 population) (from World health statistics 2018: monitoring health for the SDGs, sustainable development goals. Geneva: World Health Organization; 2018).

The use of death rates has limitations and measures that capture avoidable mortality and life-years lost are increasingly being used. Rates of avoidable mortality identify deaths that might have been avoided if good medical, preventive and health promotion services had been available, accessible and taken up and are useful for public health interventions. Rates of life-years lost reflect the relatively increased burden of premature mortality in younger people.

Morbidity

Although death is generally a certain and countable event, mortality rates do not tell us much about illness or health in a population, although 'healthy life expectancy' and 'avoidable deaths' are attempts to derive more useful mortality indicators. Illness, morbidity and health are, however, considerably more difficult to define, and hence to measure, compared with death.

Consultation rates with doctors are sometimes used as a proxy measure of illness in a population. Measured as the number of consultations over a defined period in a given population, consultation rates suffer from a number of limitations. In many countries it may be difficult to define and measure the denominator population from which the consulters came. Use of a doctor is strongly influenced by availability of doctors in a particular area and psychological, social and cultural factors strongly influence people's decision to consult (see pp. 86–87), and these may change over time.

Referral rates to hospital and hospital admission rates (by diagnostic groups) provide some information on patterns and trends in morbidity, but these also vary by referrer practice, supply of hospital services and admission and discharge practices.

Disease registers, which hold details of the identity of every person diagnosed with a particular disease (e.g. cancer), its type and its treatment, provide excellent individual, longitudinal data for research, but they are expensive to set up and to maintain and are not available in many countries.

National surveys of health are undertaken in many countries. These include the National Health Interview Survey in the USA and the General Household Survey (GHS) in the UK. The GHS, an annual national sample survey of households, asks questions about chronic and acute illnesses. It is also one of the morbidity measures used to adjust for healthy life expectancy. Although the GHS provides a regular picture of ill health, the sample size makes it difficult to examine differences in morbidity at the regional or district level.

A large number of self-report instruments (often questionnaires) have been developed to measure the impact of specific diseases and illness on health, most of which incorporate a variety of scales designed to assess the physical, psychological and social effects of the disease.

A number of instruments have also been designed to measure health and well-being more generally (Bowling, 2005). For example, the SF-36 (Box 19.3) has been shown to be reliable and valid (Box 19.4) and has become a commonly used evaluative instrument. A shorter 12-item scale has also been constructed, the SF-12, and the EuroQol group has constructed a five-item scale, the EQ-5D (see Case study).

Overall, it is important to be clear about the purpose for which measurement instruments have been designed and how this relates to their use. If using instruments in a new context or population, particularly different ethnic groups, it is important to make sure that these instruments are valid and reliable. Care should also be taken not to assume that they measure health or ill health comprehensively – they are summary indicators. Finally care should be taken when comparing the results of studies using different instruments.

Box 19.3 **The SF-36 questionnaire**

The SF-36 uses 36 questions to ask about eight health attributes:

1. Limitations in physical activities because of health problems
2. Limitations in social activities because of physical or emotional problems
3. Limitations in usual role activities because of physical health problems
4. Bodily pain
5. General mental health (psychological distress and well-being)
6. Limitations in usual role activities because of emotional problems
7. Vitality (energy and fatigue)
8. General health perceptions

Box 19.4 **Reliability and validity**

An instrument is reliable if it reproduces the same results consistently. There are different types of reliability, and a common form is test–retest reliability, which measures the stability of an instrument when used over two different time periods. Reliability can also be assessed between different users (inter-rater reliability) and when different parts of an instrument measure the same thing (internal reliability).

Validity relates to the extent to which an instrument actually measures what it sets out to measure. The main aspects of validity are:

- Face validity
- Content validity
- Criterion validity
- Construct validity
- Convergent
- Discriminant

Case study *Which health status instrument should I use?*

A study of 978 Australian patients with type 2 diabetes compared the use of three health-related quality of life questionnaires, the EQ-5D, the SF-12 and the SF-36. All three measures were found to have some limitations, but the EQ-5D generally performed as well as the SF-36 and, given its simplicity to use and its short time for completion, was the preferred option (Glasziou et al., 2007).

Stop and think

- Maternal mortality can be measured using standardized rates (dividing the number of maternal deaths by the number of women of reproductive age in a population) but increasingly also as a ratio (calculated by dividing the number of maternal deaths in a time period per 1000 live births in the same period). Why do you think the maternal mortality ratio might be more useful when comparing populations? Hint: consider different fertility rates in different countries.

Measuring health and illness

- Infant and maternal mortality rates and life expectancy are useful indicators of a country's overall health and development.
- Mortality rates need to be adjusted for the age and sex of the population.
- Disease-specific mortality rates can reveal trends in specific disease but tell us little about illness or morbidity in a population.
- Measurement of morbidity ranges from measures of health care service use to instruments measuring self-reported perceptions of illness and self-reported measures of health, well-being and functional ability.
- Considerable care should be taken when using instruments for measuring health and when interpreting their results.

20 | Changing patterns of health and illness

In the UK, the data provided on births and deaths are compiled by the Office of National Statistics, which publishes annual reports showing the incidence of disease and deaths resulting from specific causes and a variety of statistics relating to use of hospital and outpatient services. These reports are public documents and can be consulted in libraries and online.

Changes in life expectancy

Over the last century there has been a marked decline in premature death throughout the developed world. In 1845, a newborn baby girl in England and Wales had an average life expectancy of approximately 50 years. By 1930 this had risen to just over 70 years (Fig. 20.1). Life expectancies have risen slightly since then, and a baby girl born now can expect to live to almost 86 years of age. Furthermore projected figures indicate that life expectancy will continue to rise slightly, with women born in 2052 expected to live to 92 years of age. However, if a child survived into middle age, life expectancy even in 1845 was quite high. A 45-year-old woman in 1845 could, on average, expect to live to nearly 70 years of age, and in 2012 she had an average life expectancy of over 80 years.

The major cause of increase in life expectancy is a dramatic fall in the death rate for infants during their first year of life. In 1888 in England and Wales, out of every 1000 infants under the age of 1 year, 145 died. By 1930 this figure had been more than halved to 68 infant deaths, and the rapid decline continued until the present-day mortality rate of fewer than four per 1000. At the beginning of the 21st century almost all newborn babies in the UK can expect to live through childhood. In many developing countries in the world, life expectancy at birth remains below 50 years of age because of high rates of infant mortality. According to McKeown (1979), the most important factor leading to changes in infant and child mortality has been a dramatic improvement in child and maternal nutrition over the past century.

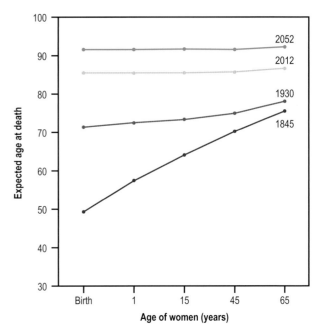

Fig. 20.1 Average life expectancy for a woman at different ages in 1845, 1930 and 2012 and projected for 2052 (England and Wales) *(from Registrar General's Mortality Statistics, 1999, with permission).*

Stop and think

- If you were going to practise medicine in a developing country today, what sorts of ill health would you expect to encounter and what sorts of intervention would you become involved in? (Once you have answered this, see spread Health: a global perspective, pp. 156–157).

Diseases that have declined

Another way to look at the changing nature of health and illness is to compare death rates for particular causes over the years. To examine the relative importance of different diseases over time, we need to take account of the fact that the population structure might also have changed over time. For example, cancers are more common in the older age groups and if the proportion of older people in the population has increased whilst the actual rate of cancer has stayed the same, we are likely to make the mistake of assuming that the rate of cancer is increasing. This could be very misleading. To calculate real changes in the rates of different diseases over time, we can calculate what are called *standardized mortality ratios* (SMRs) (see pp. 38–39). These enable us to examine changes over time and consider the possible causes of these changes (Table 20.1). Over the past century death rates resulting from nearly all causes have declined. Striking changes in

Table 20.1 **Standardized mortality ratios for selected causes of death, 1891 to 1990 in England and Wales**

Cause of death	1891–1895	1921–1925	1946–1950	1961–1965	1986–1990
Tuberculosis	867	393	157	20	4
Influenza	514	359	57	36	7
Digestive diseases	750	263	114	75	79
Diseases of the respiratory system	526	250	93	94	60
Diseases of the genitourinary system	309	226	113	60	35
Diseases of the skin, subcutaneous tissue, musculoskeletal system or connective tissue	671	381	127	97	182
Malignant neoplasms	–	–	96	103	115
Diseases of the heart	–	–	93	89	63
Cerebrovascular disease	–	100	92	95	60
Suicide	137	125	106	112	74

From Registrar General's Mortality Statistics, HMSO, 1999, with permission.

death rates have occurred for tuberculosis and influenza. SMRs for tuberculosis have changed from 867 in the period 1891–1895 to four in 1986–1990; they are, however, now on the increase. Similarly SMRs for influenza have changed from 514 in 1891–1896 to seven in 1986–1990. A significant improvement in health has been attributed to our ability to control the spread of infectious diseases and fight them more effectively when they do occur.

An important debate surrounds the explanation of changing rates of infectious disease. A great deal of medical research effort has been devoted to the identification of viruses and bacilli and to the development of vaccines and cures during the last 100 years. For example, the tubercle bacillus was first identified in 1880. The introduction of the bacille Calmette–Guérin (BCG) vaccination to prevent infection, however, did not take place until the 1950s. It can be seen in Table 20.1 that death rates for tuberculosis had

Table 20.2 **Death rates per million population in England and Wales in 1974, 1991 and 2012, by cause of death**

Cause of death	Women 1974	1991	2012	Men 1974	1991	2012
Diseases of the circulatory system	6118	4533	1118	6149	4570	1746
Neoplasms	2771	2833	1471	2244	2559	2004
Diseases of the respiratory system	1816	1043	581	1458	1054	804
Accidents, violence and poisoning	496	427	143	379	223	352
Diseases of the digestive system	292	285	247	309	361	327
Diseases of the nervous system	126	203	198	132	213	240
Diseases of the endocrine system	113	170	65	178	200	83
Mental disorders	28	145	311	47	282	266
Diseases of the genitourinary system	179	97	83	153	115	95
Diseases of the musculoskeletal system	30	44	47	83	135	35
Diseases of the blood	27	38	11	47	45	12

From Registrar General's Mortality Statistics, HMSO, 1999, & Office for National Statistics, 2014.

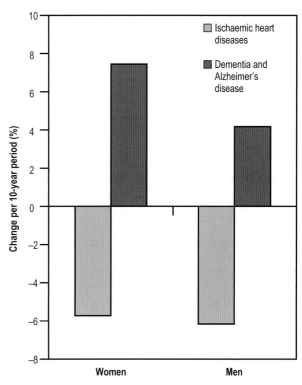

Fig. 20.2 Change in percentage of deaths caused by ischaemic heart diseases, and dementia and Alzheimer's disease, in England and Wales from 2003 to 2013 *(from Office for National Statistics, 2014).*

dropped dramatically long before the introduction of the BCG, suggesting that some other factors such as improved nutrition, public health measures and housing conditions or changes in the nature of the bacillus, must have contributed to the decline (McKeown, 1979) (see Fig. 32.1, p. 64).

Death rates for some causes have not changed a great deal over the years. The SMRs for cerebrovascular disease and suicide have shown a steady but undramatic downward trend over the last 50 years. Although the rate for suicide has gradually declined over the years, it reached an all-time high during the years of the economic depression, 1931–1935, with an SMR of 150. The only cause of death to show an upward trend over all the years it has been recorded is malignant neoplasm, or cancer. Over the last 20 years, death rates amongst women from cancers of the trachea, bronchus and breast have increased steadily, whereas amongst men death rates for cancer of the prostate have increased steadily.

Stop and think

• Bearing in mind the impact of immunization on death rates for tuberculosis, speculate on how important vaccination against HIV might eventually prove to be.

Current common diseases

Although SMRs are very useful for examining trends in the rates of disease over time, if we want to identify the most common causes of death in a population, we need only examine the rates per head of population (Table 20.2). In 1991 deaths certified as resulting from diseases of the circulatory system accounted for 47% of all male deaths and 46% of all female deaths. Treatments for these conditions are an important area of research, and survival rates are improving, as reflected in the decline in 2012 in deaths caused by diseases of the circulatory system.

An important consequence of increases in life expectancy and in the prevalence of diseases for which cures are unknown is that medical practice is increasingly concerned with the management of chronic ill health and the prevention of disability amongst a

population whose average age is on the increase. In Fig. 20.2, the decline in the incidence of deaths resulting from diseases of the circulatory system is displayed alongside the increase in the incidence of deaths from dementia and Alzheimer's disease. Although the rise in deaths caused by dementia and Alzheimer's disease may be attributable to an ageing population, it may also reflect an improved understanding of this disease, which leads to doctors more frequently recording dementia as the underlying cause of death.

Stop and think

• What implications do the changing patterns of mortality have for the demographic structure of the population and health care over the next 50 years?

Changing patterns of health and illness

• The single factor that most accounts for our improved life expectancy at birth in the UK is that at the start of the 21st century almost all newborn babies can expect to live through childhood. This has occurred largely as a result of improvements in nutrition.

• Over the last century infectious disease has declined dramatically. This may be a result of (1) changes in people's susceptibility to infection, (2) changes in the nature of the biological agents, and (3) the introduction of medical treatments.

• In 2012, diseases of the circulatory system accounted for 28% of all deaths. Malignant neoplasms accounted for 34% of all deaths.

• Compared with previous years, in 2012, deaths resulting from accidents, violence and poisoning, including suicide, were more prevalent amongst men than women.

• Regular UK statistical bulletins concerning mortality and morbidity are on the Her Majesty's Stationery Office (HMSO) website: www.statistics.gov.uk.

21 | Social class and health

In clinical practice, we are particularly concerned with the health of individual patients. When clerking a patient, we ask about occupation with an expectation that the patient's response – bus driver, publican, lawyer, computer programmer, cleaner – will tell us something about the risks associated with his or her work. We may also make an instant appraisal of the patient's lifestyle and material circumstances. Although there are significant differences between individual bus drivers and individual lawyers, there is also strong evidence that people's health is closely associated with their occupation, their occupational group and their social class.

What is social class?

Social class is a general measure obtained by combining occupational groups roughly equivalent in terms of employment relations to form occupational classes in the UK; these are an indirect indicator of education, income, standards of living, environment and working conditions. In 2001 the new National Statistics Socio-economic Classification (NS-SEC) was introduced to overcome some of the drawbacks of older Registrar General's (RG) classification. The NS-SEC is now linked to mortality and morbidity data.

Social class and health

Over the last 100 years there have been great improvements in the health of the population in most countries. However, inequalities between different sections of the population still exist; one form of increasing disparity that has received particular attention is social class inequality in health. For example, death rates for the UK can be calculated for occupational classes by combining data on birth and death certificates with occupational data collected at the decennial census. Although reproductive and adult mortality rates for each social class have been decreasing over the last 100 years, there has, however, been an increase in the disparity in mortality rates between the upper and lower social classes.

Fig. 21.1 illustrates the most recently reported gradations in life expectancy at birth from the higher managerial and professional groups to those in routine occupations. Class differentials exist in

each of the 14 major cause-of-death categories used in the International Classification of Diseases. Such differentials exist for both men and women. Only one cause of death for men, malignant melanoma, and four causes, including breast cancer, for women show a reverse trend. In Fig. 21.2 the evidence also shows that disparities in illnesses, and especially chronic illnesses, are at least as wide as disparities in death.

These facts are not challenged; controversy lies in their interpretation and in the implications of different explanations for policies of preventative or corrective action. In the 1990s the influential Research Working Group on Inequalities in Health produced the *Black Report* (Townsend et al., 1992), which started the debate about which theoretical model could best explain these social class differences. Today social class inequalities continue to be reported in many high-income countries, most recently in the UK in the Marmot Review (2010).

Recent research has tended to favour the following four explanations, which have become the matrix for current debate and research.

Cultural/behavioural explanations

These explanations stress individual or lifestyle differences, rooted in personal characteristics and levels of education, which influence behaviour and are, therefore, open to alteration through health education inputs leading to changes in personal behaviour. Cultural and behavioural explanations suggest that lack of knowledge and lack of long-term goals give fewer possibilities of making maximum use of health and other services and of taking preventive health measures. Their main focus has been on the health-risking behaviours of cigarette smoking, unhealthy diet (including alcohol consumption) and lack of exercise:

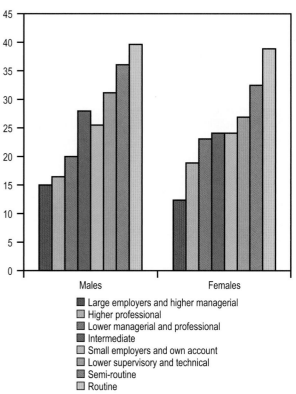

Fig. 21.2 Percentage of males and females, 45 to 64 years of age, with limiting long-term illnesses by National Statistics Socio-economic Classification (NS-SEC, 2007) *(from Office for National Statistics General Household Survey; quoted in Marmot et al., 2010).*

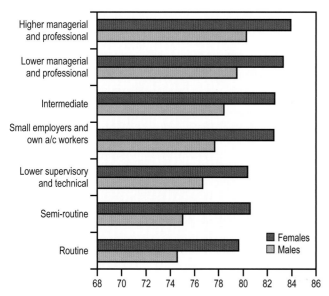

Fig. 21.1 Life expectancy at birth: by social class and sex, 2002–2006 *(from Office for National Statistics Longitudinal Study, 2011).*

- There are higher rates of smoking among manual groups, which will contribute to ill health.
- There is lower consumption of vitamin C, carotene and fibre, along with a higher dietary sodium/potassium ratio among the manual occupational classes. There are lower rates of vegetable intake but elevated rates of the consumption of saturated fats.
- People in manual occupations exercise less than those in non-manual groups.

Psycho-social model

The original ideas for these explanations relate to the deleterious effects of stress on the biological systems of the human body. Research has tended to concentrate on three spheres of life: the home, the workplace and the community. These explanations focus more on aspects of social support, and psycho-social work hazards:

- High workload combined with low control over work tasks may negatively affect the immune system.
- Poor social support within the family context may also produce high levels of psycho-social stress leading through to impaired health.

Materialist or structuralist explanations

These explanations emphasize the role of economic and associated socio-structural factors, for example, the labour and housing markets, in the distribution of health and well-being. Proponents of this explanation believe that social structure is characterized by permanent social and economic inequality, which exposes individuals to different probabilities of ill health and injury:

- Poor-quality and damp housing are associated with worse health and particularly with higher rates of respiratory disease in children.
- Low socio-economic status, low pay and insecurity produce inadequacies in diet and dietary values.
- All-cause mortality has been shown in one study to be directly related to income, with the age-adjusted relative rate of the poorest group of subjects being twice that of the richest group. The rate increased in a stepwise fashion between these extremes (Bartley et al., 1998).

Life-course approaches

There is a growing recognition that adult health outcomes cannot be understood in isolation from earlier life antecedents. This has encouraged the development of analyses that use a life-course approach. These explanations often also argue that the occupational class structure is seen to act as a filter or sorter of human beings, and one of the major bases of selection is health: physical strength, vigour or agility. In these hypotheses, health determines one's social class of destination. People in better health have greater chances to ascend the social hierarchy, whereas those with poorer health may undergo downward social mobility:

- Longitudinal studies show that low birth weight is a predictor of socio-economic disadvantage through childhood and adolescence.
- Health problems in childhood and youth can produce a downward socio-economic drift.
- The highest health risks are found among those who both grow up, and remain in, disadvantaged material circumstances.

Reducing the gap

Each of the theories mentioned previously has practical implications as to what needs to be done to reduce social class inequalities in health (see pp. 76–77). Although recent research favours a combination of materialist and behavioural approaches, where healthy or unhealthy lifestyles are seen to be linked to people's social positions, Wilkinson's (2009) ideas suggest that if we reduce income inequality whilst increasing various forms of social security provision, then social class inequalities in health will diminish. His policy focus, therefore, stresses the need for societies to develop good social security provisions for their citizens. Perhaps the most important strategy is for policies to reduce poverty, especially in families with children, strongly favoured by the Marmot Review (2010).

Regardless of interventions at a macro-level, we should also be aware of the important role doctors can play. The previously mentioned key UK reports all stressed the crucial role of the NHS at all levels for helping to reduce inequalities in health. For example, doctors can ensure that their patients are claiming the benefits to which they are entitled (Box 21.1).

Box 21.1 Evidence-based practice as recommended in: 'Working for Health Equity: The Role of Health Professionals' (Allen et al., 2013)

- Need for skills in communication, partnership and advocacy
- Practice-based skills such as social history taking and referring patients to non-medical services
- The importance of working in partnership, both within the health sector and also with external bodies
- Developing trust with local communities
- General practitioners as advocates. Again this should be on all levels: from the individual patients and their families, through health NHS Trusts and the local community, to the health profession, and also on the level of national policy change

---

Case study *The Whitehall II studies*

An influential body of work, the Whitehall research studies, analysed the health of men in the Civil Service from the 1960s to the present day. Recently Marmot et al. (2010) have analysed data from the Whitehall II study to look at self-reported health in early old age. They discovered that social inequalities in self-reported health increases with age. People from lower occupational grades aged faster in terms of a quicker deterioration in physical health compared with people from higher grades.

Social class and health

- Mortality rates for all social classes have fallen over the last 100 years.
- However, the mortality rates for the higher social classes have been decreasing faster than rates for the lower social classes.
- Morbidity rates follow a similar pattern to mortality.
- The main explanations are cultural/behavioural, psycho-social, materialist/structuralist and life-course approaches.
- High rates of disparity between rich and poor in affluent countries may strongly contribute to disparities in social class mortality rates.
- Different explanations for the relationship between social class and health imply different health, social and economic policies.

22 | Gender and health

Gender is one of the important divisions in society along with social class and ethnicity. Gender patterns existing within wider society are reflected in medicine. Health services providers need to understand gender differences and their implications for health and health service uptake to provide the most appropriate and acceptable care to patients.

Gender and sex

Social scientists make the distinction between sex and gender, whereby 'sex' refers to physical and biological differences and 'gender' refers to the social definitions of how women and men should behave under certain circumstances. Society 'prescribes' how the biological sex is transformed into the social gender. Thus biological men learn to behave in a male way and to carry out male tasks. The philosopher Simone de Beauvoir (1960) summarized this transformation as follows: 'One is not born, but rather becomes, a woman.' Every society produces norms, rules and expectations for each gender, and these differ from place to place as well as over time. Consequently what is regarded as male behaviour in one time and place can be seen as female in another. Thus society as a whole produces women and men.

Difference in mortality and morbidity

Women live longer than men, even in low-income countries (Fig. 22.1). Men are more likely to die, compared with women in the same age group, from the day they are born. Table 22.1 clearly shows differences in mortality statistics. The rates indicate that life expectancy of baby girls is higher than that of boys but that gap in life expectancy narrows at an older age. This pattern is the same for any other age group in UK and for other industrialized countries, as well as many developing countries (see. Health: a global perspective, pp. 156–157).

Morbidity statistics for Scotland indicate that women are more likely to have had an acute illness in the previous 2 weeks compared with men. This gender difference is even more profound in the over-75 age group.

Gender differences in health

Some of the gender differences in mortality, especially in babies and infants,

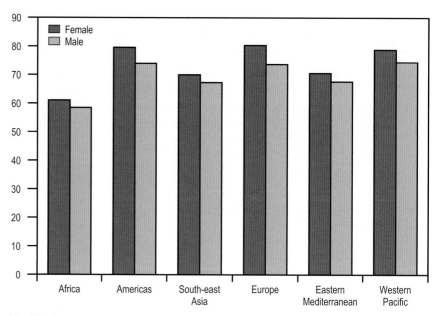

Fig. 22.1 Life expectancy at birth by gender across the globe, 2017 *(from https://data.worldbank.org/indicator/SP.DYN.LE00.FE.IN).*

Table 22.1 Selected mortality and morbidity data for men and women

	Measure	Female	Male
Live births 696,271 in 2016, England & Wales	Proportion	49	51
Life expectancy at birth (2016), UK	Age in years	82.9	79.2
Life expectancy at age 65 years in the UK	Age in years	85.9.	83.5
From Office for National Statistics, 2017.			

are related to 'natural' differences in biological and genetic make-up. However, as boys grow up to become men, social causes of death, especially those related to lifestyle, become more important. Men are more likely to be exposed to a hazardous environment than women, and many hazardous occupations in the UK are male-dominated (e.g. mining, fishing and construction work). Men are more likely to engage in more dangerous behaviour – to drink, to drive too fast, to use illegal drugs, to be involved in dangerous sports such as boxing or motor racing or to commit suicide.

At the same time many diseases that do not in themselves kill but are often chronic and disabling affect women more compared with men. Approximately two-thirds of the disabled population in the UK is female, and a large proportion of that inequality is attributed to age differences. However, not all differences between men and women can be traced back to social factors. Some of the differences between male and female mortality and morbidity rates for coronary heart disease can be linked to the use of contraceptive pills and hormones

(Committee on Health Promotion, 1996). However, men in Scotland are more likely to be overweight or obese (see pp. 106–107) compared with women.

Health service use and gender

Women are not only more likely to be ill but also more likely to use health services. Fig. 22.2 illustrates that American women – especially younger women – consult their primary care doctor more often for preventive care compared with men. This pattern generally holds for industrialized countries. Men are not only less likely to use health services, they are also more likely to delay and hence come with more serious symptoms to the consultation.

Women visit the doctor more often than men do, even if one ignores the consultations related to child-bearing (Miles, 1991), but the hospitalization rate is higher for men than for women, when maternity and gynaecological cases are excluded (Leeson and Gray, 1978).

Differences in illness patterns amongst women and men will lead to different needs for health care provision. Women

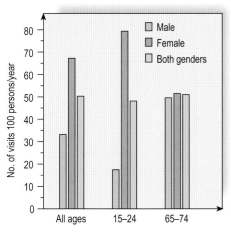

Fig. 22.2 Number of preventive care visits per 100 persons per year to primary care specialists by gender and selected ages, USA 2004 *(from Hing et al., 2006, with permission).*

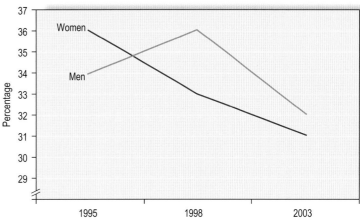

Fig. 22.3 Smoking prevalence in Scotland in women and men aged 16 years and over *(from Scottish Executive, 2005b, with permission).*

live longer than men, so consequently a large proportion of the elderly are females. The overwhelming majority of patients with hip fracture are elderly people, hence the majority of patients with a hip fracture are females, and they are more likely to occupy a bed in an orthopaedic ward. Moreover, the uptake of health care is determined not only indirectly through morbidity but also directly by social and cultural factors. Two main factors are highlighted in the following:

1. What is defined as illness in women is often a social definition instead of the purely scientific exercise of diagnosis and treatment. Childbirth, for example, helps to define women as being ill because of their biological role (see pp. 4–5).
2. Women consult family doctors more often than men do, not only for themselves but also for their children and elderly relatives (see pp. 88–89).

The first explanation is related to the fact that all societies make assumptions about what is appropriate gender-related behaviour. This is often referred to as *sexual stereotyping*. One aspect of this in Western cultures is that female socialization makes it more acceptable for women to adopt the 'sick role'.

One of the possible explanations is that women are less likely to be in full-time employment and are often paid less, and therefore they are likely to lose less income than men when they take on a sick role. There is also evidence that doctors give different emphasis to the 'same' symptoms, according to gender. For example, men's 'back troubles' are regarded more seriously, being seen as directly caused by heavy work. Women's 'back problems' are often labelled as part of general gynaecological

conditions. Similarly mental health problems in women are seen to be internally caused and thus subject to medical intervention, whereas in men these are seen as caused by external factors. In other words, men's problems are seen to be related to what they do, and women's problems are related to what they are.

Smoking

Smoking illustrates the importance of gender for the medical profession for two quite distinct reasons (see pp. 80–81). Firstly, smoking is the most important cause of preventable death. Secondly, patterns in smoking prevalence between men and women have been changing over the past three decades. It also shows that differences between men and women in health behaviour – in this case smoking – are not static. Sixty years ago it used to be 'normal' among men from all social classes to smoke, whereas only a small proportion of women smoked. Smoking prevalence among adults has fallen steadily since 1972. However, the proportion of men who smoked regularly dropped, whereas the proportion of female smokers increased in the same period. In the 1980s the proportion of women taking up smoking in their teenage years increased rapidly. In the 1990s the proportion of Scottish women smoking was, for the first time ever, greater than that of men (Fig. 22.3). The reason for this change has been sought in women's emancipation, advertising and health promotion (see: The social context of behavioural change, pp. 76–77). Furthermore, the incidence of lung cancer is increasing among women, and this is closely related to the social changes in smoking prevalence.

23 | LGBT health

Lesbian, gay, bisexual and transgender or 'trans' (LGBT) populations often experience a number of health inequalities. Biomedical explanations can account for some health disparities between LGBT people and the general population: for instance, higher rates of anal cancer among gay men can be attributed to human papilloma virus (HPV), whereas higher rates of breast cancer among lesbian women can, in part, be attributed to greater nulliparity in this population. Transgender people may also experience health disparities because of the risks and side-effects associated with hormone therapy and sex reassignment surgery. However, other disparities are largely caused by the social stigma and prejudice LGBT people experience, as well as other psychosocial factors.

The pathologization of non-normative gender and sexual identities

Historically psychological professions have pathologized LGBT people through psychiatric diagnostic categories. In 1952 homosexuality was included in the American Psychiatric Association's (APA) *Diagnostic and Statistical Manual of Mental Disorders* (DSM) and was deemed a form of arrested sexual development. Over the following two decades, evidence emerged indicating that homosexuality per se did not indicate psychological impairment, and as a result, homosexuality was declassified as a mental disorder by the APA in 1973. In its place, the DSM developed a new category of 'ego-dystonic homosexuality' to describe those persistently distressed by their same-sex attractions, although this category was also removed in 1987.

Today same-sex attractions are considered normal variants of human sexuality and not an indicator of mental disorder. The World Health Organization's International Classification of Diseases, 10th edition (ICD-10) continues to list 'ego-dystonic sexual orientation' but insists that a sexual orientation is not a disorder in itself. Meanwhile the DSM-5th edition simply indicated that although there is no diagnosable mental disorder, some non-heterosexual clients may benefit from professional support and counselling relating to social stigma surrounding their sexual orientation.

Unfortunately a minority of professionals still adhere to the view that homosexuality is pathological and advocate controversial forms of therapy known as 'conversion' or 'reparative' therapies to alter a client's sexual orientation. Awareness of these practices in the UK grew after research revealed that as many as one in six psychotherapists in the UK had engaged in efforts to change a client's sexual orientation (Bartlett et al., 2009). These forms of therapy are widely considered unethical, and in 2015, 14 UK professional associations, signed a Memorandum of Understanding objecting to conversion therapy (Box 23.1).

As in the case of homosexuality, the psychological professions have also historically pathologized transgender people. 'Trans' (or 'transgender') is an umbrella term that encompasses a wide variety of minority gender identities or those whose gender identities or expressions do not match that of the gender they were assigned at birth. The diagnosis of 'transsexualism' was first introduced into the DSM-3 in 1980 and replaced by 'gender identity disorder' (GID) in 1994. Although some trans people welcome psychiatric diagnosis because it allows them access to medical treatments such as hormone therapy and sex reassignment surgery, other trans activists have been critical of the pathologization. In 2013

GID was replaced with the category 'gender dysphoria' in DSM-5. This places emphasis more on the distress (dysphoria) often experienced by those whose gender identity does not match the gender they were assigned at birth. This new diagnostic category goes someway to recognising that psychological distress occurs within a cultural context. For example, in Samoa, a third gender called *Fa'afafine* is socially accepted, and those who identify as Fa'afafine do not experience the same distress associated with gender dysphoria in Western contexts (Vasey and Bartlett, 2007). This suggests that the distress experienced by many trans people may arise from the way that 'gender' is socially constructed.

Minority stress and health

Although most LGBT people are well-adjusted individuals, the psychosocial stress associated with being a member of a socially stigmatized minority group places non-heterosexual and trans individuals at a higher risk of psychological distress and mental illness (Meyer, 1995). LGBT individuals are often confronted by a number of psychosocial challenges rarely faced by the general population (Box 23.2). The concept of 'minority stress' is based on the idea that non-heterosexual and trans individuals are subject to chronic stress as a result of stigma (expectations of rejection and discrimination), actual experiences of discrimination and violence and internalized homophobia/biphobia/transphobia. Internalized homo-bi-transphobia can be defined as the 'direction of negative social attitudes toward the self, leading to a devaluation of the self and resultant internal conflicts and poor self-regard'.

LGBT people have been found to have higher rates of depression and anxiety and an elevated risk for suicide attempts

---

Box 23.1 UK organizations against conversion therapy

- British Psychological Society
- Royal College of Psychiatrists
- UK Council for Psychotherapy
- British Association for Counselling and Psychotherapy
- The National Counselling Society
- British Psychoanalytic Council
- The Association of Christian Counsellors
- British Association for Behavioural and Cognitive Psychotherapies
- Royal College of General Practitioners
- NHS England

Box 23.2 Psychosocial stressors

Psychosocial stressors experienced by many LGBT people include:

- Confusion over unexpected attractions to members of the same sex or feelings of gender incongruence
- Experiences of bullying, violence, threats of violence and discrimination
- Anxiety over how family and friends will respond to their sexual or gender identity
- Rejection by those not accepting of their sexual or gender identity, including family, friends and others in their community
- Stress caused by keeping one's identity/behaviour a secret
- Feelings of shame or guilt as a result of religious or cultural upbringing that condemns or stigmatises non-normative genders and sexualities.

and ideation compared with the general population. In a study of men who have sex with men (MSM), Mills et al. (2004) found that both distress and depression were associated with not identifying as gay (e.g. those who remain 'in the closet'), experiencing anti-gay violence in the previous five years and alienation from the gay community.

LGBT adolescents may be particularly vulnerable to these psychosocial stressors for several reasons. Although sexual identity formation can occur in adulthood, awareness of same-sex attractions, gender incongruence or simply feeling 'different' commonly occurs during childhood or adolescence (see spread Adolescence, pp. 12–13). LGBT young people are also likely to be living with and dependent on parents or other family who may be disapproving of non-normative genders and sexualities. Furthermore, concealing one's identity and behaviour from family members or experiencing rejection from family can cause acute anxiety and distress. LGBT people must face these unique psychosocial stressors at the same time as negotiating developmental challenges ordinarily experienced during adolescence.

Stop and think

- How can a doctor reduce the likelihood of their LGBT patients feeling judged or discriminated against?

The 'poor self-regard' associated with internalised prejudice is also considered to undermine a concern with one's own health and interfere with health behaviour decision-making, which may, in part, explain higher rates of substance use and tobacco smoking among LGBT populations.

Research by British LGBT lobbying group Stonewall suggests that bisexual men and women experience many of the same health inequalities as lesbians and gay men; there are, however, significant differences. For instance, bisexual women were more likely to report having an eating disorder compared with lesbian women, and bisexual men were more likely to have self-harmed compared with gay men. Both bisexual men and women were also less likely to be 'out' to health care professionals compared with lesbians or gay men. There is also evidence that bisexual women report poorer physical health compared with lesbian or heterosexual women and are more likely to smoke and drink heavily. One possible reason is that bisexual people may experience greater levels of minority stress because of stigmatization by both heterosexuals and the lesbian and gay community. A sense of never fully belonging in either community may result in feelings of alienation, which may, in turn, result in poorer mental health and more risky health behaviours. The minority stress hypothesis may also explain why some of these issues are more pronounced among LGBT people from ethnic minority communities. The 'coming-out' process may be more difficult for ethnic minority LGBT people as they must confront prejudice and stigma associated with both their sexual/gender identity and their race or ethnicity.

Socio-cultural and environmental factors

Although minority stress may go some way to explaining health disparities experienced by LGBT people, there may also be other socio-cultural and environmental factors.

For instance, individual risk behaviours alone cannot account for disparities in human immunodeficiency virus/sexually transmitted infection (HIV/STI) transmission rates (see spread HIV, pp. 108–109). For example, research has found that black gay men in the USA are more at risk of HIV/STI transmission compared with white gay men despite both groups reporting similar rates of unprotected anal intercourse. Social scientists have explained this by using network theory, which suggests that features of a sexual network such as the size and density of connections within the network may place individuals within them at differential levels of risk despite similar rates of risky sexual behaviour. Once STIs enter tightly connected sexual networks, they may spread more rapidly and each incident of unprotected sex within the network carries greater risk of transmission compared with the same risky sexual behaviours in larger, less densely connected networks (Mustanski et al., 2014).

Environmental factors may help explain patterns of tobacco and substance use. For instance, as 'gay bars' represent a rare social space where non-heterosexuality is the norm and cross-dressing is more socially accepted, many LGBT people may choose to socialize more in these settings where alcohol consumption, tobacco and substance use is normalized.

Cultural factors may help to explain the gendered pattern of some health disparities. For instance, gay men suffer greater body dissatisfaction and a higher prevalence of anorexia nervosa compared with their heterosexual male counterparts, whereas lesbian women have been found to be more likely to be overweight or obese than heterosexual women. It has been hypothesized that this may relate to what sociologists have termed the 'male gaze'. Western men place greater emphasis on the slenderness of their partners, resulting in more social pressure on gay men and heterosexual women to be thin compared with heterosexual men or lesbian women. However, 'gay culture' is not monolithic but consists of many subcultures, including gay men identifying as 'bears' who are typically overweight and idealize large bodies as masculine.

Barriers to effective health care

Some LGBT people may avoid or delay seeking health care because of experiences or expectations of homophobia, biphobia and transphobia from health care professionals. Health care professionals' assumptions of heterosexuality may deter LGBT people from disclosing their sexual identity and potentially lead to inappropriate advice or referrals. Concerns about disclosing one's sexual identity may prevent patients from freely discussing sexual health, and some health care professionals may feel embarrassed or feel that they lack knowledge to discuss sexual health with LGBT patients. Trans patients receiving hormone therapy may also ignore early signs of side-effects such as cardiovascular disease for fear that health professionals may discontinue hormone therapy.

LGBT health

- All health care professionals should receive training on LGBT issues.

Summary points

- Supposed 'therapies' which claim to change a person's sexual orientation or gender identity are generally considered unethical
- As members of stigmatised minority groups, LGBT people may experience psychosocial stressors with knock-on effects for their mental and physical well-being
- Socio-cultural and environmental factors may also help to explain health disparities experienced by LGBT populations
- LGBT people may experience barriers to effective healthcare due to fears of prejudice or due to health professionals lacking training on LGBT issues

24 | Ethnicity and health

It is important for health care professionals to consider their role in developing and delivering equitable health services for minority ethnic groups, which are sometimes referred to as Black and minority ethnic (BME) communities.

Race, culture and ethnicity

To monitor whether equitable access to health care is achieved, the UK government requires NHS hospitals to record the ethnicity of all patients. Ethnicity is also collected as a variable in epidemiological research. However, defining the concept of ethnicity in relation to understandings of race and culture is fraught with difficulties.

The concept of 'race' does not exist in any biologically meaningful way; genetic explanations for the differences seen in health status have long been shown to be scientifically flawed. There is more genetic variability within than between so-called racial groups, and over 99% of the genetic make-up of human beings is shared by all ethnic groups. Although there are visible differences in physical characteristics amongst people whose ancestry lies in different parts of the world (colour of eyes, skin or hair), these physical characteristics are of no major significance to health apart from genetically predisposed disorders such as the haemoglobinopathies, which have more to do with geographical conditions than with genetics. Physical characteristics are only important when values are attached to them in a society so that one group defines another as 'different' and assumes them to have particular behavioural characteristics because of the way they look. It is equally important to consider how health care professionals perceive non-indigenes because these perceptions can cloud their judgement and affect service provision and delivery.

Culture is a set of shared beliefs, values and attitudes that guide behaviour. People identify themselves as members of a group on cultural grounds; they may share similar language, religion, lifestyle and origins, and this helps them define their ethnic group. We all have ethnic identities, whether we consider ourselves to be 'Australian', 'English', 'Bangladeshi' or any combination that describes our national, cultural and social identities. Thus the concepts of 'race', culture and ethnicity, although interrelated, have different meanings.

Stop and think

• How might components of your ethnicity and culture relate to your experiences of health and illness?

Ethnicity can be identified by asking people to assign themselves to a category; in the 2011 UK census, people could place themselves in more than one national identity: for example, people could report themselves as having Scottish and British national identities. This approach attempts to capture the way people think of themselves in relation to colour of skin, continent of ancestral origin and cultural background. Other questions included country of birth and religion. These data should help in the planning of services that are appropriate in relation to religious observance and diet. The notion that this classification of populations aids planning and delivery of services is flawed because of the inconsistencies in the categories used: for example, skin colour and continent or country of origin portray different meanings and in themselves do not give accurate information to direct services and therefore perpetuate inequality. Self-classification of ethnic groups can also pose problems for those interpreting the data.

According to the 2011 Census in England and Wales, 14.1% of the people are from a BME population compared with 7.9% in 2001 (Runnymede Trust, 2012) almost doubling over the 10 years. In Scotland the BME population accounts for 4% of the total population, again doubling since the 2001 Census (National Records of Scotland, 2013). The increase in BME populations across the UK means that there is greater requirement to understand the needs of these groups when providing health and social care. Most people from the minority ethnic groups live in inner cities, and some towns or metropolitan boroughs have become known for local concentrations of people from particular ethnic origins; Leicester greatly benefited from the settlement of migrant workers who responded to the recruitment call of the 1950s and 1960s (Narayanasamy and White, 2005). People who migrated to the UK decades ago have different profiles from those who came more recently: for example, recently arrived Eastern Europeans. The health needs of these populations will differ greatly from those of Caribbean and Asian origins, who came to the UK some 60 years previously.

Socio-economic inequalities

Unemployment rates for most minority ethnic groups are considerably higher than those for indigenes, particularly amongst young people (see pp. 58–59). This inevitably affects health. Although national data on average income are not routinely broken down by ethnic group, a survey in Leicester in the mid-1990s showed evidence of lower incomes amongst people of Asian origin: the gross median weekly earnings of 'Asian' men and women were just 82% of their White counterparts. Similarly, about 19% of the white population live in 'council estates and low-income areas', whereas about 40% of Black and Indian groups and as many as 63% of Bangladeshi and Pakistani groups live in such areas (Johnson, 2003). UK Government statistics suggest that unemployment rates mirror the above pattern, with those most likely to live in 'council estates and low-income areas' having the highest levels of unemployment, indicating a rise instead of decline in BME populations (Department for Work and Pensions, 2014). However, there remain significant differences in the socio-economic experiences of sectors of minority ethnic groups.

Diversity

Patterns of health and disease are influenced by socio-economic, environmental, genetic and cultural factors (see pp. 40–41), and there are significant differences in the patterns of non-communicable diseases amongst ethnic groups. However, the major health problems of ethnic minority communities, and therefore priorities for health improvement and care, are similar to those for the majority population (e.g. cardiovascular disease and cancers). Thus although there are differences in experience of health between all ethnic groups, the major diseases of the majority are also important to minority ethnic groups. This is important when using data on ethnicity in the planning of services (Kai and Bhopal, 2003).

Comparing standardized death rates emphasizes differences: for example, in the UK, liver cancer and tuberculosis are more common in men from the Indian subcontinent but account for fewer deaths. At the same time, a UK longitudinal study of first-generation migrants found that type 2 diabetes rates were nearly three times higher in South-Asians and more than two times higher in African Caribbeans compared with people of European origin (Tillin et al., 2013).

The varied patterns in the experience of health and illness amongst different ethnic groups do not have a single explanation, as illustrated in Fig. 24.1. Genetic inheritance contributes to the aetiology of some diseases: e.g. the prevalence of sickle-cell disease and beta thalassaemia are major disorders that have higher rates amongst people of African and Asian origins, respectively. However, lifestyle and cultural factors (especially smoking and diet), exposure to poor living circumstances and the stress of racism will also contribute (Nazroo, 2003). Explanations for differences in experience of health and illness that point out the impact of socio-economic inequalities and racism are used less often by researchers, but more often by minority groups themselves. It has always been a difficult thing to prove racism: it is often said that to appreciate fully what it is like to be 'Black' in a predominantly 'White' society one should try wearing the identity.

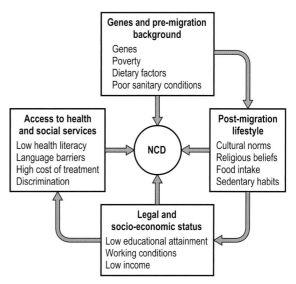

Fig. 24.1 Factors associated with non-communicable diseases in some migrants *(from Montesi et al., 2016).*

Case study *Lack of services for sickle-cell disease in the UK*

Sickle-cell disorders and thalassaemia are inherited disorders of red blood cells mainly affecting black and ethnic minority groups.

Services for sickle-cell disease, although improving, are lagging behind the numbers of cases arising in the UK. There is need for health care professionals to update themselves with the needs (see pp. 150–151) of the population for whom they provide care.

A consultant haematologist wrote in 1990:

I was hearing that not enough money goes to research on sickle cell. It's not a disease of the white people and they don't know much about it...

Debbie (17 years) wrote:

They know that I have got the disease but they don't really know too much about it, and I don't think, this is my personal view, I don't think they're interested because it's not a white man's disease, and I mean, and I can't see them really digging into this thing to get any knowledge out of it, because it is black people, and it's black people's problem (quoted in Anionwu, 1993).

What needs to accompany education is an exploration of attitudes towards provision of appropriate services at all levels of the NHS.

Experience of prejudice

'Racism' and 'institutional racism' have been defined as follows:

The term 'Racism' consists of conduct or words or practices which advantage or disadvantage people because of their colour, culture or ethnic origin. In its more subtle form it is as damaging as in its overt form.

'Institutional racism' consists of the collective failure of an organization to provide an appropriate and professional service to people because of their colour, culture or ethnic origin.

In 1997, about 25% of white people said that they were prejudiced against minority ethnic groups, and between 20% and 33% of people from a range of minority ethnic groups reported being worried about being racially harassed (Coker, 2002). This fear is not unfounded; reported racist incidents in London

increased from 11,050 in the year ending March 1999 to 23,345 by March 2000 (Coker, 2002). It is inevitable that racism that contributes to adverse mental health amongst BME groups (Wallace et al., 2016) will result in physical health morbidity applying the concept of 'holism'. To focus on mental health impact of racism could be misconstrued and neglect the effects of the 'person' as a whole and that of the family unit.

Unequal provision of health care

For a range of reasons, some related institutional racism, many health care services are inappropriate for the needs of minority ethnic populations. For example, health services have been concentrated on issues that are seen by health care professionals to be of special relevance to particular ethnic groups, whereas people themselves may not attach such significance to them. In the UK, this led to health education on rickets or fertility control, whereas until recently haemoglobinopathy services have been largely ignored (see Case study).

The other criticism is that the methods by which health issues are brought to the attention of minority groups are often inappropriate. For example, recent policies to increase fruit and vegetable intake and decrease the proportion of fat in the diet all too frequently miss out foods often eaten by minority ethnic groups. Therefore there is a risk that health education messages (see pp. 76–77) do not reach (some) ethnic minority groups.

Ethnicity and health

- 'Race' does not exist in any biologically meaningful way.
- Ethnicity is a complex concept, linking cultures, history, language and so on. We all belong to an 'ethnic group'.
- Ethnic minority groups are at increased risk of being poor, principally through the effects of racism and negative discrimination.
- The major diseases and health problems of most minority ethnic groups are the same as for the general population.
- There is evidence of unequal and inappropriate provision of health care services for ethnic minority groups. Involvement of ethnic minority groups in planning services and policies can make these more effective.

25 | Quality of life

Quality of life (QoL) is a popular concept. The definition and accurate measurement of QoL are still widely debated. As successive generations live longer, healthier lives and are more likely to die from a chronic illness or disability than from an infectious disease, health care providers are increasingly aware of the importance of assessing the value of health care interventions to those who receive them. Clinical trials routinely assess whether treatments/drugs, procedures and therapies make a significant difference to the patients' QoL. Economists can use QoL information to determine whether treatments are affordable to the health care service. Many different terms are used to describe QoL (Box 25.1). This chapter focusses on physical and mental health aspects of QoL, well-being and standard of living.

Standard of living and 'objective' indicators of well-being

There is a relationship between average income and QoL. Easterlin found that in the poorest global countries, subjective well-being (SWB) increases as gross domestic product (GDP) rises, but only up to a point. When a country's income reaches a certain level, further increments are no longer associated with SWB improvements; the so-called Easterlin paradox. Thus standard of living alone is not an adequate measure to assess personal well-being.

'Objective' well-being refers to people's material goods and can relate to income and economic development (e.g. owning a television or fridge) and to statistics such as changing divorce rates. Objective well-being indicators suffer from similar problems to those of standard of living; for instance, we cannot assume that divorce necessarily damages QoL. Divorce means different things to different people – a personal disaster or a blissful release. Well-being and QoL are subjective states that are only loosely related to size of income and possessions; hence, overall, subjective measures of QoL and well-being are preferable.

Subjective well-being

SWB was initially defined as 'central to a person's experience containing measureable positive aspects, and…global or overall assessment of that person's life'. Later the definition was expanded to include negative feelings, thinking about life satisfaction and emotional reactions to life events. A review found that although the components of the SWB model are important, how they relate to each other is still speculative (Busseri and Sadova, 2011).

It is now much clearer how SWB relates to QoL because positive feelings, negative feelings, cognitions and life satisfaction are often assessed by QoL measures. New research shows that SWB is subsumed within QoL, and some QoL scales can measure both concepts (Skevington and Boehnke, 2018). Happiness (or positive mood) is a key component shared by SWB and QoL but does not explain a significant part of both concepts. Box 25.1 shows that positive affect alone is insufficient to account for QoL entirely because other dimensions are also globally important. However recent cross-cultural research shows that SWB is subsumed within the QoL concept, so both measures are not needed (Skevington and Boehnke, 2018)

What is important to a good quality of life?

Despite personal idiosyncrasies, socio-demographic features and cultural characteristics, there is some global consensus about the life qualities that most people value. A World Health Organization (WHO) collaboration agreed upon a methodology that could be used simultaneously in diverse cultures, and the findings were pooled. After defining the concept (see page. 51), patients, health care professionals and community members identified important QoL concepts and proposed suitable questions that were later tested in a cross-cultural survey before selection for the WHOQOL-100 questionnaire. Questions (items) were culturally adapted during translation to ensure acceptability. The WHOQOL Group confirmed 25 aspects of QoL that are important to both sick and well adults living in diverse cultures and assessed by the WHOQOL suite of measures (Box 25.2) (Skevington, Sartorius, Amir and the WHOQOL Group, 2004).

Box 25.1 Concepts used to describe well-being and quality of life

- Standard of living/gross domestic product (GDP) per capita
- Objective well-being (e.g. material assets, divorce rates, city infrastructure)
- Subjective well-being
- Quality of life
- Life satisfaction
- Happiness, positive feelings, mood, affect, contentment
- Negative mood, feelings or affect (absent)
- Personality traits (e.g. depression, anxiety, aggression)
- A worthwhile life
- Meaning and purpose in life
- Symptoms (absent) including their intensity and frequency
- Survival (e.g. life expectancy)
- Hedonia
- Eudaimonia

Camfield, L., Skevington, S. 2008. On subjective well-being and quality of life. J Health Psychol 13 (6), 764–775.

Box 25.2 Twenty-five dimensions of quality of life (QoL) found to be important to 15 cultures across the globe, included in WHOQOL measures

General overall quality of life and health

Physical QoL	Psychological QoL	Social QoL	Environmental QoL
Pain & discomfort	Positive feelings	Personal relations	Physical safety & security
Energy & fatigue	Thinking, learning, memory & concentration (cognitions)	Social support	Home Environment
Sleep & rest	Self-esteem	Sex life	Financial resources
Mobility	Body image & attractiveness		Access to health & social care
Activities of daily living	Negative feelings		Opportunities for information & skills
Dependence on medication & treatment	Spiritual, religious & personal beliefs		Opportunities for recreation & leisure
Working capacity			Physical environment
			Transport

Defining quality of life

Many published definitions of QoL are orientated towards health. The general public tends to define it in terms of health failures or physical and mental problems. This problem-centred approach has historically been reflected both in QoL definitions and questions included in a broad spectrum of measures. However, although questionnaires that address symptoms and dysfunction are useful to clinicians, a negative orientation is not always attractive to patients who see a more balanced life.

To disclose the positive side of life to a clinician may be seen as unimportant. Consequently the clinical agenda downplays a balanced view of QoL, so positive psychology cannot be readily used to maintain or improve health. Some recent definitions pose QoL as a positive and negative state of well-being. As indicated by the WHO definition of health, it is not simply the void left when illness and disability are absent, but a tangible, measurable of health that is often overlooked.

The WHO defines QoL as:

"An individual's perception of their position of life, in the context of the culture and value systems in which they live, and in relation to their goals, expectations, standards and concerns. It is a broad ranging concept, affected in a complex way by the person's physical health, psychological state, level of independence, social relationships, and relationship to the salient features of his/her environment"

(The WHOQOL Group, 1998).

The WHOQOL Group later added spiritual QoL covering spiritual, religious and personal beliefs. The WHOQOL definition of QoL addresses whether we have met our goals, expectations and standards, as well as having concerns, and suggests these judgements that make comparisons impact on our view of QoL. For instance, when expectations match experience, there is no impact on QoL, but if the experience is worse than expected, then this impact can be measured. Uniquely, the WHO sees culture as a 'lens' through which people interpret life events. This analogy serves to explain the many different meanings attached to QoL.

This cross-cultural definition of QoL chimes well with previous definitions, sharing common agreement that a person's perceptions of his or her QoL are vital. Most of this information is not readily observable. For example, it is difficult to know what QoL is like in relation to sleep by inspecting electro-encephalography (EEG) readings or by documenting sleep onset, duration, waking, medication intake and so on. It is better to ask a QoL question such as 'How refreshing is your sleep?' Otherwise incorrect assumptions may be made about the QoL of a patient who states sleeping 12, 3 or 8 hours a night. A carefully phrased QoL question can provide accurate information. This is especially necessary when QoL is largely invisible: for example, in personal relations and in one's purpose in life.

QoL has been assessed by observing what patients actually do: for example, grimacing in pain; but this gives only a practical answer. Few of the important aspects of QoL in Box 25.2 can be observed because they are the results of internal thoughts, feelings and physiological or psychological states. A paradox here for QoL assessment is that patients with significant health and functional problems do not necessarily have poor QoL. People with severe disabilities may report good QoL despite having difficulties with activities of daily living and being socially isolated (Albrecht and Devlieger, 1999). This is because these issues have very different *meanings* for different people. A systematic review of studies of proxy judgements by spouses, carers and health care professionals shows that even knowledgeable observers are less accurate judges of another person's QoL (e.g. Crocker, Smith and Skevington, 2015). In summary, the best way to find out about a person's QoL is to ask him or her.

Stop and think

- How refreshing was your sleep in the last two weeks?
- What could you do to make it more refreshing, if you need to?

Quality-adjusted life years

The quality-adjusted life-year (QALY) takes account of quantity and quality. This arithmetic estimate is based on life expectancy and the expected quality of each remaining life-year, when a patient in particular diagnostic group receives a certain treatment. This index ranges from 'perfect health' with no problems (1) through increasing levels of problematic health and disability, to death (0) and states worse than death (−1). This is not ideal because defining perfect health is not objective. When adjusted for the cost of treatment, QALYs provide a cost-utility ratio that assists in sharing out a limited budget. The QALY is the common currency used by health commissioners to decide how to distribute health resources (Phillips and Thompson, 2001 www.evidence-based-medicine.co.uk).

Case study

Susan is 28 years old and was diagnosed with breast cancer. She was considering the effect of treatment on her QoL and was anxious about feelings of mutilation and altered body image. She was aware that the physical effects of chemotherapy and radiotherapy might be nausea, vomiting and diarrhoea, tiredness and loss of libido. The hospital was 20 miles away and getting there involved taking two buses. She was confused because she knew that radioactivity caused cancer and therefore radiotherapy might be dangerous.

Hospital staff discussed breast reconstruction and how to cope with possible hair loss. She was reassured that tiredness was to be expected. She was offered help with travel expenses from a hospital fund. Leaflets explaining the procedures gave her more confidence about safety and efficacy. She was encouraged by the survival rates when cancer was detected early, and was aware that her sister had survived for more than 5 years since her breast cancer diagnosis. Susan started making plans for the future.

Consider the impact of psychosocial support on Susan's QoL:

- Look at Box 25.2 and identify the most important aspects of QoL in your own life now.
- How do you think these aspects of your QoL will have changed when you are 70 years old?

Stop and think

- Can you only know about someone's quality of life by what they tell you?

Quality of life

- QoL has many different definitions and lots of related terms.
  - Which definition will you chose, and why?
  - How will this definition guide the type of measure you might use?
- QALY analyses require careful appraisal and use.

26 | Media and health

The mass media are a rich source of information about health: presenting ideas about everything from the symptoms of disease or the risks of different behaviours to the validity of scientific research or trustworthiness of the medical profession (Seale, 2003) (Fig. 26.1). That is why so much money is now spent on trying to affect media representations through direct health education initiatives, advertising and public relations (Williams and Gajevic, 2013). However, the media's role is not straightforward. A direct impact may be evident when, for example, uptake of a vaccination declines after media coverage questioning its safety (Boyce, 2007); however, people are not unreflective media consumers, ready to absorb any message indiscriminately.

Research into how people actually respond to the media shows that we may engage with media facts, images, stories, characters and plots in different ways, depending on how it relates to our own lives, including social and economic contexts, the ease with which we can change our behaviours and the ways in which any particular media representation relates to our self-image, aspirations, group identity and networks (Boyce, 2007). Sometimes the same media representations can generate diametrically opposed responses. For example, the British soap opera 'Brookside' included a storyline about a businesswoman, Susannah, successfully standing up to a man who complained about her breast-feeding in a café-bar. This storyline was welcomed by middle-class breast-feeding women, who felt inspired by it. Reactions were strikingly different among the young working-class women in this research. Susannah's strength of will did not fit with these women's self-perceptions – 'You need to be confident, which I'm not' – and they pointed out that if breast-feeding in a café-bar might cause a scene, then trying to do it in the local burger joint would be likely to be even more controversial. For these working-class women, this episode *reinforced* the fact that breast-feeding in public was ill advised, rather than encouraging them to think of it as an option (Henderson et al., 2000).

Perhaps the mass media's most significant role may be in how they cultivate underlying common-sense understandings of the world – reflecting and helping to create ideas about what is normal and sometimes also promoting stereotypes by, for example, portraying people with mental illness as violent, thus encouraging fear and stigma (Philo, 1999). Fictional programmes may be particularly important – their power to provoke identification with particular characters can engage people's

empathy but can also mislead. The drama and human interest potential of stories about 'inherited' breast cancer, for example, generated many fictional TV representations and helped raise its profile but has also made many people overestimate the role of genetic risk factors (Henderson and Kitzinger, 1999).

However, it is easy to exaggerate the power of fiction. Scientists and policy-makers sometimes blame science fiction (sci-fi) for making the public worry about human cloning (for stem cell research purposes). Actually sci-fi may be used to *discredit* anxieties more often than to *underwrite* them. People are shame-faced about fears that 'sound like a sci-fi film'; they are more likely to back up their concerns about human cloning with reference to Nazi eugenics or news stories about rogue states misusing science or an international trade in organ transplants. It is profoundly unhelpful if scientists/policy-makers dismiss public concerns as simply a result of watching too many horror films (Haran et al., 2007).

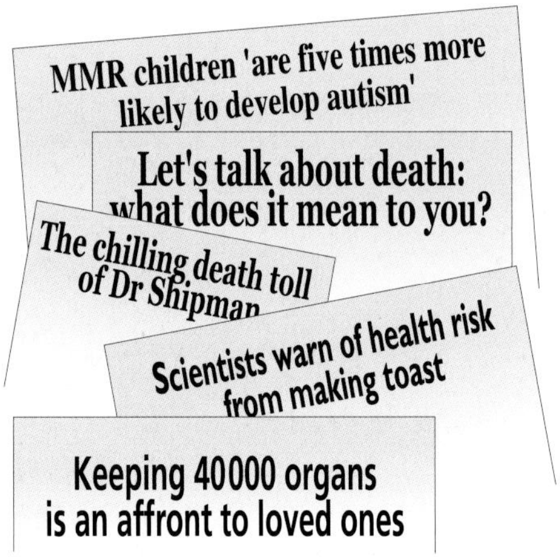

Health and social issues

Newspaper reports and both factual and fictional television may also open up ways of thinking, talking and acting around health issues – breaching taboos, for example, about sexual health (and talking about safer sex) or about particular diseases such as bowel and testicular cancer (helping to overcome reservations about seeking testing) or enabling conversations about mortality itself (including planning for the end of life). In the 1980s, for example, the media, played a vital role in putting AIDS and safer sex on the public agenda (Miller et al., 1998), and in more recent years, increasing discussion of death in the media is helping to reflect and fuel a social revolution to confront our own mortality. At the same time, however, underlying tendencies (e.g. the idea that medicine can 'win' every battle and that new research will eventually lead to cures for almost everything) can nurture common assumptions about how to approach ill health. Misleading media stereotypes about certain conditions can also leave individuals and their families ill-equipped to face devastating conditions for which modern medicine has few solutions. Research on media representations of 'brain death' and of the permanent vegetative state, for example, highlights the gaps and errors in mainstream media representations of such conditions and/or hype about what new neuro-technologies will deliver (Samuel and Kitzinger, 2013).

Medicine and the media

The medical profession is also acutely aware of how the profession as a whole is represented in factual and fictional media. Doctors may be heroes in fiction, but intense public attention has also been given to scandals such as the Alder Hey hospital use of children's organs, the doctor turned mass-murderer Dr Harold Shipman, or the controversy about the 'Liverpool Care Plan' for end of life (Watts, 2013). The mass media also have a crucial role to play in the development of scientific and medical research. In the field of human genetic research, for example, public acceptability is increasingly important. The ground was prepared for changing legislation on stem cell research and hybrid embryos, for example, by intense media lobbying. Interestingly, the resulting coverage, although arguably 'balanced' around the 'rights of the embryo' debate, excluded wider social and political questions and gave little opportunity for explorations of ambivalence (Williams et al., 2003).

MMR children 'are five times more likely to develop autism'

Let's talk about death: what does it mean to you?

The chilling death toll of Dr Shipman

Scientists warn of health risk from making toast

Keeping 40000 organs is an affront to loved ones

Fig. 26.1 Headlines promote powerful messages about health.

Understanding how the media represent all aspects of health and illness is important for medical students. In-depth research on audience responses to media representations suggests that the relationship with public attitudes is more complex than might at first appear. It is important to go beyond personal impressions and anecdotes to take into account the diversity of the media and of audiences and to consider the implications of the associated research.

In a recent review on patient health enabling technologies and social media it has been noted that there are six areas relevant to participatory health. These include: media sharing platforms, web-based platforms, patient portals and crowd sourcing websites, medical avatars and other mobile health technologies. There are some benefits that relate to improvement in cross-cultural values, patient empowerment, awareness raising in clinician and patient. However, ethical concerns are raised in the need to de-identify individual patient data, and the potential commercialization of patient data collected by agencies that offer information and advice. Hence the tension between participatory approaches and maintaining privacy is ongoing and requires careful attention by the patient and health authority (Househ et al., 2018).

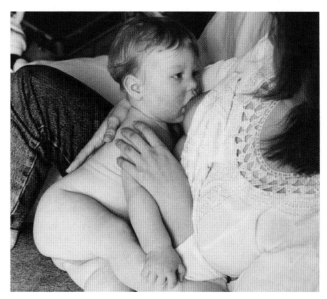

Fig. 26.2 Representations of infant feeding can impact on public attitudes and women's experience.

Case study *Infant-feeding in the media*

A systematic content analysis of 1 month's UK press and TV coverage showed that the overall pattern of coverage implies that breast-feeding is odd or problematic, whereas bottle-feeding is largely normalized, associated with 'ordinary' families and problem-free feeding.

- Breast-feeding is rarely shown (Fig. 26.2). There was only one scene on TV of a baby on the breast and nine scenes involving breast pumps (not in use), but 170 scenes with babies on bottles.
- Babies' bottles have become a routine and iconic way of visually representing babyhood.
- Whereas a baby may be bottle-fed in a background scene on TV, breast-feeding, where it does feature, is on the foreground as a focus for debate.
- Breast-feeding is used to characterize particular types of women (e.g. middle-class 'earth mothers').
- Bottle-feeding is used to symbolize positive male involvement in fatherhood.
- Problems with breast-feeding are highlighted, whereas difficulties with bottle-feeding are rarely mentioned. For example, there was only one reference to potential difficulties associated with bottle-feeding ('hassle' of bottle-washing) but 42 references to problems attributed to breast-feeding (sore nipples, saggy breasts, sleepless nights).
- Routine mass-media coverage rarely acknowledges the health implications of bottle-feeding. There was only one oblique reference within the entire sample to the potential disadvantages of formula milk (Henderson et al., 2000).

The media and health

The mass media can:

- Put new health issues on the public/policy agenda or help raise their profile.
- Provoke debate about the ethics of scientific and medical developments.
- Invest public hopes in particular types of scientific research (e.g. stem cell research) as promising cures.
- Convey factual information and advice.
- Promote or challenge stereotypes (e.g. about people with schizophrenia or about who is likely to contract HIV).
- Cultivate common-sense understanding of health and illness and support ideas about what constitutes appropriate behaviours.
- Play a key part in short-term health 'scares' (whether that be about using the contraceptive pill or about a threat such as Ebola virus infection).

However, media influence is not straightforward or all-powerful:

- There is a large gap between what we know and what we do.
- Wider social issues are often more important than health messages on their own.
- The impact of media representations varies depending on format (e.g. fictional versus factual programmes) and the type of narrative, vocabulary, images and associations used.
- The impact will vary depending on how much the public trusts the sources of the story (e.g. government scientists).
- Different audiences may respond to the same programme or report quite differently depending on their identities and the context of their own lives.

Stop and think

- How do media representations influence how you think about your own health or how you respond to patients? Have the media influenced your images of the type of person liable to engage in particular risk behaviours?
- If you were going to design a campaign to promote a health-enhancing behaviour, what media factors would you take into account?
- With the inexorable rise of social media, how could you use this approach to improve your practice and care of your patients?

27 | Housing, homelessness and health

Housing affects health directly and indirectly. Lack of adequate housing causes both mental and physical ill health. It can make existing health problems worse and delay recovery from illness (Fig. 27.1). Lack of adequate housing has detrimental social and economic consequences that reduce people's opportunities to protect and promote their own health. Energy-inefficient housing contributes to fuel poverty and is damaging to the environment and has consequences for the health of the whole population.

Housing and health

In Victorian Britain, concerns about housing conditions causing ill health led to programmes of slum clearance. This commitment to improving public health by changing harmful social conditions contributed to the decline in infectious diseases and increases in life expectancy (see pp. 42–43).

The 1950s and 1960s saw rapid growth in public-sector housing. The focus on quantity rather than quality brought problems such as dampness and lack of sound insulation and privacy, as well as social isolation. Research evidence emerged during the 1970s and 1980s showing the negative health impact of these 'new' housing problems, but health policy focussed on individual behaviour as the cause of ill health rather than social conditions such as housing.

The late 1980s and 1990s saw a decline in the availability of affordable housing and a rise in the numbers of homeless people who were roofless or in temporary accommodation. In the early 21st century the economic downturn and welfare cuts have meant that homelessness continues to be a problem. Concerns about energy efficiency, the environment and fuel poverty have also begun to reinforce the centrality of housing to public health.

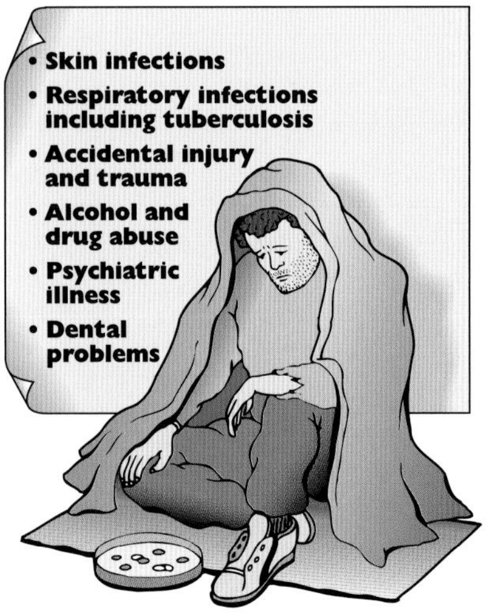

Homelessness and health

The term 'homeless' is often used to describe people who are 'roofless' and living on the streets and those living in temporary accommodation. People who are homeless are exposed to extreme environmental hazards such as damp, cold and noise, as well as overcrowding, risk of violence, risk of accidental injury, poor hygiene and poor access to health services. Fig. 27.1 shows the main illnesses associated with homelessness.

Housed but homeless

Social policy currently distinguishes between people who have permanent accommodation and the homeless. A broader definition of homelessness is the problem of a lack of an affordable, decent and secure place to live. This definition means that people may be seen as homeless if their housing is overcrowded or deprives them of resources that are necessary to maintain or protect health.

The health impact

Poor housing can affect health both directly and indirectly (Box 27.1). There are three main models used to explain the impact of housing on health.

The direct effects of lack of adequate housing can be explained using a *medical model* (see spread 1, pp. 2–3) whereby specific aspects of the environment have physical effects that lead to specific symptoms or illness.

A second model of illness is the *general susceptibility model*, in which aspects of the environment act as stressors that make people more susceptible to illness. Specific features of the environment are not linked to specific illness as they are in the medical model. This model takes some account of the indirect effects of housing on health.

In both models researchers have to rule out the possibility that associations between housing and health occur as a result of other factors. The two most common artefact explanations that have to

be ruled out are those of confounding factors and downward drift (Box 27.2). If researchers have data on other social conditions and past health and housing history, statistical techniques can be used to take account of these factors and assess the independent contribution of housing to health.

A third model that can be used to understand the health impact of housing is a *socio-economic model*. This holistic model recognizes that it is important to understand the experience of living in inadequate housing, the impact on daily life and the compound effects of different aspects of inadequate housing and other conditions of social deprivation.

> ### Box 27.1 Lack of adequate housing: effects on health
>
> **Direct effects**
> - Exposure to physiological effects of the environment or harmful agents fostered by environmental conditions
>
> **Indirect effects**
> - Exposure to poor living conditions in childhood may have consequences for health in later life
> - Causes stress or discomfort, which increases general susceptibility to physical illness and emotional problems
> - Exacerbates or delays recovery from existing health problems
> - Undermines social relationships
> - Makes it difficult or stressful to get on with the tasks of daily life
> - Makes it difficult to access other resources that are necessary to sustain or promote health
> - Can drain other household resources, including income, which protect and improve health
> - Has an impact on energy efficiency and the environment, which, in turn, has an impact on public health

---

> ### Box 27.2 Key problems in establishing the links between lack of adequate housing and ill health
>
> **Confounding factors**
>
> Lack of adequate housing is frequently associated with other factors that are known to cause ill health such as unemployment or low income.
>
> **Downward drift**
>
> People in poor health drift into poor housing or homelessness because of the consequences of ill health.

- Skin infections
- Respiratory infections including tuberculosis
- Accidental injury and trauma
- Alcohol and drug abuse
- Psychiatric illness
- Dental problems

Fig. 27.1 Illnesses associated with homelessness.

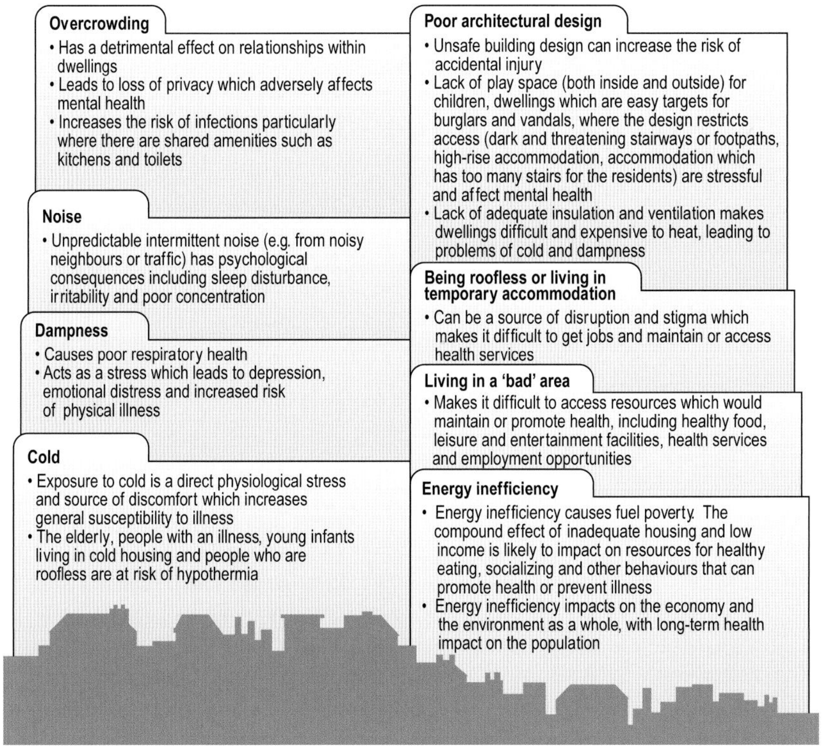

Overcrowding
- Has a detrimental effect on relationships within dwellings
- Leads to loss of privacy which adversely affects mental health
- Increases the risk of infections particularly where there are shared amenities such as kitchens and toilets

Noise
- Unpredictable intermittent noise (e.g. from noisy neighbours or traffic) has psychological consequences including sleep disturbance, irritability and poor concentration

Dampness
- Causes poor respiratory health
- Acts as a stress which leads to depression, emotional distress and increased risk of physical illness

Cold
- Exposure to cold is a direct physiological stress and source of discomfort which increases general susceptibility to illness
- The elderly, people with an illness, young infants living in cold housing and people who are roofless are at risk of hypothermia

Poor architectural design
- Unsafe building design can increase the risk of accidental injury
- Lack of play space (both inside and outside) for children, dwellings which are easy targets for burglars and vandals, where the design restricts access (dark and threatening stairways or footpaths, high-rise accommodation, accommodation which has too many stairs for the residents) are stressful and affect mental health
- Lack of adequate insulation and ventilation makes dwellings difficult and expensive to heat, leading to problems of cold and dampness

Being roofless or living in temporary accommodation
- Can be a source of disruption and stigma which makes it difficult to get jobs and maintain or access health services

Living in a 'bad' area
- Makes it difficult to access resources which would maintain or promote health, including healthy food, leisure and entertainment facilities, health services and employment opportunities

Energy inefficiency
- Energy inefficiency causes fuel poverty. The compound effect of inadequate housing and low income is likely to impact on resources for healthy eating, socializing and other behaviours that can promote health or prevent illness
- Energy inefficiency impacts on the economy and the environment as a whole, with long-term health impact on the population

Fig. 27.2 Features of inadequate housing that are detrimental to health.

Stop and think

- What are the possible health consequences for a family with young children living in damp and overcrowded conditions?
- How might health care services meet the needs of homeless people?

A range of factors associated with housing have been shown to cause physical illness and discomfort as well as depression and emotional distress (Fig. 27.2).

It's very noisy right by the motorway but we couldn't open the windows anyway because of all the break-ins. The walls are damp and there's mould on our walls, our clothes and shoes. It's freezing cold most of the time and in winter we all huddle into the one room. The kids are always sick and I'm at my wits' end.
(Hunt, 1997).

Households with low incomes are often more likely to live in poorly constructed, least energy-efficient housing – they live in fuel poverty. *Fuel poverty* means that a household will spend at least 10% of its net income on heating the home to an acceptable level. A greater proportion of lower incomes is spent on energy costs and this may still not alleviate the problems of cold and dampness. Poor housing is seen to compound the problems of living on a low income, rather than low income being seen as a potential confounding factor in the relationship between housing and health.

Working in the home

There are fitness standards for formal work environments such as offices (see pp. 56–57), but not for domestic housing. People who are not in formal employment may spend substantial amounts of time in housing environments that would not meet the minimum occupational health standards. Carrying out housework such as child care, cleaning and cooking is particularly stressful in poor conditions.

Housing and health services

Health care professionals must consider the extent to which patients' illness or distress is the result of their living conditions. Health care professionals are sometimes asked to comment formally on this in assessments of medical priority for rehousing or assessments for community care (see pp. 154–155). The move to day-case interventions and early discharge from hospital makes it even more important that health care professionals know about patients' housing conditions and ensure that poor living conditions do not exacerbate illness or prejudice recovery.

Case study *How do cold houses affect health?*

An independent review by Marmot et al. (2011) looked at the impact of cold homes and fuel poverty for people's health. The review found that between 2004 and 2010 the number of fuel-poor homes in England increased significantly from 1.2 million to 4.6 million. A cold home is seriously detrimental to health and can lead to a number of health problems and even death. The review found that people of all ages are adversely affected by cold homes:

- Approximately 40% of excess winter deaths were attributable to cardiovascular diseases and 33% to respiratory diseases.
- Minor illnesses such as colds and flu increase in cold homes, and existing problems such as rheumatism and arthritis are exacerbated.
- Twice as many children in cold homes are likely to suffer from respiratory problems compared with those in warmer homes.
- Adolescents who live in a cold house have a fivefold increased risk of mental health problems.

There is an economic, social and health cost of inadequate housing and a clear need to address health inequalities in housing. The review recommended more investment in energy efficient housing, which would bring benefits to the labour market through opportunities in construction in addition to health benefits.

Housing, homelessness and health

- The housing environment affects health directly and indirectly.
- Overcrowding, noise, dampness, cold, poor design and poor neighbourhood are detrimental to health.
- Being housed does not necessarily imply having a home.
- Housework is often carried out in conditions that would not satisfy Health and Safety at Work standards.
- Provision of adequate, affordable housing is an important component of a policy for health.

28 | Work and health

The United Nations Universal Declaration of Human Rights states that 'everyone has the right to work'. Does this imply that work is 'good' for us and for our health? Is all work good for us? Table 28.1 summarizes some of the characteristics of work that have been identified as important for health and also itemizes those hazardous conditions that can lead to ill health and injury. The United Nations International Labour Organization (ILO) tells us that two million people worldwide die each year from work-related accidents and disease. The 'right to work' is, therefore, complemented by ILO's commitment to 'adequate protection for the life and health of workers in all occupations'.

The 21st century world of work is changing. The health of working people will be affected by these changes, which include increased use of information technology; increase in small businesses; falling trade union membership; more women and older people in the workforce; intensification of work; 24-hour society (e.g. call centres); increased demand for flexibility; more temporary/short-term contracts; growing inequality in skill levels; downsizing; privatization of state-owned industries. Globalization of industry is accelerating and can lead to the export of health and safety risks from the developed world to the developing world (see pp. 158–159). The ILO estimates that the fatal injury rate for established market economies is 4 per 100,000 workers, whereas for Asia it can reach a high of 23 per 100,000 workers.

Work-related ill health and injury

Discovering accurate information regarding the extent of work-related ill health and injury is difficult. In the UK there is systematic underreporting. The government accepts that less than half of non-fatal incidents reportable by law to the Health and Safety Executive are, in fact, reported (Health and Safety Executive, 2000). As well as official reporting mechanisms, data come from a number of sources, including voluntary reporting schemes by occupational physicians and regular Labour Force surveys at both UK and continental European levels. The latter indicate that 2.9% of UK workers report taking time off work because of work-related

ill health. The UK rate is lower than those of many other European countries, including the EU-27 average (5.5%), Germany (3.9%), Spain (4.2%) and Poland (11.8%) (Health and Safety Executive, 2014).

Accidents

At the turn of the 21st century, the UK government launched a strategy to address the continuing toll taken by workplace injury and ill health. One of the targets of the strategy *Revitalising Health and Safety* (Health and Safety Executive, 2000) was to reduce fatal and major injuries by 10% by the year 2010. Sadly, in their policy document of 2009 – *The Health and Safety of Great Britain* – it was admitted that the country's safety performance had stalled (Health and Safety Executive, 2009). Figures released for the year 2013–2014 showed that 133 workers died in that year as a result of work injuries. In 2013–2014, 629,000 injuries occurred at work, according to the Labour Force Survey, a rate of 2140 per 100,000 workers (Health and Safety Executive, 2015). It is important to recognise that risk of accidents is not uniform but is concentrated in certain industries (e.g. construction, agriculture, and recycling) and among certain groups (e.g. young workers).

Occupational ill health

A less visible but more extensive problem is that of work-related ill health and disease (Fig. 28.1). Common work-related conditions are back injuries and other musculoskeletal problems, respiratory conditions such as asthma and bronchitis, work-related dermatitis and psychological conditions. With changes in the working environment, some conditions decline – for example, bladder cancer in the rubber industry – but others increase, for example, dermatitis and occupational asthma caused by exposure to a wide range of substances, including latex in disposable gloves, and stress-related conditions. Deaths resulting from work-related disease are over 20 times those from work accidents. The majority of these deaths are a result of occupation-related cancers. Recent research has indicated that 5% of all cancer deaths and 4% of cancer registrations each year in the UK are caused by work. Of particular concern is the fact that this burden of death does not fall equally amongst groups but is concentrated in skilled and unskilled manual workers.

Table 28.1 Summary of psychosocial and organizational hazards

Category	Hazardous conditions
Content of work	
Job content	Lack of variety or short work cycles, fragmented or meaningless work
Workload/work pace	Overload or underload, high levels of time pressure. Machine pacing
Work schedule	Shift working, night shifts, inflexible work schedules, unpredication hours
Control	Low participation in decision-making, lack of control over workload
Environment and equipment	Inadequate equipment, availability. Poor environment: lack of space, excessive noise
Social and organizational context of work	
Organizational culture and function	Poor communication, low levels of support for problem-solving
Inter-personal relationships at work	Social or physical isolation, interpersonal conflict
Role in organization	Role ambiguity, role conflict
Career development	Career stagnation or uncertainty. Under- or over-promotion
Home–work interface	Low support at home, dual-career problems

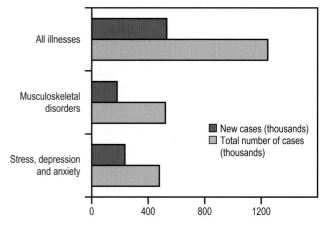

Fig. 28.1 Estimated 2013–2014 total and new cases of self-reported work-related illness by type of illness, for people working in the last 12 months (*from Labour Force Survey*. <www.hse.gov.uk/statistics/).

Responsibility for health at work

There is an apparent conflict for employers in the implementation of a healthy and safe environment. Creating such a positive work environment can cost both time and money. This must, however, be balanced against the greater cost of not taking action, including sickness absence, increased turnover, compensation costs, damage to morale and industrial relations and, most importantly, the personal cost to the individual worker. Employees too may be caught in an economic conflict and may ignore health and safety in some situations, for example, where pay is related to speed or levels of production.

The law places the responsibility for workplace health firmly with the employer, although employees too have duties to take care of themselves and others and to follow health and safety rules. Most accidents are caused by systems failures. Two independent studies have found that in only about 18% and 11% of cases, respectively, was the employee responsible for the accident, and even in these cases part of the cause may have been lack of training, low morale or pressure of work.

Another key group is the trade union. Research has shown that workplaces with a union presence show a 24% reduction in workplace injuries and that workers in unionized workplaces are less likely to have a fatal injury (Organisation and Service Department, 2011).

Stress at work

Stress is now the second largest cause of work-related ill health and sickness absence in Europe, next only to back problems and other musculoskeletal conditions. Research has highlighted the hazardous elements (listed in Table 28.1) that can result in work-related stress (Leka et al., 2004). Evidence of the link between stress and ill health is growing. Research has shown that job insecurity leads to increased self-reported ill health and clinical symptoms, with those at the lowest levels of the company being the worst affected. The introduction of new technology can lead to psychological distress, particularly among lower-paid, less-skilled and older workers. There is clear evidence of links between stress and coronary heart disease but conflicting evidence about which stress factors are most implicated. Overtime work is associated with high blood pressure. It is known that stress can suppress the immune system (Segerstrom and Miller, 2004).

It is now accepted that organizational solutions (primary prevention) aimed at addressing the causes of stress are more effective than interventions targeted at individual coping skills (secondary prevention) or counselling (tertiary prevention), although the best employers will provide all three. Factors that potentially lead to stress are now included in those which employers must risk-assess.

Work–life balance

A problem reported by workers throughout Europe is difficulty in achieving a healthy balance between work and life outside work. This is exacerbated in the UK because it has the longest working hours in Europe. Women bear the brunt of this. Even when working full-time, women still carry much higher levels of responsibility for the home, including care of children and other dependants. However, there is now clear evidence that financial well-being and physical well-being are strongly linked to paid employment. Domestic labour can be routine, boring, unpaid and undervalued. However, when women choose to enter paid employment, they are consistently paid less compared with men, and this means that childcare costs take a proportionately higher percentage of their income. There is now pressure on employers to consider the introduction of family-friendly policies to address this issue: for example, flexible working hours, working from home, term-time working, job sharing and subsidized childcare. In the case of parents and carers, employers are under a legal obligation to consider requests from employees for flexible-working.

Stop and think

- When making diagnoses and considering causes of ill health, it is important for doctors to think and ask about work as well as biological and social factors. Did you know that approximately 8% of patient visits to GPs are about work-related conditions? More people will be suffering from some condition caused or made worse by work (Weevers et al., 2005).

Case study

The relationship between work and health is complex, long-term service workers may reach an 'understanding' with their employers:

'When Monica developed psoriasis, she had been working at a bag factory for 21 years. She explained how she negotiated time off to contain the disruption at work:

'... I was the only one that got paid when I went to hospital, coz I used to have to go regular, like three times a week for the ultraviolet. The governor used to pay me when I went to the hospital. Like he used to go like, "Don't tell anyone". It was a crappy job but it was work, you know. They treated me good. As I said, I had a lot of friends. (Monica, White English, 50–54 years old)' (Qureshi et al., 2014).

Work and health

- Official figures for occupational death, injury and disease underestimate the total amount of occupational ill health.
- It is crucial in occupational health to prioritize prevention.
- Worldwide trends in employment have important implications for occupational health and safety.
- High-demand and low-control jobs create stress, and ill health.
- One major issue facing all workers but particularly women is finding a balance between demands at work and at home.

29 | Unemployment and health

We are now in the era of what has been called 'liquid capitalism', and we are witnessing increased part-time employment, more flexible work patterns and more self-employment. At the same time unemployment over the life course will become a more common experience for a sizeable section of the population. Unemployment will be especially high amongst young men (Office for National Statistics (ONS), 2013a). There will be more chronic unemployment and more workless households. Medical professionals are increasingly being faced with having to deal with the health effects of unemployment (Ferrie et al., 2001).

The evidence and mechanisms

Unemployment is a stressful life event that can cause ill health, both mental and physical (Fig. 29.1) and even mortality (Table 29.1). Research has also been able to capitalize on the volume of work carried out since the 1990s, which gives more attention to the mechanisms that cause ill health. One way to summarize the research evidence is by considering casuality and the possible links between unemployment and ill health and mortality (Fig. 29.2).

The stress pathway – psychological morbidity and mortality

Stress is strongly associated with lowered mental well-being and becoming unemployed is a serious stressful life event. A meta-analysis by Karsten and Moser (2009) of over 300 studies

found significant differences between the unemployed and employed. The unemployed ranked significantly lower on several indicators of mental health, including mixed symptoms of distress, depression, anxiety, psychosomatic symptoms, subjective well-being and self-esteem.

One of the most important series of studies on psychological well-being was carried out by Warr (1987) on different subgroups of the unemployed from redundant steelworkers to men attending unemployment benefit offices. Again all of his studies showed significant differences in mental health indicators between employed and unemployed respondents. Importantly these studies also threw light on some of the factors that moderated the negative impact of unemployment:

- Those committed to their work and who became redundant were found to be particularly disadvantaged.
- Age and length of unemployment were likely to be inter-correlated, and so older people were less likely to become re-employed and were more likely to be sick. The middle-aged unemployed had the lowest well-being scores.
- Although they found gender differences, with men having higher rates of psychological morbidity than women, this was thought to be related to personal commitment to their work. When the variable of personal work involvement was held constant, the sexes were equally affected.

Death rates have also been found to rise in times of economic depression; unemployed people have higher death rates than the

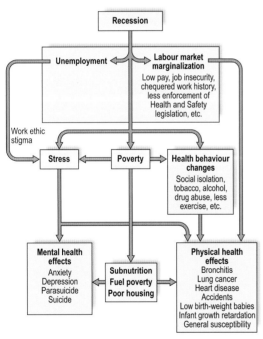

Fig. 29.1 How might unemployment lead to poor health?

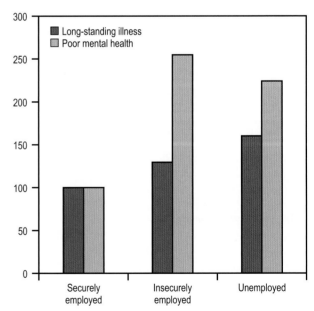

Fig. 29.2 Effect of job insecurity and unemployment on health *(from Social Determinants of Health (2008)).*

Table 29.1 **Frequencies, numbers of deaths and corresponding percentages for levels of economic position**							
	Scotland				**England and Wales**		
Variable	Frequency	Percent	Deaths	Percent[1]	Frequency	Percent	Deaths	Percent[1]
Economic position								
In work	62,856	65.5	6003	9.6	132,252	68.3	11,384	8.6
Unemployed	5600	5.8	1213	21.7	10,841	5.6	1802	16.6
Retired	6487	6.8	2195	33.8	13,104	6.8	3826	29.2
Permanently sick	8726	9.1	3346	38.3	2705	6.8	4668	36.7
Other inactive	12,294	12.8	1610	13.1	24,810	12.8	2591	10.4

[1]Death percentages are expressed as a proportion of deaths against all members in that group.

Source: Scottish Longitudinal Study; England and Wales. ONS Longitudinal Study in Health Statistics Quarterly (2009).

employed; and death rates rise with the increasing duration of unemployment (Waddell and Burton, 2006). The causes of death that predominated among the unemployed were malignant neoplasms (particularly lung cancer), accidents, poisonings and violence (particularly suicide). The stress pathway was implicated in some of these causes of death.

Association or cause?

Any cross-sectional analysis comparing groups of employed workers with unemployed men and women shows that employed people are healthier despite occupational hazards (see spread Work and Health, pp. 58–59). These studies point towards the health condition of the long-term unemployed (for more than one year), amongst whom there are likely to be far more health problems than amongst the short-term unemployed. Such studies cannot, however, tell us whether these effects are caused by unemployment. Selection processes operate: individuals may have become unemployed because they had health problems to begin with. It is also difficult to separate the direct effect of unemployment from any indirect effect of poverty, bad housing conditions, geographical location and social class. Although most research produces correlations between unemployment and health, the establishment of causality requires studies over time, looking at workers before termination of their employment and monitoring them through and after redundancy.

Ferrie et al. (2001) considered the health effects of privatization after one civil service department was sold to the private sector. Eighteen months after privatization they analyzed two groups: (1) the insecure re-employed and unemployed; and (2) those permanently unemployed. Group 1 showed significant increases in minor psychiatric morbidity and consultations with a general practitioner (GP). Within group 2, levels of long-standing illness were significantly different, but not the rest of the measures. This demonstrates that both re-employment and unemployment were associated with increased minor psychiatric morbidity and that being permanently out of paid work was associated with long-standing illness.

Death rates are elevated among the unemployed. A longitudinal prospective study on 49,321 Swedish men (Lundin et al., 2010) not only corroborated these findings but also discovered that a substantial part of the unemployment association was confounded by health-related risk factors such as crowded housing, alcohol and tobacco use, psychiatric diagnosis and police/childcare contact.

Relative poverty- or health-related behaviour

The work of Waddell and Burton (2006), Wadsworth et al. (1999) and Weich and Lewis (1998) stress the interplay between unemployment itself and linked financial elements (Fig. 29.2). Psychological health is seen to be affected by financial problems, which increase the frequency of stressful life events. Mental health is also affected by decreasing social activity and participation and diminishing social support. Although alternative social networks may eventually be formed, these may involve groups that have withdrawn from the norms and values of mainstream society. They may, thus, be more likely to indulge in health-damaging behaviours: tobacco and alcohol use, drug-taking and bad diet. In terms of physical health, the 'stress pathway' involving physiological changes (e.g. raised cholesterol and lowered immunity) is believed to be the main mechanism. The importance of relative rather than just absolute disadvantage has also been highlighted in the recent literature. Work by Wadsworth et al. (1999) looked at a longer timeframe, focussed on younger age groups and considered the effects of today's increasingly fluid labour market. They concluded that 'prolonged unemployment

early in the working life of this population of young men was likely to have a persisting effect' on their future health. This has obvious implications for the importance of targeting our efforts towards reducing unemployment among the young.

Policy implications

So how can we mitigate the worst effects of unemployment upon health? Fig. 29.2 shows the centrality of poverty within the unemployment and health nexus. Government policies directed at alleviating economic disadvantage can cushion the worst health-related effects of unemployment. Research carried out by Wilkinson and Pickett (2009) and Bambra and Eikemo (2008) in different European countries demonstrated the moderating health effects within those countries with the best social security provision. But, of course, GPs and hospital doctors have their own part to play in giving advice to patients to reduce secondary health effects related to stress and disadvantageous behavioural change and to ensure that they also claim the benefits to which they are entitled.

Stop and think

- Social scientists are now predicting rapidly increasing trends towards flexibility in the world's labour markets. They also believe that detrimental health effects will be particularly bad for young people. What do you think?

Case study

The personal effect of unemployment

The following two quotes are from men who had experienced long-term unemployment and lived in the most disadvantaged circumstances. These extracts highlight how men describe certain health behaviours, which lacked any sense of moderation or control, in terms of release and reward, as well as a means of escape:

'When I go for a drink, I don't really feel like its enjoyment ... I feel it's a need to get pissed, a need to get stoned ... You kind of feel shit that you've got no job ... no money, so you try to look for an escape from that and then because it costs you money to do that so you end up on this downward spiral... People say you drink and smoke and take drugs ... because you like to have fun, but it is not about that at all ... It is a form of escapism ... You numb your brain with certain chemicals and things and that is the escapist aspect of it' (Chris, age 28 years).

'It's like with the drugs ... It was a lousy, lousy time and the reason I took up smoking the grass was I got out of the situation I was in ... We were struggling, really struggling ... It shuts out the hurts ... and everything else ... for most people, that's what it is, it's just a way out' (Bob, age 39 years)

From Dolan, 2010, p. 598.

Summary *Unemployment and health*

- All cross-sectional studies show the employed to be in better health than the unemployed. Longitudinal studies strongly suggest that the contrast is caused by unemployment rather than by selection within the labour market.
- The main causes of mortality among the unemployed are malignant neoplasms (particularly lung cancer), accidents, poisonings and violence (particularly suicide).
- Relative poverty, social isolation, lack of self-esteem and damaging health-related behaviours are the major factors associated with the production of ill effects among the unemployed.

30 | Labelling and stigma

We all use labels to name and describe things. Such labelling can have both positive and negative associations: for example, the 'good doctor', the 'caring nurse' or the 'lazy medical student'! Labelling and its associated idea of stigma are useful in understanding the importance of the *social* consequences of medical diagnosis. We are particularly interested here in the way neutral medical labels acquire negative and stigmatizing connotations. Labelling and stigma are important for medical practitioners for two reasons. Firstly, negative labels are often applied by the public at large to people with particular diseases such as epilepsy, schizophrenia or psoriasis, which are thought to signify some moral failing, social disgrace or separation from normal society. Such beliefs may be rooted in superstition, fear and ignorance, but they are quite common. Secondly, medical practitioners act as important arbiters of the labels that get applied in much of what they do.

Doctors and labelling

A medical diagnosis, as well as being a scientific way of identifying a disease and differentiating it from others, is also a social label with potentially powerful negative consequences. For example, a psychiatrist in diagnosing mental illness is doing more than prescribing a course of treatment. Such a diagnosis may result in significant restraints on liberty if institutional care is involved. General practitioners sign sick notes and declare people unfit to work and eligible to receive financial benefit from the state. A chest physician may be called upon to assess the degree of loss of lung function in a man with asbestos-related illness who is making a claim against his former employer. In each of these three examples the medical diagnosis is also an important social label with social consequences and moral and financial implications.

The medical diagnosis is a biological or medical explanation of some underlying pathology in the body or mind. However, that diagnosis has social effects that go well beyond biology and may have significant social and psychological consequences for the person and perhaps his or her family and employer.

Stop and think

- For yourself, immediate or extended family what diagnoses have resulted in some negative consequences?
- What attempts were made to mitigate these?

Social reaction

The behaviour of the public is strongly influenced by medical labels. Think of the types of reaction that are often made to diagnoses of cancer. But it is not only life-threatening illnesses that produce strong reactions. For example, knowing that someone has epilepsy, or has a mental illness, can strongly affect the way others respond to them. People react not just to the biological pathology but also to what they regard as its social significance. When the social significance of the label carries a strongly negative connotation, this is an example of what sociologists and psychologists call *stigma*. The two terms – labelling and stigma – are not interchangeable because some labels are highly positive. However, in the context of medical work, it is the negative attributions by self or others that are of particular significance.

The case study shows that an important distinction needs to be made between the presence of some deviation from normality – in this case the presence of unrecognized coronary heart disease – and the social reaction to the subsequent diagnosis – the change in the man's behaviour and the response of his wife and the insurance company. Sociologists have called this distinction *primary deviation* and *secondary deviation* (Lemert, 1951). Primary deviation is some kind of physical or social difference of an individual or a group. Secondary deviation is the response of self and others to the public recognition – the label – of that difference.

This idea of primary and secondary deviation was originally developed in a classic text about crime by Edwin Lemert (1951). Lemert observed that many people commit crimes. He also noted that for the vast majority of people this is only a brief excursion into things such as petty shoplifting, under-age drinking, pilfering in the office, fiddling their expenses or speeding in their car. The point was that these activities did not lead to a life of crime. Indeed, the vast majority of people who have at one time or another transgressed the law actually regard themselves as morally upright citizens. For most people, in other words, their law-breaking has no long-term effects because it is not detected and it is not punished and very few others know about it. Their law-breaking is the primary deviation since a deviant act has been committed. Secondary deviation occurs if and when the general public, the courts and the police respond to an individual as a criminal and that person's whole life gets caught up in that social role. Career criminals are classically involved in the reinforcement of their own secondary deviation.

Stigma

The term 'stigma' is most usually associated with the work of Erving Goffman (1968a) in another classic text. He was particularly interested in the public humiliations and social disgrace that may happen to people when highly negative labels are applied. He made the distinction between *discreditable* and *discrediting* stigma. A discreditable stigma is one that is not known about by the many people with whom the person with the stigma comes into contact every day. Only the person with the stigmatizing condition and a few close intimates will know about it. A discrediting stigma, on the other hand, is one that cannot be hidden from other people because it is obvious and visible. People respond to the condition rather than to the person (Fig. 30.1).

A good example of a discreditable stigma is a patient who has had a mastectomy or an ileostomy (see pp. 118–119). To people in the street, such patients look quite normal when they are fully clothed. Apart from their closest friends and relatives, their doctor and the few other people they might wish to inform, theirs is a hidden stigma. Other people do not react to it because it is not obvious and they therefore do not know about it. Individuals with a mastectomy or an ileostomy may go to great lengths to conceal their physical difference – say, by not going to a swimming pool and never getting undressed in front of strangers. The existence of mastectomy or ileostomy will be very important to them and will have an effect in their own thoughts, feelings and behaviour. To other people, because it cannot be seen and is therefore not known about, it is irrelevant (Kelly, 1991).

In contrast, someone with an amputation, or who is in a wheelchair, or who has lost an eye does not have the option of

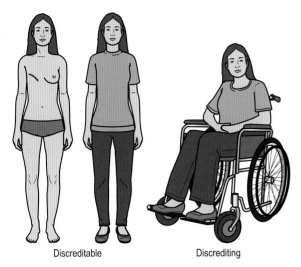

Discreditable   Discrediting

Fig. 30.1 Discreditable and discrediting stigma.

concealing these things from others very easily and people respond on the basis of the visible difference rather than the person (Fig. 30.1). What this means is that for some disabilities and diseases, individuals have little control over the publicly available information about them. As that information may be the basis of judgements, both positive and negative, and these judgements can have profound social and psychological effects, they are important medical issues.

Felt stigma and enacted stigma

Sometimes a distinction that is sometimes made is between *enacted* stigma and *felt* stigma. Enacted stigma is the real experience of prejudice, discrimination and disadvantage as the consequence of a particular condition, say epilepsy. However, the research shows, at least in the case of epilepsy, that such frank negative stigmatization and labelling is thankfully relatively rare (Scambler and Hopkins, 1986). However, it is the fear that such discrimination might occur – which is defined as felt stigma – that can be so worrying. This is why the degree to which people feel able to be in control of information about themselves is so important. In epilepsy, for example, the worry may stem from the fact that the disease is not well controlled, and the concern is about having a seizure in public.

Stop and think

- What are likely to be the primary and secondary deviations as a consequence of screening for disease? Note: no screening test is 100% accurate.
- What are some examples of screening tests that might produce stigma?
- Not all medical conditions carry negative labels. Patients with the common cold, chickenpox, measles and influenza or who fracture their leg playing soccer, do not generally attract stigmatizing labels, and the social response of the general public is usually unremarkable. Indeed, such illnesses may attract sympathy. Why do these illnesses attract sympathy?
- Problems such as alcoholism, schizophrenia, syphilis, HIV/AIDS and epilepsy, however, frequently do attract highly negative labels. What is the reason for these conditions attracting negative labels?
- Are smoking-related diseases and obesity stigmatized conditions?
- What are the implications of the existence of groups of illnesses that are stigmatized for the provision of care?
- Do you think that treatment decisions and decisions to fund certain drugs are linked to issues of stigma?

Case study *Negative labels applied to self: the case of coronary heart disease*

A middle-aged man has begun to experience the early symptoms of angina. He does not know what the pains are, and he merely assumes they are typical for a man of his age and are caused by his playing vigorous games of cricket with his grandson. So long as he believes his pains are the harmless consequences of ageing, he will do nothing to alter his behaviour; indeed he continues to smoke and to drink alcohol as he has done for the last 40 years. A biological abnormality is present that could be medically detected but has not been yet and the disease has not yet reached a point where it is significantly debilitating. Therefore it has had no social consequence for the man or his family.

However, let us assume this man goes for a routine insurance medical exam because he wants to alter his pension plan. He describes his symptoms, and the doctor suspects heart disease. After investigation, coronary heart disease is diagnosed. The medical label is applied, and treatment can begin. But let us also imagine how the man feels. He is now a patient who thinks of himself as a 'cardiac case'. He is very frightened. He immediately stops smoking. He also gives up drinking and goes on to a low-fat diet. He becomes extremely concerned about overexertion and gives up playing cricket with his grandson. His wife also becomes anxious and discourages him from digging the garden and insists that he sit in an armchair at home. Finally, he is unable to get additional insurance and alter his pension. We can see that this man's life has been transformed, even though biologically speaking his angina is no worse now than it was before he had his medical check-up. However, his own behaviour, that of his wife and, indeed, that of his insurance company have all changed as a consequence of the medical label.

Labelling and stigma

- In the social and behavioural sciences, labelling refers to the social response of individuals and groups to physical, psychological or social characteristics and particularly differences in others.
- Medical diagnoses are an extremely important example of labels in this sense, and doctors are key people in some labelling processes through the act of diagnosis.
- Not all labels are negative, but some medical ones certainly are.
- Primary deviation refers to the fact of biological, physical or social difference.
- Secondary deviation refers to the social response of the individual and others to the difference.
- Stigma is a particularly negative form of labelling.
- Fear of stigmatization is a very powerful force affecting people's behaviour.
- Stigma and labelling may play a part in some medical decision-making.

31 | Perceptions of risk and risk-taking behaviours

The identification of risk factors for disease is crucial for prevention. We know that social as well as biological factors are implicated in the patterning of ill health. However, People's lifestyles and health-related behaviours also have a very important role in both preventing and causing disease and ill health. Those behaviours that are deleterious to health can be termed *risk-taking behaviours* because of the known risk they pose for an individual's health. There has been a growing emphasis – in health promotion policy and initiatives – on individuals' responsibility for their own health and the promotion of behaviour change to reduce an individual's risk of disease and ill health (see pp. 72–73).

This has brought with it an emphasis on self-control, on moderation in behaviour and on the provision of information to inform people of the risks to health associated with certain lifestyles and behaviours. However, it is important to recognize that individuals' potential for control over their lifestyles, behaviours and health is limited by the social and economic circumstances in which they live and which shape their lives (see pp. 42–43). Understanding people's own perceptions of risk and the contexts within which their risk-taking behaviours occur is important for doctors and others who may be assessing a patient's risk of disease and encouraging a healthier lifestyle.

Perceptions of risk

Ignorance is often considered to be a major barrier to following lifestyle advice, although there is much evidence to suggest that the lay public are well aware of the publicized risks to health such as the relationship between smoking and lung cancer or the range of risk factors associated with heart disease. In fact, research suggests that knowledge itself is not a powerful predictor of behaviour.

People may view a range of risks very differently. For example, *Salmonella* infection from eggs was viewed as very risky when this was highlighted in the media, although the chances of infection were small. However, the longer-term risks of cholesterol and heart disease were not viewed in the same way (Frankel et al., 1991). These different perceptions of risk may influence behaviour in different ways, with reactive lifestyle changes around egg consumption occurring quickly but modification of diet to prevent heart disease being much harder to achieve.

People have a tendency to believe that the likelihood of personally experiencing a negative event, including illness, is less than objectively measured standards would predict, but more for a positive event. Furthermore they believe that their chances are more favourable than those of other people. These respective concepts are called 'unrealistic *absolute* optimism' and 'unrealistic *comparable* optimism' (Weinstein, 1980; Shepperd et al., 2013). Factors regarded by individuals as decreasing their risk include perceptions about their behaviour (e.g. engaging in preventive health behaviours or seeking appropriate help) and psychological attributes (e.g. the personality type who does not let things get you down, or holding 'health-conscious' values). These are both associated with perceived controllability of the event. Environmental or hereditary factors are perceived differently; beliefs that contribute to unrealistic optimism include the belief that if the problem has not yet appeared, there will be an exemption from future risk; that the problem is perceived as preventable through individual action; that the hazard is perceived as infrequent; and that there is a lack of experience with the hazard (Weinstein, 1987).

There are, however, different practical implications in relation to health-related behaviour. On the one hand, unrealistic optimism may weaken intentions to engage in health-promoting behaviours and/or to avoid in health-damaging behaviours. For example, the tendency to under-estimate the harms of smoking and to over-estimate one's ability to quit may weaken any intention to avoid smoking (Weinstein et al., 2004). On the other hand, unrealistic optimism may strengthen intentions to take preventive action because it enhances self-efficacy and belief in the controllability of negative events (Weinstein and Lyon, 1999). The relative importance of the positive or negative aspects of unrealistic optimism will depend very much on the nature of the health problem – compare a patient recovering from a heart attack, for example, with an intravenous drug user. It is important to understand an individual patient's risk perception as individuals are unlikely to engage in health-protective behaviours or avoid health-damaging behaviours unless they perceive themselves to be susceptible (Weinstein, 2000).

Stop and think

- Examine briefly your own behaviour (e.g. consumption of alcohol or lack of exercise).
- In what way do you think you might demonstrate unrealistic optimism in your own potential health-damaging behaviour?
- What prevents you from changing your behaviour?

Differences between lay and expert perceptions of risk in relation to health can be better understood when lay knowledge is viewed in the context of people's lives and experiences. It is important that lay perceptions of risk are not just seen as wrong or based on ignorance but rather as embedded in particular social and cultural circumstances, as examined in the following example.

Example 1: lay understanding of heart disease

A large, in-depth study of people living in south Wales investigated lay explanations of heart disease. This research took place during a large campaign to prevent heart disease (Davison et al., 1992). The results showed that people had their own explanations for the causes of heart disease, which drew on, yet differed from, the publicized lifestyle risks. In this 'lay epidemiology', people drew on a range of knowledge and experience to explain who was a candidate for heart disease (Box 31.1). This included lifestyle factors, heredity, social environment

Box 31.1 People who may be identified as coronary candidates

- Obese people; people who do not take exercise and are unfit
- Red-faced people; people with a grey pallor
- Smokers
- People with a heart problem in the family
- Heavy drinkers
- People who eat excessive amounts of rich, fatty foods
- Worriers (by nature); bad-tempered, pessimistic or negative people
- People who are under stress (e.g. because of work, unemployment, bereavement, family life and so on)
- People who suffer strain through hard manual labour, working conditions, overindulgence in 'unhealthy' lifestyle behaviours)

Source: Davison et al., 1991, with permission.

such as work, physical environment such as climate and a degree of randomness attributed to luck and chance.

This demonstrates that people understand the range of risks associated with heart disease, not just those associated with lifestyle. However, people are also well aware, from their personal observations, that those at high risk of getting heart disease do not always suffer from it and that sometimes those at low risk do. People know that predicting who will actually get ill is difficult for those conditions that are multifactorial (i.e. caused by several different factors). Any attempt to over-simplify this with an emphasis on behaviour such as eating is likely to be sceptically received, as lay people's own experience and knowledge tell them that the process is more complicated and less certain than that.

Risk-taking behaviour

Just as it is important to understand lay perceptions of risk, risk-taking behaviour must also be examined in the context of individuals' lives. Risk-taking behaviours often do not take place in isolation, but in interaction with others. This can explain why some people engage in behaviours that are considered to be, even by themselves, detrimental to health. The importance of social context in understanding risk-taking behaviour is illustrated through two different examples: men's risk-taking behaviour after a friend's accidental death (see Example 2 in the following section) and prenatal smoking (see Case study).

Example 2: men's risk-taking behaviour after the death of a friend

In Western countries, accidents are the leading cause of death for men aged 15 to 40 years (see pp. 44–45). A study of men who had experienced the death of a friend in a 'risky' activity (an outdoor or extreme sport, over-dosing, motor vehicle accident or fight) (Creighton et al., 2015) demonstrated the importance of the social and cultural context in shaping such behaviour. These men's perceptions of and engagement with risk-taking behaviour after a friend's death were explained in relation to the social practices and ideals within specific social reference groups – practices that produced and affirmed particular masculine identities. For example, continuing with extreme sports after a friend's death from the same or similar activity was typically framed in terms of 'living for the moment', where the possibility of death was accepted, normalized and in some cases valorized. Whilst those who had lost a friend from an overdose – arguably a more stigmatized cause than extreme sports – displayed a greater tendency towards reining in their risky practices and realigning their identities to a social reference group associated with different masculine identities.

Stop and think

- Why might knowledge of risk factors for ill health, or even death, not influence an individual's behaviour?
- In what ways are individuals constrained in their actions?
- Think of some 'risky' or 'unhealthy behaviours' that you, your friends or family engage in. What explanations can you think of for this?

Practical applications

Recognition of the social context of risk, in terms of both perceptions of risk and risk-taking behaviours, is important for doctors as they become involved in public health and health promotion as well as in dealing with individual patients. Doctors should try to elicit people's own explanations and treat these as reasonable and based on experience. This should lead to greater understanding and empathy between doctor and patient (see pp. 94–95). Similarly, account must be taken of the circumstances within which people live and how this may influence their behaviour. Doctors should take care to avoid 'victim-blaming', where those who engage in behaviours considered damaging to their health are deemed to be irresponsible. Often such behaviour can be considered a rational response to poor social conditions or the only choice in a situation where the individual has little control.

Case study *Pregnant women and smoking*

A qualitative study of women with current or recent experience of prenatal smoking (Naughton et al., 2013) found that all interviewees were aware that smoking during pregnancy was 'harming the baby', leading to most experiencing cognitive dissonance (see pp. 72–73). Whilst such feelings provided motivation to quit, most relapsed early on. This meant that the women drew upon social and contextual influences to resolve their dissonance. For example, similar to the lay epidemiology that Davison et al. (1992) described, many referred to an awareness of others (or themselves from a previous pregnancy) having had a 'healthy' child despite smoking during the pregnancy. Some mentioned reassurance from what was said – or not said – during consultations with midwives. Others highlighted the potentially damaging impact on themselves and the baby from stress that would be brought on by them not smoking.

Perceptions of risk and risk-taking behaviours

- The concept of a risk factor for disease is important for both professionals and the lay public.
- Risk perceptions and risk-taking behaviours are part of a wider social context, including both social conditions and social interactions.
- These may constrain the choices that individuals can make; risk-taking behaviours should be seen, at least in part, as socially determined.
- Promoting healthy behaviours means more than encouraging individuals to change. People's own risk perceptions must be understood.

32 | What are disease prevention and health promotion?

The goals of disease prevention and health promotion are to preserve and promote good health in society by preventing disease and minimizing its consequences. It is useful to distinguish between three types of prevention, usually referred to as primary, secondary and tertiary prevention. The distinction between these three prevention types is that each has a different goal. See Table 32.1 before you read on.

Primary prevention: disease incidence

The incidence of disease is measured in terms of the number of new cases of disease occurring in society, usually during a specified time period, such as one year. Primary prevention can be undertaken whenever the cause of disease has been identified.

Perhaps the best-known form of medical intervention in primary prevention is mass immunization. Over the years, immunization has been introduced against poliomyelitis, tuberculosis, measles and many other diseases. However, since it usually takes several years of medical research before a virus is identified and a vaccine developed, the impact of immunization on disease incidence is sometimes very small. Poliomyelitis immunization is probably one of the few medical interventions to have had a demonstrable primary prevention effect in the last century (Fig. 32.1). Health education and broader public health measures that help people avoid contact with viruses and bacteria may be particularly valuable early interventions.

The major causes of death in developed countries today are diseases of the circulatory system and neoplasms (see pp. 40–41; and pp. 156–157). These diseases have been linked to particular behaviours such as smoking tobacco, excessive alcohol consumption and a diet high in fat. Fig. 32.2 demonstrates the dramatic impact that behaviour change can have on an individual's survival rate. Specifically, the

chance of a 50-year-old smoker living until the age of 80 years is 25%, whereas a smoker who has quit at age 50 years has almost double the chance of reaching the age of 80 years.

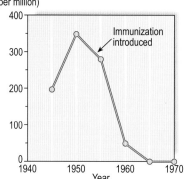

Fig. 32.1 Poliomyelitis notifications before and after introduction of immunization: England and Wales *(adapted from McKeown, 1979, with permission).*

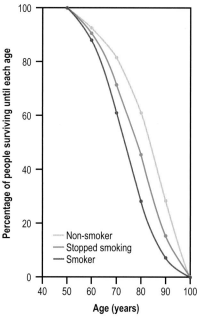

Fig. 32.2 Increase in survival to specific ages after stopping smoking at age 50 years *(reproduced from Doll et al., 2004).*

Secondary prevention: disease prevalence

Prevalence refers to the number of people who have a particular disease at any one time. Clearly if diseases are left untreated and new cases are occurring all the time, the prevalence of a disease will increase. Although doctors are continually involved in secondary prevention, from time to time campaigns are mounted to increase the likelihood of doctors detecting particular diseases: for example, skin cancer may go unrecognized by patients and doctors unless specific efforts are made to identify it during consultations. Some forms of secondary prevention such as screening for diseases, including colorectal cancer, require the participation of practically all people in society if those with the disease are to be detected and the screening programme is to prove cost-effective. Similarly immunization programmes for infectious diseases require maximum participation to reach and maintain herd immunity. Efforts to persuade people to take part may, therefore, be seen by some as efforts to compel people to participate in secondary prevention programmes, and doctors delivering these services need to be aware of potential reservations patients may have (see pp. 66–67).

Tertiary prevention: adverse consequences of disease

As a result of increased life expectancy there is increasing concern for the care of people who survive treatment: for example, heart disease, cancer or stroke. This means ensuring that patients experience the best possible health for the longest possible period of time after diagnosis. Tertiary prevention is concerned with a wider range of health indices than either primary or secondary prevention. For instance, tertiary preventive interventions might have as their goals the reduction of disability and promotion of psychological well-being.

Table 32.1 **Goals of prevention**				
Type of prevention	**Focus**	**Distal goal**	**Proximal goal**	**Behavioural goal**
Primary prevention	Incidence	Prevent new cases of AIDS	Prevent HIV infection	Use of condoms during sexual intercourse; safe injection practices for IV drug users
Secondary prevention	Prevalence	Reduce cases of cervical cancer	Early identification of precancerous cell abnormalities	Regular screening (i.e. Papanicolaou (Pap) test every 2 years)
Tertiary prevention	Impact	Minimize disability in children with cerebral palsy	Identify nature and extent of disability	Uptake and maintenance of skills training

IV, Intravenous.

Table 32.2 Levels of intervention to achieve behavioural change: alcohol consumption

Level of intervention	Example of intervention	Impact of intervention on individual behavioural change
Governmental legislation/policy	Minimum pricing to establish a baseline price for alcohol Value added tax (VAT) Labelling of alcoholic content Minimum age for purchasing and consuming alcohol	Increasing the cost of alcohol and making people aware of the alcoholic content of a beverage make people less inclined to purchase and consume large amounts.
Social/environmental	Mass-media campaigns (e.g. Dry January (challenge people to give up alcohol for 31 days); Alcohol Awareness Week (local authorities and other organizations get involved) Work place screening of alcohol intoxication Alcohol-free events	Challenge and a sense of community facilitate behaviour change and increase self-efficacy to avoid alcohol in the future. Health education provides knowledge and skills to aid behaviour change. Societal and environmental changes to make alcohol consumption difficult.
Individual	Opportunistic screening and history-taking by doctors to assess risk and provide motivation and alcohol reduction advice Mobile apps have been developed for individuals to track their alcohol intake	Motivational interviewing can be used to increase willingness to change. Tracking alcohol consumption on a mobile device, can help individuals monitor and reduce consumption.

Exercise and rehabilitation programmes may be provided in medical settings and during follow-up care to enable stroke survivors to walk and acquire control over a range of movements (see pp. 118–119). Early detection of incurable diseases is also a focus of tertiary prevention: for example, early detection of Alzheimer's disease can improve quality of life and optimize functioning. Palliative care facilities focus entirely on pain management and psychological adjustment.

Chronic conditions that are genetically acquired or acquired during childhood or early adulthood are also a focus of tertiary prevention. These conditions cannot be cured, but much can be done to minimize the extent to which they result in disability or distress: for example, a person with asthma.

Levels of intervention

The success of prevention and health promotion depends upon the ability of the health care system to deliver preventive interventions to people who believe themselves to be in good health, and on the extent to which people engage in interventions. To bring about behavioural change, it is important to acknowledge the cultural and social processes that influence behaviour (see pp. 70–71). The social-ecological approach (see pp. 76–77) to health promotion provides a theoretical framework for understanding the dynamic interplay between the individual, social/environmental and broader governmental/societal levels outlined in Table 32.2. The social-ecological approach suggests that when these interventions are combined, rather than considered in isolation, we can directly influence behavioural change.

Strategies to change behaviour occur at many different levels (Table 32.2). Action by governments is important in facilitating behavioural change among both doctors and patients. For instance, in 1990 the British government changed the GP

contract to encourage greater participation in preventive health care. One target for change was in primary and secondary prevention of heart disease. GPs were offered financial inducements to encourage them to screen patients diet, smoking habits, exercise and blood cholesterol levels and to offer appropriate treatments or behavioural change clinics to help people to modify their lifestyles. Governments may also seek to prevent disease by imposing taxes on substances that cause disease such as tobacco and alcohol to limit their consumption: for example, in 2014, legislation was passed in England and Wales to set a minimum price per standard drink to discourage excessive consumption of alcohol.

A second level of change concerns attempts to modify the social environment or commonly held views about health and health-related behaviours. Community- and organizational-level interventions such as media campaigns can do a great deal to assist individual behavioural change. People are very much influenced in their behaviour by what they see or believe others do and by what they think will be approved or disapproved of by others (see pp. 52–53). For example, the 'Dry January' campaign, in which people try to give up alcohol for a month, increasing awareness and providing support.

Doctors' advice can be very effective in motivating people to change. Many preventive behaviours require people to acquire new skills and confidence in their ability to control or promote their own health. It is on the development and delivery of effective behaviour change strategies that much of primary and tertiary prevention depends (see pp. 72–73).

Dilemmas in disease prevention and health promotion

For many years, prevention has been organised as a specialty of public health

medicine. A shift towards prevention requires that all health care professionals, including school teachers, social workers, prison officers, acquire new skills in behaviour change.

Some forms of prevention rely upon the participation of everyone in society to make them cost-effective such as screening and immunization. These considerations question how we distinguish between education, persuasion and compulsion. Health promotion considers autonomy to be important, yet strongly encourages individuals to make the 'correct' decision about their health, which undermine this autonomy. Other forms of prevention now rely on the detection of foetal abnormalities. Genetic screening has raised concerns about the ethics of parental choice and society's view of those with genetic disorders (see pp. 68–69).

Stop and think

- Make a case for spending money on disease prevention and health promotion?
- What ethical issues are associated with preventive programmes?
- What skills do doctors need to practise preventive medicine and health promotion effectively?

What are disease prevention and health promotion?

- Primary prevention refers to the prevention of disease incidence.
- Secondary prevention refers to the prevention of disease prevalence.
- Tertiary prevention refers to the prevention of disease impact.
- Preventive efforts occur at many levels: governmental or societal policy, social or environmental and individual.
- Health promoters need to provide informed choice to individuals making health-related decisions.

33 | Health screening

Health screening plays a valuable role in the prevention of illness and the promotion of health. For those who screen positively, there is the possibility of early diagnosis or early identification of risk, with the resulting benefits of early medical intervention. Those who screen negatively are likely to benefit from reassurance. However, the usefulness of health screening may be limited if the uptake rate is low or if no benefits are obtained by patients who screen positive. In addition, there may be disadvantages to patients if the techniques simply serve to increase their anxiety or, in some areas, result in over-treatment.

Patients can be screened for the presence of existing disease (e.g. phenylketonuria, breast cancer), for precursors of disease (e.g. cervical cytology, HIV test, tests for chromosome abnormality) or for risk factors for disease, which may take the form of negative health behaviours (e.g. smoking, poor diet) or biological or genetic factors (e.g. hypertension, Huntington's disease, *BRCA* gene mutations in breast cancer).

Screening: process and results

Usually those found to be positive will go on to have further tests that will determine whether the first result was a true or false positive. Since no screening test is perfect, there will always be a number of false positives and false negatives, and the number will depend on the sensitivity and specificity of the test. Fig. 33.1 shows the four possible outcomes of screening.

Uptake of screening

No test achieves 100% uptake by the relevant population. Doctors may fail to offer the test and patients may not accept it if offered. Research suggests that doctors may not offer a test even when it would be appropriate, perhaps when they think the test is ineffective or the patient would not take the appropriate actions (e.g. change diet, adopt safer sex procedures), or they may simply forget to offer the test. If a test is not offered, the patient will be unable to make an informed decision. Furthermore the benefits of some screening programmes such as mammography for breast cancer have been questioned, and the surrounding controversy makes it difficult to provide patients with definitive information to inform their decision-making (Biller-Andorno and Jüni, 2014). That said, how best to facilitate informed choice in relation to screening remains unclear (Biesecker, Schwartz and Marteau, 2013).

Patients offered a test may refuse to take it because it is incompatible with their health beliefs (see pp. 70–71); for instance, they may not think they are susceptible to the condition being tested. Thus women were more likely to have amniocentesis if they thought they were likely to have a baby with Down's syndrome; uptake of the procedure was related to *perceived* risk,

but not to *actual* risk as indicated by the maternal age. Patients may also decide not to have a test: for example, declining a faecal occult blood test for colorectal cancer because the test is unpleasant or difficult.

Adverse effects for those tested

Patients show high levels of anxiety when being screened and awaiting results. Informing the patient that the test is negative lowers anxiety more effectively than telling them to assume the result is normal if they hear nothing more. However, even communicating a negative result can have adverse effects. A false-negative result can be harmful if it prevents the patient from receiving appropriate treatment or advice on lifestyle; a false-negative HIV test might result in the patient putting his or her partner at risk by sexual transmission and remove the motivation to adopt safer sexual practices. Similarly a true-negative result can also be harmful: for example, a patient with a familial risk of type 2 diabetes may be reassured by a negative diabetes test and may fail to make the necessary preventive changes to diet and exercise, thereby increasing the risk of developing the disease in the future.

Testing positive

After a positive screening test result, there are further stages of tests, results and medical management. Each of these involves further social and behavioural processes, as shown in Fig. 33.2.

When the initial test result is positive or ambiguous but is followed by a clear negative result – i.e. the patient has received an initial false-positive or invalid result – patients may continue to be anxious long after being told the negative result.

If the result is a true positive, patients' reactions will tend to vary with the implications of the results, depending on the seriousness of the condition and the available preventive or curative medical treatment. Nevertheless there may be unexpected reactions: for example, individuals found to be positive for genetic diseases such as Huntington's chorea or polyposis have reported feeling relieved, perhaps because their uncertainty was reduced.

When screening identifies people at risk of disease, there may be adverse effects of labelling the individual and it has been found that they may respond as if they are ill rather than just at risk (see pp. 60–61). Studies of people shown on screening to have hypertension have found that they subsequently show higher levels of distress, report more symptoms, take more time off work and participate less in social activities. The level of distress is affected by the way in which the diagnosis is communicated: for example, those informed that they were hypertensive and given leaflets describing hypertension as 'the silent killer' were more anxious months later than those fully informed that it was a risk factor and reassured about management (Rudd et al., 1986).

Implications of a positive result

For some test results, such as Huntington's chorea, the result carries no specific implications for action in a clinical context, although the recipient may choose to make relevant plans for the future. For other tests, such as genetic tests with a probabilistic rather than certain result, there may be continued uncertainty and

	Result	
	+	**–**
Actual state of patient **+**	True **+**	False **–**
–	False **+**	True **–**

Fig. 33.1 Four possible outcomes of a screening test.

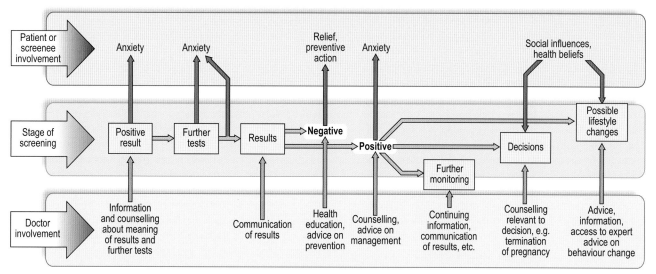

Fig. 33.2 Schematic outline of health screening and the social and behavioural factors involved – the process after a positive result.

further clinical monitoring will be required. For yet others, such as hypertension, appropriate medical management may reduce the likelihood or severity of the condition.

Other positive results may require the recipient to make critical decisions (e.g. whether to terminate a pregnancy) or to consider changes in behaviour and lifestyle (e.g. reducing fat intake or practising safer sex). Whilst there is ample evidence that many people will make these changes successfully, a substantial number will attempt to change but fail. The overall success of the screening programme may be limited by failures to change behaviours in those screening positive.

Role of doctors in screening

Doctors may play key roles at every stage (see Fig. 33.2 and list later in this section). The results of screening, both in terms of successful detection and management of clinical conditions and in terms of the potential adverse effects for those tested, depend on the doctors' behaviours. The role of doctors in screening includes:

- Offering screening: inviting individuals to attend without raising unnecessary fears
- Counselling about screening: giving information about procedures, potential benefits and limitations, and checking comprehension, thereby enabling individuals to reach an informed decision
- Providing health education: before screening (e.g. for serum cholesterol or HIV); after positive screening (e.g. for risk factors for cardiovascular disease)
- Communicating results that may be complex: providing enough information to enable patients to understand; achieving a balance between raising unnecessary anxiety and giving inappropriate reassurance
- Advising on decisions after positive results: giving information to enable informed choice and consent
- Clinical management: varies depending on the type of screening
- Assisting individuals to make necessary lifestyle changes (e.g. quitting smoking, improving diet, increasing exercise, taking medication, safer sex, repeated screening or monitoring)

Case study

Mrs Green had been alarmed to be recalled for further tests after blood tests suggested something might be wrong with her baby. She had taken a long time to conceive, and this was a much-wanted child. Although Mrs Green thought the pregnancy might already show, she felt she could not tell her friends at work until she got the result of the amniocentesis and could be sure the baby was all right. After the amniocentesis, the obstetrician said there was nothing to worry about as the test result was normal. However, Mrs Green continued to be concerned: why had the original test been positive? Surely that indicated something was wrong; after all, 'there's no smoke without fire'. If one test was positive and one was normal, how could the doctors be sure which one was right? Her continuing anxiety led her to be on the lookout for signs that things were going wrong even after the birth of her normal healthy baby.

Health screening

- For any screening test, a substantial number of those offered the test do not accept – a result of poor information, social influences or, in some cases, good decisions.
- Screening may have adverse effects, especially raised anxiety, which may persist even when the result is normal.
- The way in which results are communicated can affect the impact of the results on the individual.
- Those being screened require information and counselling before and after screening.
- For some tests, those being screened may need health education and advice on behaviour and lifestyle change.
- People do not always succeed in making lifestyle changes without further professional assistance.

34 | The social implications of the new genetics

Developments in molecular genetics have major implications for society and individuals, doctors and patients. The knowledge and techniques that have arisen from the development of recombinant DNA affect profoundly how we think about and deal with health, risks to health, disease and illness (Cunningham-Burley and Boulton, 2000; http://www.sponpress.com/books/series/GANDS/). These developments influence the social, cultural, ethical and personal realms as well as the biological realm and have ethical implications around confidentiality, autonomy, informed consent and individual choice. Hence social and ethical implications are widely debated, especially around how this knowledge may be used (Nuffield Council on Bioethics, 1993; http://www.who.int/genomics/en/).

Genetic services and genetic counselling

There has been a growth in specialist genetic services offering genetic counselling. In the UK and other countries, genetics centres offer 'genetic counselling' to individuals or families with, or at risk of, conditions which may have a genetic basis and is undertaken by a clinical geneticist or genetic counsellor. Their main role is to provide accurate information about a genetic condition and genetic testing (where available) to help people make an informed decision about their options in a non-directive manner. However, complex ethical and moral issues can arise: for example, around the nature of 'non-directiveness' and how/whether to alert any at-risk relatives. The emergence of direct to consumer testing has raised considerable concerns because there may be limited or no genetic counselling, sparking debates about paternalism in mainstream health care.

Predictive testing: Huntington's disease

Huntington's disease (HD) is an autosomal-dominant neurodegenerative disorder that leads to a gradual deterioration of mind, movement and mood over 10 to 15 years. Those who inherit the changed gene will develop the disorder usually between 35 and 55 years of age ('late adult-onset'). The disorder is fatal and untreatable, although there are guidelines for standards of care. Definitive predictive testing has been available for adults since 1993. At first glance the provision of predictive testing within families known to be at risk of HD may seem to be desirable, with benefits such as relief from uncertainty, information to make future plans and more informed reproductive choices. However, the possibility raised by predictive testing brings with it specific concerns about the rights of individuals to know or not know their genetic status, the rights of family members to information and the psychological impact of a positive result. Thus after two decades, less than 25% of those at-risk seek testing, ranging from 3% to 25% (Tassicker et al., 2009). Those who have the gene fall into three different groups who want to:

1. Be tested to plan their lives or avoid passing the gene on to children
2. Obtain an early diagnosis (they are already suspecting symptoms)
3. Establish that they are free from the disease (they are past the age when symptoms are likely to develop)

People have not come forward for testing considered that: firstly, a positive test result would have implications for their children, who may have inherited the disorder. Secondly, as there is no effective treatment testing may not bring any medical benefits. Thirdly, some people were worried about the loss of health insurance. Lastly, some felt that the completion of their own childbearing removed any reason to have the test. Whilst the number of those who test remains low, more young people (aged 16–25 years) may be seeking testing, raising concerns about their 'maturity' to test, informed decision-making and other issues related to testing young people for adult-onset genetic conditions (Forrest Keenan, McKee and Miedzybrodzka, 2014). Interestingly both positive and negative results can cause distress as those found to be free of the disease may experience survivor guilt or feelings of 'not belonging'. The certainty provided through testing is not always welcomed. Families have lived with uncertainty in terms of the risk status of its members, and this uncertainty forms a crucial part of identity and experience (Richards, 1993). Thus information is not always desired by those at risk, and an individual's right to refuse to be tested must be preserved. The situation is even more uncertain in relation to genetic susceptibility (see Case study).

Carrier testing for recessive disorders: beta-thalassaemia

Beta-thalassaemia is an inherited blood disorder. If both parents are carriers of the trait, there is a one-in-four chance of passing the disease on to their child, whilst the carriers themselves remain free from the disease. The disease can be fatal without treatment, which is complex. Knowledge of carrier status makes possible greater reproductive choices, particularly the use of prenatal diagnosis and the abortion of affected foetuses, where this is personally and culturally acceptable. In Cyprus, where the trait is common, the Orthodox Church insists that people are aware of their carrier status for beta-thalassaemia when they marry. Where both partners are carriers, the couple then use prenatal diagnosis and abortion to avoid the birth of an affected child. Abortion is accepted on these grounds, but not on others. This has virtually eliminated the births of children with beta-thalassaemia in Cyprus. Screening for carrier status can raise a range of other issues, too: for example, screening for sickle-cell trait in the USA demonstrated that stigma can be attached to carrier status, leading

---

Case study

Susan is 32 years old and has two young daughters. Her mother died from breast cancer at the age of 56 years. She thinks that other female relatives may have had breast cancer. Susan had not really given her risk of breast cancer much thought and certainly viewed herself as a healthy person. However, when her older sister was diagnosed, she began to think it might be 'in the family'. She had read that susceptibility genes had been identified (*BRCA1* and *-2*) for some familial breast cancers and that a test was available to those at risk. She wondered whether this could explain her family history and what the consequences of that would mean. Would she want to be tested? How would she discuss this with her sister? What might happen to her – would she have to have both her breasts removed, or would she just have regular check-ups? After worrying about all these things for several weeks, she decided to see her GP. On the basis of her family history, the GP referred her to a clinical geneticist to assess her risk and discuss management strategies, as well as social/ethical issues such as insurance and other relatives who may be at risk.

to further discrimination of Black people (see pp. 48–49). Where people do not perceive themselves to be at risk, because they have little direct knowledge of the disease or 'do not want to know', uptake has been low: for example, with testing for cystic fibrosis carrier status. Even with the introduction of newborn screening programmes uptake rates in relatives can remain low.

Stop and think

- Will research into the genetic basis of disease lead to geneticization, where other causes are ignored?
- How can we avoid the stigma and discrimination that those with genetic disease may face?
- What sort of information (and genetic counselling approaches) will help informed decision-making for patients?

Understanding susceptibility to common diseases

Most diseases are multifactorial in aetiology, involving the interaction of genes with each other and with the environment. Research may lead to tests to identify genetic susceptibility to a range of common diseases in individuals. One major research investment is the UK Biobank (www.ukbiobank.ac.uk), where 500,000 healthy volunteers aged between 40 and 69 years have contributed genetic, lifestyle and medical histories so that researchers can study why some people develop certain diseases. The sample will be followed up through their medical records. The study aims to improve the prevention, diagnosis and treatment of common diseases such as cancer and heart disease. In recent years the possibility of whole genome sequencing (WGS) and whole exome sequencing (WES) has become a reality and is likely to be integrated into mainstream clinical care soon. This will raise additional questions, not least about whether individuals want to know, or should be told, the results of incidental findings.

Population screening

Population screening for susceptibility to disease could be beneficial where treatment or lifestyle modification improves health outcome. With the development of pharmacogenetics, treatments may become better suited to an individual's genotype. However, population screening raises ethical and other concerns (Willis, 2002). Firstly, screening whole populations to identify individuals with genetic susceptibility to common diseases is commercially attractive to corporations developing tests and treatments. Secondly, like other screening, those not considered at high risk may view themselves as invulnerable to disease, whilst those at high risk may not necessarily be helped, especially if lifestyle modification is difficult or treatment options limited. Thirdly, population screening may lead to a view that genes determine health. The geneticization of disease may result in neglect of other solutions such as social and environmental interventions and the belief that such information is more definitive and certain than is actually the case. Nevertheless specific screening programmes may be very useful where early intervention in those identified at risk will help improve outcomes.

Limits to the use of genetic technology and genetic explanations for disease

Two general issues are relevant to the application of knowledge gained from research into the genetic components of diseases and behaviours: eugenics and individual choice.

Eugenics

Concerns about eugenic control of populations are sometimes raised. The identification of genes implicated in disease can quickly lead to the availability of tests such as those for HD and beta-thalassaemia. Where such testing aims to provide people with the information to make informed decisions (e.g. greater choice in relation to reproduction to not pass on the disease to their children), this can mean aborting affected foetuses. The elimination of disease in this way may add to the stigma and discrimination currently experienced by those with disabilities in our society and may affect the resources available for their care. Concerns also relate to the potential increase in the number of tests available and, therefore, the range of diseases that may be deemed serious enough for interventions of this kind.

Individual choice

Many of the concerns expressed about eugenics are muted by individual choice in democratic societies. The rights of individuals to choose whether to be tested and whether to have an abortion are considered paramount: there should be no coercion. Whilst the preservation of individual choice is important, it is crucial to recognize that decisions are not made in a social vacuum. There may be subtle rather than overt pressures on individuals to conform to what is regarded as the obvious or right decision; or people may not have sufficient information to make informed decisions. Where there are inequalities, discrimination and concerns about the costs of care, the extent of choice available to individuals is culturally and socially constrained.

Practical application

Those involved in health care should be aware of the developments in genetics and their effects on both patients and society. Within consultations, it is important to discuss social and ethical issues and consider the context within which decisions are made so that patients can make informed, autonomous choices, particularly about genetic testing. Doctors should work towards ensuring that the possible negative outcomes of genetics (e.g. increased discrimination, stigma and inequality) are minimized. This can be achieved through open and public discussion and by actively promoting regulation and control of those institutions influenced by genetic research and its application – insurance, employment and health care provision. Research into the social implications of the new genetics is also integral to informing policy and practice.

Social implications of the new genetics

- Research into the genetic basis for disease can lead to applications in clinical practice, but we need to consider the ethical and social consequences.
- Genetic testing raises important social and ethical issues for individuals, doctors and society, which need to be discussed openly.
- Decisions taken by patients and doctors should be understood within their social, cultural and economic context; these may vary across cultures and social groups.

---

35 | Health beliefs, motivation and behaviour

Unhealthy behaviours such as physical inactivity, poor diet, smoking and excess alcohol intake are associated with increased risks of premature death, disease and disability. To encourage and support individuals to engage in health-promoting behaviours it is important first to understand the factors that determine health behaviours. A number of modifiable social–cognitive variables play a key role in determining the adoption and maintenance of health-promoting behaviours. Social–cognitive factors include an individual's attitude, perception and beliefs about their social environment, their health and health behaviour. Over the years, several influential social–cognitive models have been developed.

The health belief model

The Health Belief Model (HBM; Rosenstock, 1974) was the first model to identify the importance of an individual's attitudes and beliefs about health behaviour in determining future health

behaviour. There are four key factors stated in the HBM influencing whether an individual will engage in health-promoting action (Fig. 35.1): (1) *perceived susceptibility* of contracting a disease/condition; (2) *perceived severity* of the disease/condition in terms of the implications the individual believes it will have on their life (e.g. death, disability, occupation and family life); (3) *perceived benefits* taking action; (4) *perceived barriers* to taking action (e.g. action may be perceived as being unpleasant, painful, inconvenient or expensive). Health-promoting behaviour would be initiated when an individual experiences *cues to action*, which are internal or external events that set the process in motion.

Since its conception the HBM has been applied to explain a range of different health behaviours such as exercise, smoking and adherence to medical treatment. The development of the HBM advanced theoretical thinking; however, in its original form, the HBM did not include constructs that could capture an

individual's level of *motivation/intention* to act and *self-efficacy* (confidence in one's ability to take action). These have been shown to be powerful indicators of an individual's health actions.

The protection motivation theory

In the 1970s the protection motivation theory (PMT; Rogers, 1975) emerged as a theoretical model based on the HBM, but with a focus on motivation (Fig. 35.2). According to the PMT, *protection motivation*, an individual's motivation or intention to act, is the proximal determinant of health-related behaviour and is influenced by two main cognitive appraisals. The first is the individual's appraisal of a potential threat (e.g. tuberculosis), which is determined by the individual's *perceived vulnerability* and the *perceived severity* of the threat (similar to the HBM). The second is the individual's coping appraisal, which is determined by the individual's evaluation of how effective a response (e.g. immunization) is in reducing the threat (*response efficacy*) and the confidence they have in their ability to execute this particular response (*self-efficacy*).

The PMT, including the constructs of motivation and self-efficacy, was recognized as an advanced theoretical model describing the factors that influence an individual's health-promoting behaviours. Since motivation is fundamental to health behaviour the model presumes that when an individual's motivation is high, this will lead to corresponding behaviour. However, evidence shows that despite good intentions people often do fail to translate their intentions into actual behaviour. This has been named, the 'intention-behaviour

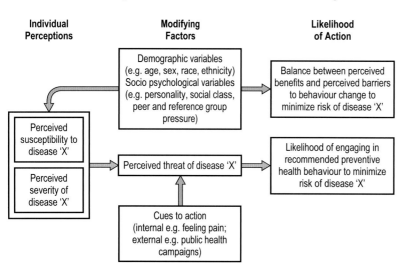

Fig. 35.1 The Health Belief Model.

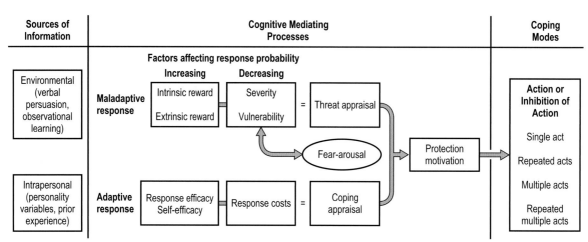

Fig. 35.2 Protection motivation theory.

gap'. Although the PMT is useful, it does not address the psychological processes by which motivation/intention is translated into action. Intentions are important but are not sufficient for explaining health behaviour.

The health action process model

Recently there has been a distinction made between motivational and volitional phases involved in health-related behaviour change. The Health Action Process Approach (HAPA) model (Schwarzer, 1992) states that behaviour change is a process whereby individuals pass through motivational and volitional phases acting on one's intention (Fig. 35.3). Specific cognitions are important during the motivational phase; *risk awareness* (perceived severity and susceptibility of the threat), *outcome expectancies* (perceived consequences of the threat) and *self-efficacy* (confidence in one's ability to initiate behaviour change). Once individuals are motivated and have formed an intention to act, they progress to the volitional phase where processes including *planning, self-regulation* and *self-efficacy* help

to translate intentions into behaviour. Self-efficacy in this phase is needed for maintaining the newly adopted behaviour and for recovery from relapses.

Interventions using social–cognitive models have been effective in changing cognitions and motivation but less effective in changing actual behaviour. Literature reviews have shown that interventions based on theoretical models that account for motivational and volitional phases of behaviour change, (e.g. HAPA model) are more effective in changing health-related behaviour. The HAPA model's key strength is the inclusion of specific strategies that can be used to encourage behaviour change in practice (see Chapter 38).

The utility of social cognitive models for changing health behaviours in practice

Theoretical models of behaviour are important when designing interventions to change health behaviours as theoretical models represent the hypothesized causal determinants of behaviour. They provide information about the mechanisms of behaviour to be targeted. Furthermore, interventions using theoretical models add to a cumulative evidence base. A number of theoretical models focussing on health beliefs and motivation have been developed to understand, predict and change health-related behaviours. However, some theoretical models have become outdated (e.g. the HBM, the Theory of Planned Behaviour). Empirical tests have concluded that these models are no longer state of the art indicating some progress in theorizing (Sniehotta, Presseau and Araujo-Soares, 2014).

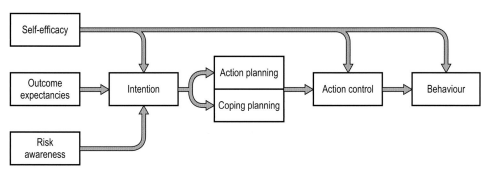

Fig. 35.3 Health Action Process Model.

36 | Changing cognitions and behaviour

Cognitive processes have a crucial impact upon whether one conducts a behaviour that may have a positive or negative impact upon one's health (Matarazzo, 1984). Multiple models have been developed to understand and target cognitive constructs to change behaviour, including the Health Belief Model (HBM) and the Theory of Planned Behaviour (TPB). The HBM proposed that behaviours are influenced by the costs and benefits of the behaviour, one's perception of susceptibility and severity to the related illness, (internal and external) cues to action, perceived control over the behaviour and motivation to conduct the behaviour (Abraham and Sheeran, 2005; Becker and Rosenstock, 1987). In an intervention designed to increase mammography attendance amongst women over 35 years old, Champion (1994) demonstrated that information-only or HBM-specific counselling interventions individually had little effect. However, when both interventions were combined to provide information and alter cognitions, the intervention was up to four times more effective than control. Additionally, the TPB proposed that whether one conducts a behaviour is due to one's attitude towards a behaviour, whether it is socially normative and perceptions of control relating to that behaviour, in addition to whether one intends to conduct it. By developing interventions that target TPB-based constructs, interventions have successfully brought about changes for behaviours such as exercise, testicular self-examination and protective sexual health behaviours (Ajzen and Driver, 1991; Ajzen, 1991; Ogden, 2012). Therefore interventions designed to change cognitions may successfully influence behaviour change.

Contradictions and change

In response to noting that people are motivated to seek consistency in their beliefs, Festinger's (1957) Cognitive Dissonance Theory (CDT) proposed that being aware of two inconsistent cognitions (e.g. beliefs or attitudes) causes an aversive psychological state that motivates elimination of one belief through cognitive change. In addition, behavioural commitment must be present as inconsistencies without implications are unlikely to cause dissonance (Beauvoid and Joule, 1996). An 'Action-based Model' (Harmon-Jones, Amodio and Harmon-Jones, 2009) has been proposed to account for those occasions where dissonance interferes with effective and unconflicted action that causes negative arousal. The consequence is that cognitions are brought into line with behavioural commitments to reduce CDT. For example, increased awareness that smoking enhances one's susceptibility to serious illness may facilitate a smoker to experience cognitive change.

Stone et al. (1994) demonstrated the relevance of CDT to health promotion in the form of condom use through comparing four intervention conditions: (1) information provision only; (2) a (commitment-inducing) talk with information provision and health education; (3) a discussion on (awareness-inducing) recollection of past failures; and (4) a combined commitment- and awareness-inducing condition. After the intervention, all participants were given an opportunity to buy condoms. Fig. 36.1 shows that generating commitment and increasing awareness of one's past failures led to greater condom purchase levels than the other three strategies. CDT may be used to interpret these results. The combined condition (based upon CDT) would find it difficult to negate the belief that condom use was worthwhile. This would be as a result of persuasion of the importance of condom use combined with increased awareness of their own past failures

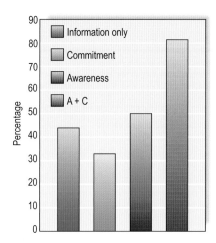

Fig. 36.1 Cognitive dissonance and health promotion. Percentage buying condoms. *A*, Awareness; *C*, commitment *(from Stone et al., 1994, with permission).*

resulting in cognitive dissonance. One may try to resolve dissonance through distancing from one's past failures and affirming the intention to use condoms in the future. This might resolve the cognitive contradiction created by the 'awareness' condition. Furthermore, more people in the combined group took the opportunity to buy condoms than people in the awareness group (82% versus 50%); this demonstrates that providing information is important but in isolation may not be enough to take action (as only 44% of the information-only group bought condoms).

Hence perceived behavioural control was high, as condoms were made easily available; however, this is not always the case. For example, smokers may find it difficult to distance themselves from their past smoking and therefore not resolve to quit. Instead they may resolve dissonance to change beliefs about their future susceptibility to illness. For example, they may convince themselves that their genetic make-up will protect them from the risks of smoking or that other risks mean that they will die prematurely whether or not they smoke (see pp. 62–63). Thus it is critical to take account of perceived barriers and perceived control when attempting to assist people in changing their behaviour (see pp. 72–73). In some cases this may mean that people are required to learn new skills before they can change their behaviour (e.g. how to cook tasty nutritious meals).

How people process persuasive messages

When communicating information it is important to consider that people are not passive recipients of information. They may actively engage in information processing, with existing cognitions influencing how new information is processed. Effective communication has a dynamic nature that involves demonstrating an understanding of current conditions, presenting new information in a way that relates to ones' existing cognitions. If existing cognitions do not incorporate new information, then communications need be presented in a persuasive way that develops new cognitions (Marteau, Dormandy and Mitchie, 2001). The Elaboration Likelihood Model (ELM) (Petty and Cacioppo, 1986) proposed that the extent to which one *cognitively elaborates* upon persuasive messages may vary, with people taking either the central or the peripheral processing route. Central processing involves thinking about message content and evaluating the

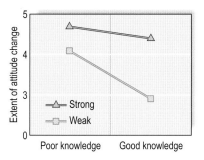

Fig. 36.2 Prior knowledge and the effect of argument strength on persuasion *(from Wood et al., 1985, with permission).*

people have confidence in their ability to change and can do so in a supported and graded manner. Where this is not possible, people may reject health promotion messages and reaffirm attitudes associated with health-risking behaviours (see pp. 24–25; pp. 62–63 and pp. 74–75).

Stop and think

- Imagine you want to encourage an overweight patient to do more exercise. What would you say to them? Why might giving this person free gym membership not increase the amount they exercise?

Case study

Steven is an obese 55-year-old gentleman living with type 2 diabetes. He has been intending to lose weight for a few years and has had short periods of improved nutrition but overall has struggled to manage his weight. Steven was previously provided with information from the Dietetics Service as to positive changes he could make to improve his nutrition and diabetes control, but as he has not experienced medical complications, he has struggled to maintain changes. As a consequence of previously struggling to manage weight, Steven has reluctantly agreed to attend a health psychology clinic. A diary was completed to understand his current behaviour. Discussions explored what he feels are the physical, mental and emotional pros and cons of maintaining unhealthy eating habits and making changes. The staff explained to Steven his long-term illness susceptibility and severity if he maintains or changes his eating habits. The staff were concerned that his anxiety was associated with lapses of unhealthy eating and emphasized that this was a normal process. Plans were made for coping with lapses and overcoming barriers that he may face (e.g. ordering a half portion of a take-away meal). Steven was advised to attend a diabetes group to receive peer support from people experiencing similar difficulties and attend a 6-week nutrition group programme to receive tailored information and practical lessons. Realistic plans were made to gradually change Steven's eating habits in a sustainable manner. Steven began his new nutrition lifestyle changes the next day.

arguments in terms of existing knowledge, with this approach being most likely to lead to long-term attitude and action changes. However, if one is unwilling or unable to provide the cognitive resources required for central processing, one may use peripheral processing to make decisions without proper understanding or evaluation of arguments, which is less likely to be sustained as new information is not linked to existing knowledge and beliefs. For example, if individuals are under time pressures or feel an issue is not relevant to them, they may make decisions based simply on what they feel about the message, or use simple rules to make decisions such as expertise-accuracy (e.g. 'The Doctor is an expert, so she must be right') or consensus-accuracy (e.g. 'If the majority agrees, it is probably right').

To persuade people of health-promoting messages (see pp. 64–66), one must have the opportunity and motivation to engage in central route processing, lack of knowledge and understanding of the message can be important barriers (see pp. 92–93). Whereas central processing should result in dismissal of weak arguments, peripheral processing is more likely to result in persuasion caused by a lack of evaluating arguments. For example, the Wood et al. (1985) experiment compared the impact of messages containing weak and strong arguments on people who had either good or poor prior knowledge. Fig. 36.2 shows those with good pre-existing knowledge required strong arguments to change their attitude; however, those with poor pre-existing knowledge – assumed to be engaging in peripheral processing – were equally persuaded by weak and strong messages.

Encouraging people to take greater responsibility for their health is an important aim for health care services. This will be facilitated when people develop good knowledge: for example, knowledge of how their body works, what symptoms mean and how medication has its effect. Presenting well-informed people with well-argued messages that appear relevant to them, in a manner that allows them to concentrate on and revisit presented information, will enhance cognitive processing and persuasion. Persuading people of a new position and then contrasting this with their current behaviour can generate cognitive dissonance and thereby motivate change. However, behaviour change is only likely to follow from attitudinal and motivational changes when

Changing cognitions and behaviour

- Cognitive dissonance theory proposes that being aware of two inconsistent cognitions causes an aversive psychological state, which we are motivated to eliminate.

- Attitude change may be prompted by cognitive dissonance but if behaviour change is thought to be difficult, people may reject health promotion messages rather than change their intentions.

- People may process persuasive messages using the central or peripheral route. Central route processing is more likely to lead to enduring attitude change and action.

- Providing information alone is unlikely to change behaviour, but knowledge is important to central route processing of health-relevant messages. Hence information, motivation and behavioural skills are all crucial to successful behaviour change.

37 | Helping people to act on their intentions

If an individual is not motivated to adopt or maintain a specific health behaviour, a first step towards encouraging them is to increase their motivation to act (pp. 76–77). However, even when individuals do intend to change their health behaviours, they often fail to translate their intentions into action. This discrepancy is called the 'intention–behaviour gap'.

The intention–behaviour gap

A key study examining the relationships between motivation/intention and behaviours identified four patterns of association in relation to attendance at cervical screening (Sheeran and Orbell, 2000):

(1) inclined actors (i.e. those who intend and subsequently act);
(2) inclined abstainers (i.e. those who intend but do not subsequently act);
(3) disinclined actors (i.e. those who do not intend to act but subsequently do so); and
(4) disinclined abstainers (i.e. those who do not intend and do not act) (Fig. 37.1).

When followed up a year later, 57% of the women who intended to attend cervical screening had not translated their intention into action. Similar findings have been demonstrated across a range of other health behaviours (e.g. exercise, condom use).

Strategies to bridge the intention–behaviour gap

There are a number of strategies that individuals can use to translate their good intentions into action. Some of the key strategies include self-efficacy, planning and action control and are specified within the Health Action Process Approach (HAPA) model (pp. 70–71) (Schwarzer, 1992). These volitional processes are described in more detail later.

Self-efficacy

Self-efficacy refers to one's perceived capability to adopt and maintain new behaviour and manage relapse (Bandura, 1986). Self-efficacy is required throughout the whole behaviour change process. Three different types of self-efficacy are distinguished in the HAPA – task self-efficacy, maintenance self-efficacy and recovery self-efficacy – which reflect the self-regulatory challenges at different stages of the change process. To progress, individuals may require different phase-specific self-efficacy from each other at any one time. An individual's perceived self-efficacy influences the difficulty of tasks they will select (if given a choice) as well as the amount of effort and persistence they have towards achieving a task. Self-efficacy also influences the type of goals individuals will

form and how they will respond to stressors and setbacks when trying to achieve their goals (Bandura, 1986).

There are four key methods that can be used for increasing an individual's self-efficacy: mastery experience, vicarious experience, verbal persuasion and physiological states (Bandura, 1986). Self-efficacy can be increased by direct mastery experience of the task itself. Vicarious experience refers to the observation of people who are considered role models succeeding at a given task. This can increase an individual's belief that they may also possess the capabilities to master the task. A third technique to increase self-efficacy involves verbal persuasion from influential people such as parents, partners and friends or authority figures (e.g. doctors, managers and coaches). Verbal persuasion can be used to strengthen beliefs about initial capability and also to encourage sustained effort and perseverance. Doctors are in a unique position, in many respects, with their patients to encourage and persuade changing health behaviour because they are credible figures and have received training in communication skills. Finally, self-efficacy is influenced by physiological states. Positive emotions can boost self-efficacy, whereas periods of low mood or anxiety may decrease beliefs about capability.

Stop and think

- Try to think of ways that you could use these principles of increasing self-efficacy when you are with patients who would benefit from improving their health behaviour such as reducing sugar or alcohol consumption. What techniques have you learnt in your communication skills training to increase your attempts to persuade behaviour change?

Planning

There are two different types of planning – action planning and coping planning. Both have the function to improve the frequency and/or intensity of behaviour change. Action plans are intentional, prospective goal-directed responses that are put into motion when relevant opportunities arise: i.e. a person plans to do X when situation Y is encountered (Gollwitzer, 1999). Individuals who are prompted to form action plans, stating how, when and where they would perform a health behaviour are significantly more likely to act in line with their intentions than those who did not make such plans. There is strong support for the effectiveness of forming action plans for translating intentions into action compared with simply forming intentions alone. For example, women instructed to form implementation intentions to attend medical follow-up appointments were significantly more likely to attend than controls who were not instructed to make such plans (Sheeran and Orbell, 2000). Effects have been found when interventions encouraging the formation of simple action plans as brief as one minute (Sniehotta, Araújo-Soares and Dombrowski, 2007). A patient may form an action plan to take their medication as instructed (how) when at home (where) in the morning while they are having breakfast (when). This helps the patient to act in these specified contexts because aspects of the environment prompt intended actions that may have been forgotten or postponed. Prompting people to make both action plans and coping plans have been shown to be the most effective in changing behaviour (Kwasnicka, Presseau, White and Sniehotta, 2013). Coping planning refers to specific plans formed to shield new behaviours from distractions, barriers or high-risk situations where relapse is likely to occur. Action plans may be particularly

Screening behaviour at 1 year follow-up	I intend to attend cervical screening within the next year	
	Agree	Disagree
Undertaken screening	Inclined Actors 16%	Disinclined Actors 7%
Not undertaken screening	Inclined Abstainers 22%	Disinclined Abstainers 55%

Fig. 37.1 Patterns of association between motivation/intention and behaviour (modified from Sheeran and Orbell, 2000).

useful for helping individuals to *initiate* behaviour change, whereas coping plans may be required to *maintain* behaviour change.

Volitional help sheets are planning-based tools that can help engage individuals in planning. These sheets ask individuals to link problematic situations (e.g. binge drinking) to other appropriate behavioural or cognitive responses (e.g. avoidance of alcohol). A list of potentially problematic situations pertaining to the behaviour to be changed is followed by another list with appropriate behavioural or cognitive responses to these situations. Subjects are typically required to connect the situation to a response. Volitional help sheets can help people adhere to the outlined temptation–behavioural response plan.

Action control

Action control refers to the self-regulatory strategies people required when they plan to adopt or maintain a new behaviour. Self-regulatory processes involve self-monitoring behaviour to identify whether the current behaviour matches a previously set behavioural goal. If there is a discrepancy identified, effort is needed to initiate change to achieve the goal behaviour. As a result, action control processes are important throughout the behaviour change process. An individual may experience self-regulation failure in social or emotional situations, when resources are weakened (e.g. in times of stress), when situational demands are high or when competing behaviours are habitual. Asking individuals to self-monitor their behaviour has been shown to be effective in changing a number of health-related behaviours and can in practice easily be facilitated with self-monitoring diaries, apps or devices (e.g. to monitor physical activity). For health care providers this is an under-rated technique to encourage change in health behaviour. The mere cataloging of a health-related behaviour using pencil-and-paper diaries or mobile phone check-lists with reminders to complete can assist important health improvements.

Goal hierarchies

Lack of time is one of the most highly cited reasons people give for not doing the things they intended to. In some instances this may reflect that the individual had more pressing intentions, which took priority. As a result the intention–behaviour gap can be influenced by the presence of competing goals. It is important to acknowledge that individuals may have specific goal hierarchies and pursue a number of goals that may conflict or facilitate with a goal to change a health behaviour. Many individuals who engage in unhealthy behaviour engage in several unhealthy behaviours, which emphasises the need to consider how these behavioural goals are related to each other (e.g. giving up smoking may lead to increased weight).

Stop and think

- Mr Patterson is a 55-year-old patient who has type 2 diabetes. He tells you that each day when he wakes up he has every intention to improve his diet and physical activity levels in line with the recommendations you gave him at his previous appointment. However, he never manages to achieve this and is starting to feel disillusioned. What might you say to help him make changes to Mr Patterson's dietary and physical activity behaviours?

Helping people to act on their intentions

- Despite good intentions, people fail to translate these intentions in actual behaviour.
- The intention–behaviour gap may be bridged by prompting individuals to make specific plans, encouraging them to self-monitor their behaviour and enhancing their self-efficacy.
- Self-monitoring and self-evaluation in relation to specific goals is needed for action control.
- Individuals who make specific plans about how, when and where they will perform a behaviour and who have plans for how they will cope with potential problems seem to be more successful in achieving their health-related goals.
- Self-efficacy can be increased by encouraging mastery and vicarious experiences, verbal persuasion and limiting negative physiological states that dampen self-efficacy.
- It may be important to consider the relationship between different behavioural goals and assess whether they conflict or facilitate with the goal behaviour.

Case study

Cardiac rehabilitation patients who had been advised to increase their physical activity were at random allocated to either standard care, an action-planning and coping-planning condition or an action-planning/coping-planning plus self-monitoring condition. Two months after discharge, the planning group reported more physical activity than the controls but did not differ from the self-monitoring group. A further 2 months later, the self-monitoring group reported higher levels of activity than both standard care controls and the planning group. The study, reported by the health psychologist Sniehotta, is interpreted as evidence that planning might be more effective to initiate changes whereas self-monitoring is required to sustain these changes.

38 | The social context of behavioural change

Social context or milieu refers to the immediate physical and social setting in which people live, work and relax. It includes most aspects of daily living including power and politics, income and educational opportunities, family and work colleagues among other factors. Those interactions can take place directly, in person, or indirectly through communications via the media. Societal factors are important determinants of health and health behaviours (Fig. 38.1).

The social context of individual behaviour

There are two aspects of social context: firstly, the social context in which individuals behave in a certain way; and secondly, the way society influences its citizens' health behaviour. The social context in which many of us live has seen rapid socio-cultural changes, including transformations in the nature of employment; availability and aggressive marketing of cheap, highly processed food containing large quantities of fat, sugar and salt; and growth of sedentary leisure time facilities. We all operate within a social and economic context that may not be supportive of individual behaviour change programmes, and we need to appreciate this when considering choice in behaviour change interventions.

Behaviour prediction models such as the Health Belief Model (see Chapter 35, pp. 70–71) are based on the assumption that individuals think rationally about costs and benefits before engaging in particular behaviour. This model has some predictive power in certain health domains for highly specific preventive behaviours such as cancer screening. The model is based on an assumption that influencing behaviour is simply a matter of targeting people's thoughts (attitudes/beliefs). This was conceived to work on the basis that attitudes *cause* behaviour in a fairly unproblematic way, which empirical research suggests is wrong. Interestingly advertising companies had long recognized that their campaigns would only be effective in altering the consumption habits of a small percentage of the targeted audience. Early health education initiatives had unrealistic expectations about their impacts and, importantly (unlike advertising campaigns designed to, say, switch the consumer's allegiance to another brand of soap

powder), they were often aimed at altering behaviour that was *pleasurable* such as smoking. Further, in some cultural contexts, hazardous behaviour may be valued and engaged in precisely because of the associated risk (Bunton and Burrows, 1995): for example, a cigarette brand named Death Cigarettes has sold successfully.

Behaviour becomes habitual when it becomes automatic, independent of conscious thought. Since people are less likely to attend to information associated with habits (that are experienced as pleasurable, e.g. smoking, drinking alcohol) and exhortation or persuasion is therefore far less effective as a behaviour change strategy (Ioannou, 2005; Blue et al., 2016).

Understanding 'unhealthy' behavior in a social and economic context

Behaviours such as smoking occur in a social context that, for the smoker, is a web of interdependent causes and associated and varied cultural meanings. A classic study that illustrated the importance of investigating the context and complexity of the role played by smoking in people's lives was that by Hilary Graham (1987). She argued that parents (mothers) caring for children and managing the financial and organizational burdens of domestic life considered this to be an extremely stressful experience and used smoking as a coping strategy to deal with the stress. One of her participants said:

> After lunch, I'll clear away and wash up and put the telly on for Stevie [her son]. I'll have a sit down on the sofa, with a cigarette… It's lovely, it's the one time in the day I really enjoy and I know Stevie won't disturb me. I couldn't stop, I just couldn't. It keeps me calm. It's me [sic] one relaxation, is smoking
> **(Graham, 1987, p. 172).**

Smoking actually enabled this carer to be a more effective mother. Graham termed this phenomenon 'the responsibility of irresponsible behaviour'. Nicotine does act neuropharmacologically to reduce stress in the short term. Behaviour change is constrained by social circumstances and

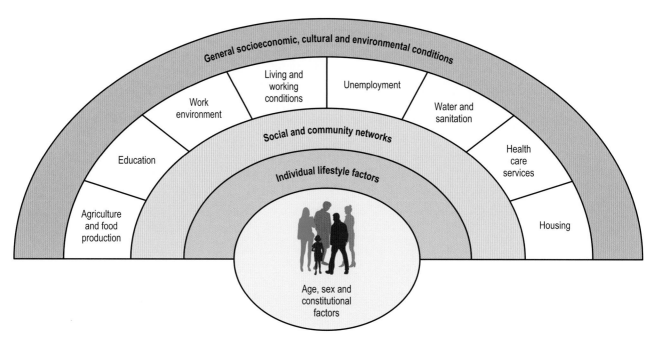

Fig. 38.1 Layers of Influence Model *(from Dahlgren and Whitehead, 1991).*

reveals reasons behind social class differences in health behaviour (and outcomes (Marmot Review Report, 2010)); for example, why working-class mothers (with fewer material resources) may find it harder to give up smoking than middle-class mothers. The role played by smoking in Graham's respondent's life by focussing solely on isolated psychological factors such as her attitude towards, or knowledge about, quitting the habit is simplistic.

Case study

Mrs Berry, a 34-year-old mother, visited her GP about the weight of her 14-year-old son. Whilst she had tried to improve meals and encourage him to eat more healthily, he refused to do so, and she knew that outside the house he was buying junk food. He also spent most of his time in sedentary pursuits – watching TV or playing computer games. Dr Hall recalled a study in which young people's love of technology – specifically of their personal cell phones – had been used to help them quit smoking. Researchers had texted messages to them such as: 'write down four people who will get a kick outta u kicking butt' every day for 6 weeks. This strategy had proved really successful in changing behaviour and in engaging the target audience's interest. Dr Hall wondered whether a similar project could be set up on resisting junk food and to taking up exercise.

If smoking cessation appears much more complicated once we begin to examine it in context, consider obesity (see spread, pp. 106–107).

Tools employed to change social attitudes and behaviour

Mass education campaigns directed at people's attitudes have been commonly used for population behaviour change goals by governments. Yet, despite its popularity, this approach has had limited success in changing behaviour (see spread media, pp. 72–73).

Sometimes the state might implement external incentives to achieve the desired health behaviour – subsidies (for gym membership or reduced priced healthy food), taxation (on alcohol and tobacco) or legislation (speed limits or a ban on smoking in public places). There is also debate about the acceptability of state intervention to prohibit practices such as smoking or drinking in the private sphere.

'Healthy choices'

The UK government's approach to population health improvement has typically presented people as having maximum freedom and the capability to choose a healthy lifestyle and, as a consequence, placed considerable emphasis on an individual's responsibility for their own health. However, there are some problems with this individualism as the World Health Organization's (WHO) Commission on the Social Determinants of Health's review concluded that material, environmental and political conditions continue to play significant roles in generating health inequalities within and between nations (WHO, 2008).

Clearly governments have conflicting interests: whilst wishing to promote individual control and choices around health issues, supporting economic growth can lead to pollution and unhealthy working and living conditions all with negative health consequences. In addition, most governments receive vast revenues from the sale of tobacco and alcohol, and it is perhaps not surprising that they allow companies producing such products to advertise themselves at events that would appear counter intuitive from a health perspective (e.g. by sponsoring sports events). The 'look after your own health' philosophy has also spawned a burgeoning health industry that encourages the purchase of 'health' products from yoghurt to gym membership as the means of achieving health. The tensions governments experience in trying to, on the one hand, offer citizens the kind of information they need to 'choose' healthy options and, on the other hand, attempt to control the choices that are available, is well illustrated in relation to obesity. Food manufacturers are now required to provide information about fat, salt and sugar levels, yet the advertising on TV of 'junk' food is banned around programmes aimed at young children. The overall context in which we play out our behaviour is thus ultimately determined by political and economic considerations.

The role of health professionals

Health professionals by virtue of their role and day-to-day clinical practice have some knowledge about the lives of the people they treat or care for. In these roles they can operate as powerful influences on individuals (e.g. by advising patients to alter their behaviour), on local government (e.g. by supporting community self-help groups) and on national government (e.g. by recommending a reduction in the amount of alcohol that drivers may legally consume) through their professional associations. For example, the Ontario Society of Nutrition Professionals in Public Health lobbies the Canadian government to consider a basic income guarantee for all citizens as a policy option (OSNPPH, 2015).

Stop and think

- Which would you support: a health warning about saturated fats on packets of butter and cheese or increased tax on those products?
- What would be your reasons for this choice that might convince a policy maker?

The social context of behavioural change

- Social context of behavioural change refers to (1) our individual efforts to stop a damaging (or start a beneficial) behaviour and (2) overall societal influences upon how we behave and think.
- Attempts to effect mass behaviour change may be more successful if the behaviour and cultural attitudes associated with it and its socio-economic determinants are targeted.
- The idea that individuals can exercise choice over their health status can deflect attention from environmental/material explanations of health inequalities.
- Health professionals have a role in supporting people to change their behaviour. Health professional bodies can also play a role in raising awareness of health damaging social and economic policies amongst their membership and the general population to help create supportive environments that are conducive to health behaviour change.
- Trying to influence behaviour always has ethical implications.

39 | Illegal drug use

Illegal drug use is common, particularly amongst younger people, and this has created extensive concern. The UK has one of the highest drug-use prevalence rates in the world, with perhaps 300,000 problematic drug users and over 11 million people who have ever used an illegal drug. Rates of use have been falling recently, but the variety of drugs used has increased, and survey data may not reflect use accurately. Fig. 39.1 shows the most widely used types of drugs in the UK in 2006, before the rise of 'legal highs'. Some forms of drug use such as cannabis smoking, which is as common as tobacco smoking amongst younger people, are ceasing to be unusual or deviant in the UK, and many illegal drug users, particularly the more moderate ones, probably suffer few problems, just like many alcohol drinkers. This is no reason for complacency because as prevalence has increased, drug-related problems have increased and diversified. Whereas 20 years ago drug services mostly saw heroin or cocaine users, these days people who seek help for drug-related problems commonly include people whose primary problems are one (or more) of the following:

- Cannabis abuse or dependence (Box 39.1), usually with alcohol and occasional use of other drugs. There are more people dependent on cannabis than on all other drugs combined (Dennis et al., 2002).
- Heroin or opiate abuse or dependence, sometimes combined with benzodiazepines and other drugs, and typically involving drug injection.
- Cocaine or crack cocaine abuse or dependence. The likelihood and severity of cocaine dependence have sometimes been

overstated (Ditton and Hammersley, 1996). Yet cocaine is becoming even more prevalent, potentially leading to more widespread problems.

- Amphetamine abuse or dependence.
- Psychotic or delusional symptoms related to drug use. This is more likely for people with pre-existing mental disorders and is most commonly found with amphetamines or cocaine (Farrell et al., 2002), although it can also occur with cannabis or hallucinogens such as LSD. People already vulnerable to schizophrenia may have symptoms triggered or worsened by illicit drugs, most commonly cannabis.
- Overdose, most commonly on opiates, alcohol or benzodiazepines, or mixtures of such drugs.
- Use of a wide and rapidly changing variety of chemicals that are not currently illegal and are often bought online. These include many with similar effects to existing drugs such as cannabis or MDMA, but with unknown risks and long-term effects on health.

People who seek help for drug problems often have other psychological, social and physical health problems (Table 39.1), which may also need attention (Orford 2000; Dennis et al., 2002; Farrell et al., 2002).

Treatment

Drug users seeking help include some who are doing so mainly because of the concern of other people. Many drug users have mixed feelings about use, which they enjoy and find beneficial in some way and can sometimes fail to recognize the development of a problem as quickly as others do. Techniques for motivational enhancement (Miller and Rollnick, 1991) can encourage users to consider frankly the costs and benefits of use. This is particularly useful in the form of brief interventions for people who are not dependent and are appropriate in primary care (Dunn et al., 2001).

Treating drug dependence is difficult. It can take a decade before drug-dependent individuals stop, during which time they typically have repeated involvement with health care and other services. They will usually have tried to stop or moderate their use several times. Relapse management is an important component of any competent antidrug treatment. Users should also be provided with the information and means to minimize the harm their drug use causes. Information also benefits users who are not dependent (Box 39.2). For opiate users, methadone or buprenorphine maintenance can allow users to stabilize their lifestyle and reduce the problems related to a criminal, drug-injecting lifestyle. Ideally, prescribing should occur in a way that makes it difficult for people to abuse their prescribed drugs or sell them on the black market and it should occur with regular, competent counselling, for example, from the community pharmacist doing the dispensing.

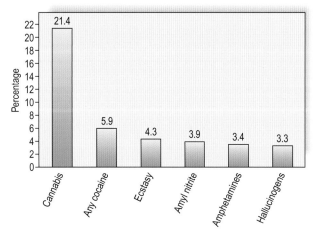

Fig. 39.1 Percentage of 16- to 24-year-olds reporting use of the most prevalent drugs in the previous year, 2005–2006 *(adapted from Home Office 2005/06, with permission).*

Box 39.1 **Diagnosing drug problems**

The Diagnostic and Statistical Manual of Mental Disorders, fourth edition (DSM-IV; American Psychiatric Association, 2000) recognizes two forms of drug problems:

- Drug abuse: involves use over at least 12 months, with repeated problems interpersonally, or in social roles such as education or work, or legal problems, or dangerous behaviour linked to use and significant concern about those problems, but without dependence
- Drug dependence: can additionally involve unsuccessful attempts to quit, classic signs of addiction, such as increased tolerance (taking higher doses over time) and withdrawal symptoms, spending excessive time seeking and taking drugs, and having difficulty controlling intake

Table 39.1 **Situations where drug users may require special psychological attention**

Situation	Special problems
Maternity care/ obstetrics	Maintenance or reduction of prescribing and counselling may be required to minimize harm to mother and foetus
General practice	Can be disruptive and deceptive
May require specialized support services
Internal medicine	May fake pain to obtain painkillers
Casualty	Overdose, violence related to the drugs trade

Education
- Hazards of injecting (especially equipment-sharing)
- Safer sex
- Getting sterile equipment and condoms
- Cleaning equipment
- Avoiding overdose
- First aid

Direct action
- Hepatitis B and C immunization
- Provision of sterile injecting equipment and condoms
- HIV testing (with counselling)
- Substitution of oral methadone

Adapted from Department of Health, 1991.

Case study

Mike is a 23-year-old drug injector with a history of criminal convictions and drug misuse going back to age 14 years. Two years previously he had been discharged from a residential detoxification programme for using drugs. He told the GP that he was now highly motivated by having a steady partner and a newborn daughter but cannot give up heroin. The GP prescribed methadone and established a good relationship with Mike. With the prescription his general health improved and his previously hostile approach to NHS staff decreased. He was also referred for dental treatment because of numerous caries caused by neglect and a sugary diet; the pain of these had previously been concealed by high drug doses.
Unfortunately 6 months later Mike was arrested for burglary. He denied involvement and the GP testified in writing on his behalf, but as a persistent offender he was nonetheless convicted and sentenced to 2 years. In prison his maintenance regime was replaced by a rapid reduction of methadone dose. Mike was unable to manage and began to inject again occasionally, sharing a syringe. As a result he contracted hepatitis C. On release he was determined to stop injecting. However, his GP was now reluctant to prescribe methadone as Mike had not used opiates regularly in prison. This, and a serious quarrel with his partner, led Mike to resume heavy drug use and crime for some months. He returned to the GP requiring treatment for a large abscess from a repeated injection site. He is now back on methadone, requires regular monitoring for liver damage from hepatitis C and has re-established a relationship with his family, although he no longer lives with his daughter's mother.

No single treatment works best. A good relationship between the therapist and the patient is very important with the aim of enabling clients to change themselves (see pp. 132–133). Cognitive–behavioural approaches (see pp. 138–139) can help, particularly in changing negative drug-related behaviours such as harmful injecting. Motivational interviewing is frequently used to help clients make change themselves and prepare for the almost inevitable difficulties and relapses (Miller and Rollnick, 1991). Involving the client's relatives in family or systemic therapy can also be helpful, particularly for younger drug users. The Minnesota model of treatment using a '12-steps' approach and focussing on abstinence can also work. When treatment is evaluated, only 20% to 30% will quit or reduce drug use and stay that way for 6 months or more. Treatment needs to be extended over weeks or months, rather than necessarily being intensive or residential. Alleged higher success rates tend to be resulting from biased selection of patients or weak measures of outcome. Treatment is more difficult when the client has little social support, a chaotic lifestyle and also has other major psychological, health or social problems. Most substance users modify or quit drug use without treatment, leaving a residue of people with severe problems who require extensive help; however, encouragingly, recovery rates from substance-use disorders are higher than from most other mental health disorders (Orford, 2000).

For people under 18 years of age, abuse or dependence may not be clearly diagnosed and it may be better simply to describe them as having drug problems.

Stop and think

- Should illegal drugs be regulated, or should they remain illegal? Many of the harms of illegal drugs are caused by the fact that they are illegal, hence sold by a dangerous industry – one of the largest in the world – in unsafe ways and unsafe forms with no controls over who uses when and how (RSA, 2007). Attempts to stifle use have not been effective.
- Should cannabis products be allowed for medical use, or is this simply a ruse to permit cannabis intoxication? Possible uses for cannabis may include to alleviate the symptoms of multiple sclerosis; to manage chronic pain; to reduce nausea and loss of appetite with cancer and chemotherapy and to manage anxiety.

Illegal drug use

- Illegal drug use is quite common and complicated by 'legal highs'.
- Much illegal drug use is not a medical problem, but most drugs do cause occasional acute problems, even deaths.
- There are a number of different common patterns of drug problem.
- The dependent drug user may take a long time and repeated attempts to stop. Before stopping he or she may benefit from help with:
  - Harm reduction, including substitute prescribing such as methadone for heroin or advice on safe injecting.
  - General medical care.
  - Life problems as well as drug dependence.

40 | Alcohol use

Alcohol is the most widely used recreational drug in the Western world. Although many users come to no harm, its use can cause medical, psychological and social problems. The management of alcohol should be a major public health and public policy issue, but historically people have resisted alcohol regulation (Anderson and Baumberg, 2006; Measham, 2006).

Medicalization of alcohol problems

Between about 1850 and the late 1950s alcoholism came to be considered a disease caused by some biological reaction to alcohol. This reaction was supposed to be permanent, so the only palliative treatment for alcoholism was permanent abstinence. Still widely believed, this idea is faulty:

- Many problem drinkers come to harm from drinking but are not alcoholics. The most notorious contemporary example is the rise in binge drinking, mirrored in the UK by a rapid rise in liver cirrhosis. Average personal intake in Europe, excluding abstainers, is in excess of recommended safe limits (Anderson and Baumberg, 2006); we all drink unhealthily, and it is counterfactual to stigmatize alcoholics.
- Even dependent drinkers have some control over their drinking, and some people with severe alcohol problems can moderate their drinking to problem-free levels, often without help (Heather and Robinson, 1983).
- Some very heavy drinkers survive unchanged for 30 years or more.

Alcoholics Anonymous (AA) emphasizes abstinence, as do some professional treatments. Other treatments include monitored detoxification for severely dependent drinkers, counselling (see pp. 98–99) to enable the patient find methods of coping other than drinking, or therapeutic communities where patients stay off alcohol and undertake group therapy. Given a choice, some patients opt for abstinence and some for moderating their drinking. Occasional relapses to heavy drinking are common, even amongst those trying to abstain, and patients are taught to expect and cope with this. Controlled follow-up studies suggest that approximately 80% of people treated for alcohol dependence by any method have relapsed within 2 years. Alleged better rates tend to be a result of bias (e.g. treatment programmes that only admit people who have virtually stopped drinking already) or poorly controlled research.

The 12-steps approach

AA (www.alcoholics-anonymous.org.uk/) consists of groups of recovering alcoholics who provide one another with mutual support to achieve complete abstinence. Their philosophy is the famous '12-steps approach', which requires that alcoholics surrender to a higher power (or God), admit their wrongs and try to rectify them. People who are heavily dependent, have religious or spiritual feelings and accept abstinence as a goal are likely to benefit most from this approach. AA has less to offer people who are not dependent. Doctors often suggest AA as a supplement to treatment.

Drinking problems and government advice

Even quite moderate drinking increases morbidity (Table 40.1) and mortality. Consequently the UK government advises that women should not regularly drink more than 2 to 3 units of

Table 40.1 **Alcohol, disease and possible benefits**	
Disease	**Beneficial effects**
Liver disease – fatty degeneration, fibrosis, acute alcoholic inflammation, cirrhosis	1–2 units per day may reduce the risks of coronary heart disease
Cardiovascular disease – hypertension. Heavy drinking increases stroke risk and coronary heart disease	Red wine lowers cholesterol levels
Cancer – oesophageal cancer, possibly stomach cancer	Small occasional dose of alcohol may serve as a sedative or tranquillizer
Neurological disease – Korsakoff's syndrome, alcoholism	

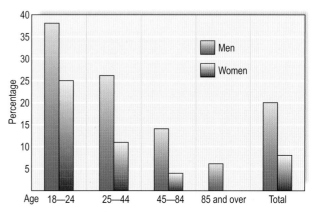

Fig. 40.1 Percentage drinking above safe limits – note that some of all age groups drink heavily *(from Lader and Meltzer, 2001, with permission).*

alcohol a day, men should not regularly drink more than 3 to 4 units of alcohol a day and pregnant women or women trying to conceive should avoid drinking alcohol (National Alcohol Strategy, 2017). A unit or standard drink is usually defined as a half-pint of beer, a small glass of wine or a standard measure of spirits. However, many people, especially young men, drink above these limits (Fig. 40.1), often as a result of going out a few nights each week (Hammersley and Dittan, 2005).

At the legal limit for driving (England and Wales: 80 mg alcohol in 100 ml blood. Scotland has recently reduced to 50 mg/100 ml), reactions are slowed by about 20% and thought is impaired. People who are drunk may generally behave in risky, antisocial or foolish ways without adequately considering their actions. This causes some of alcohol's pleasurable effects – people are more likely to dance, flirt or converse. Unfortunately drunkenness also contributes to quarrels, violence, disorder, suicide, fires, road-traffic accidents, other accidents, child abuse and other problems. It is also quite easy to overdose on alcohol, which can kill through respiratory depression.

There is currently great social concern over links between alcohol and violence and disorder and there are initiatives to manage this such as banning the consumption of alcohol outside and the use of plastic glasses to reduce injuries. However, increasingly liberal licensing laws in the UK have probably led to increased alcohol consumption (Measham, 2006), worsening a major public health problem.

Controlling the nation's consumption

Increasing the price of alcohol by taxation can reduce national consumption, which, in turn, reduces alcohol-related problems.

Another approach is to control the price of alcoholic drinks. Nowadays more drinking occurs at home and alcoholic beverages can be purchased at large discounts in supermarkets, encouraging excess consumption. In 2012 Scotland attempted to introduce a modest minimum price of 50 p per unit of alcohol, but this was appealed unsuccessfully by the Scotch Whisky Association after a 2017 court verdict writing. Alcohol advertising in the mass media may influence children, but it has little effect on consumption levels. However, the portrayal of alcohol in TV programming and writing is predominantly positive (or melodramatically negative), and there is scope for using mass media more skilfully to promote safer drinking. Other approaches try to change the way people drink by:

- Education about safe levels and risks. This may have helped change society's attitude to drunk-driving. A simple message to drink less may offset people's tendency to treat safe limits as 'allowances'.
- Continued control over where, when and by whom alcohol may be consumed, with licensing laws. For example, decreasing under-age drinking may require a reduction in tolerance of violations of existing law.
- Manipulation of the physical and social settings where drinking problems are common: for example, the banning of alcohol on football trains and at football grounds to prevent disorder. A major barrier to such changes is a widespread indifference to and minimization of alcohol-related problems (Measham, 2006). The health professional's role is to raise the profile of alcohol-related problems, by routinely taking alcohol histories and treating alcohol use as a priority health care issue.

The role of medicine

Alcohol consumption has a direct impact on patient care. At peak times, up to 70% of all admissions to accident and emergency units are related to alcohol consumption, and the total cost of alcohol misuse to the health service is estimated to be in the region of £1.7 billion a year. The medical profession can:

- Be aware of the contribution that alcohol can make to illness and injury in general practice and hospital specialities (see Table 40.1 and Box 40.1).
- Counter the drinks industry's promotion of its products.
- Press for better controls on the sale, marketing and pricing of alcohol.
- Routinely ask patients about their drinking and relate this to illness and disease.

Box 40.1 **Alcohol in medical practice**

Alcohol abuse can play a role in:
- Depression
- Anxiety and other psychiatric problems
- Problems of the digestive system
- Cardiovascular problems
- Neurological problems, apparent dementia and headaches
- Abuse of other drugs and medicines
- Family problems
- Falls and accidents
- Obesity
- Insensitivity to anaesthetics and pain relief

- Advise patients of safe drinking levels and suggest that they adopt these levels.
- Monitor patients' drinking, and praise and encourage reduced drinking.
- Serve as a role model by drinking moderately, within safe limits.
- Be aware of and refer to local specialized alcohol treatment services.

Alcohol use

- Alcohol is often involved in many health, psychological and social problems.
- Alcohol use should be a routine part of history-taking.
- Some people require treatment for dependence.
- Others require advice to moderate their drinking.
- Drinking beyond two to three drinks per day, 14 a week (women) or 21 a week (men) is not unusual, but it endangers long-term health.
- Society tends to be complacent about the health risks of alcohol.

Stop and think

- Some students and doctors drink excessively. Could you, or your colleagues, benefit from cutting down? How might you go about this? Doctors often drink as part of medical school culture, to cope with stress and to relax, although drinking can end up worsening the stress and work can be affected by drinking or hangovers. What other methods of coping might be more constructive?

Case study *Brief intervention with a heavy drinker*

Ralph is 35 years old and a travelling salesman. He presented with frequent abdominal pains, which he attributed to stress. From examination and tests there was no evidence of physical abnormality and non-specific gastritis was diagnosed. When Ralph attended the GP again to discuss the test results, the GP asked him to go through the previous 7 days and list all the alcohol he had consumed (a retrospective drinking diary). Ralph was drinking over 50 units of alcohol a week – about 2 pints (4 units) or equivalent at lunchtime and a further 2 pints in the evening to relax.

GP: *You don't drink that much a day, but it's steady. Now the recommended safe limit for men is 21 units a week – that's about 10½ pints of beer a week.*

Ralph: *Is that all? How much did I get through last week then?*

GP: *A bit too much, 58 units. I think that your stomach pains are made worse by your drinking. I'd like you to stop for a week or so and see what happens to your pain.*

Ralph: *I can't give up drinking! It goes with the job. A lot of my clients wouldn't stand for it if I didn't have a couple with them.*

GP: *I'm not suggesting you give up forever, just for a week to see what happens, then maybe try and cut down a bit. Try not to drink every day, or have some soft drinks sometimes, or low-alcohol beer.*

Ralph: *That's going to be hard, but I guess I have to, don't I, doctor, if it's affecting my stomach and that?*

GP: *Yes. Come back and see me after you've stopped for your week. If you want to know more about cutting down then there's a good book, Let's Drink to Your Health! (Heather and Robinson, 1996).*

Ralph now has the advice of the doctor as a motive for cutting down and as an excuse when he feels social pressure to drink.

41 | Smoking, tobacco control and doctors

The global picture

Smoking is the largest preventable cause of premature death and disability in the UK and the world and the largest cause of social inequality in health in most high-income countries. Cigarettes kill half of lifetime users. Half of these deaths occur in those under 70 years of age. Smokers on average lose 10 years of life. In 2011 tobacco killed almost six million people. Nearly 80% of these deaths were in low and middle-income countries. By 2030 eight million people will die each year from tobacco use (Eriksen et al., 2012). Death rates are higher in men than women as men have a longer history of smoking. In countries such as the UK, where women have smoked for several decades, the gap is closing rapidly. Globally in 2011 around 600,000 non-smokers died from exposure to second-hand smoke (SHS).

The costs of smoking in the UK

Smoking affects health throughout the life course. Each year approximately 100,000 people in the UK are killed by smoking – nearly one-fifth of all deaths (Action on Smoking and Health (ASH), 2014a). Most die from lung cancer, chronic obstructive lung disease (bronchitis and emphysema) or coronary heart disease. Smoking is also a risk factor for other cancers (e.g. mouth, larynx, liver, bladder, cervix), strokes, miscarriage, cot death, infertility, impotence, osteoporosis and many other diseases. Breathing in other people's smoke, SHS, causes around 12,000 deaths in the UK each year (ASH, 2014b). Children are particularly vulnerable. SHS increases their risk for diseases such as pneumonia, bronchitis, glue ear and worsens asthma (Royal College of Physicians (RCP), 2010).

The NHS spends over £2 billion a year treating diseases caused by smoking (ASH, 2014c). This includes hospital admissions, GP consultations and prescriptions. The total cost to society in England is estimated to be around £12.9 billion a year including lost productivity because of premature deaths and sick leave (£4 billion), smoking breaks (£5 billion), social care of older smokers (1.1 billion) and fires caused by smoking (£391 million). Scotland has set a target to become a tobacco-free country (i.e. adult smoking rates below 5%) by 2034.

Smoking and inequalities

Smoking in Great Britain has declined since the 1970s. In 2013, 22% of men and 19% of women smoked cigarettes (Office for National Statistics (ONS), 2014). This decline has been faster in affluent groups than in poorer groups. Smoking is a major cause of inequalities in health, accounting for over half of the excess deaths as a result of inequalities in Scotland. The more disadvantaged you are, the more likely you are to start smoking and the less likely you are to quit. In 2013 people in routine and manual occupations (29%) had twice the smoking rate of those in professional and managerial occupations (14%) (ONS, 2014).

The tobacco industry

Tobacco companies are in business to make profits. They need to recruit young smokers to replace the 50% of their adult customers who die from using their product. They need to keep their customers smoking as long as possible by reducing motivation to quit and maintaining nicotine addiction. They achieve this

Case study *Smokefree legislation in the UK*

In 2004 Ireland became the first country in the world to implement a comprehensive ban on smoking in enclosed public spaces. Scotland introduced similar legislation in 2006 and the rest of the UK in 2007. The Scottish First Minister described it as the largest single step in generations that Scotland had taken to improve its health. The legislation aimed to protect non-smokers from breathing in second-hand smoke (SHS) whilst at work. It was also hoped that the legislation, and accompanying media campaigns, might influence social norms about smoking, encouraging smokers to cut down or quit, and reduce children's exposure to smoking in public. Studies evaluating the UK legislation have shown significant positive public health impacts. In the year after the ban these included:

- Reduced children's and adults' SHS exposure, no displacement of smoking into the home
- Reduced smoking consumption in adults and increased quit attempts
- Improved children's health: for example, 18% reduction in asthma hospital admissions in Scotland and 12% reduction in England, reduction in pregnancy complications in Scotland
- Improved adults' health: for example, 17% reduction in heart attack admissions in Scotland, 5% reduction in asthma hospital admissions in England

through manipulating the marketing mix (promotion, price, product, place) to appeal to different smokers and expanding their markets in low- and middle-income countries.

FCTC – a global tobacco control strategy

The WHO Framework Convention on Tobacco Control (FCTC) came into effect in 2005 and has been ratified by 180 countries. This is the first international treaty on public health and is based on evidence from around the world on what are effective tobacco control polices. It commits governments to take action to protect citizens from the harm caused by tobacco, including:

- Increase taxation of tobacco products and combat smuggling: the level of smoking is highly related to price. The cheaper the price, the higher is the level of consumption. For every 1% increase in the real price of cigarettes there is around a 0.5% decline in adult consumption. The decline is even greater in young people. Tobacco tax can be used (hypothecated) to pay for other elements of tobacco control and to address factors (e.g. disadvantage) that make it difficult for smokers to quit.
- Ban tobacco advertising, promotion and sponsorship: tobacco companies argue that they do not target young people. Research studies and the companies' own confidential documents show that this is not the case. Banning tobacco promotion reduces smoking. Many countries, including the UK, have introduced comprehensive bans. Bans must include direct advertising and sponsorship, including at point of sale and packaging; indirect promotion such as putting cigarette brand names on other products, e.g. clothes (brand-stretching) and paying for cigarette brands to appear in films (product placement) and other media, including the internet.
- Protect people from tobacco smoke in workplaces, public transport and indoor public places: people have the right to breathe smokefree air. As well as reducing exposure to SHS, smokefree policies increase motivation to quit and reduce uptake (see Case study).

- Promote and strengthen public awareness of tobacco control: relevant education on prevention, cessation and SHS. For example, young people need to be aware of the health effects, how quickly addiction occurs, and have the motivation and skills not to start.
- Regulate the content, packaging and labelling of tobacco products: this includes requiring large rotating health warnings on packaging and prohibiting misleading descriptors such as 'light' or 'mild'. This is important in low-income countries where there is little awareness of the health effects. Warnings should include visual images, which can be powerful, particularly where literacy levels are low. Following Australia's example, several countries, including the UK, are planning to bring in mandatory plain or standardized packaging for cigarettes and tobacco.
- Promote cessation and adequate treatment for tobacco dependence: two-thirds of smokers want to quit. Cessation support greatly increases success rates. This could include mass-media campaigns, quitlines, group or one-to-one support and providing pharmacotherapy such as nicotine replacement therapy (NRT). The evidence on the effectiveness of e-cigarettes as a cessation aid is, as yet, limited.
- Prohibit sales to children: even in countries such as the UK, where it is illegal to sell cigarettes to under-18s, surveys show that young smokers still buy cigarettes directly from shops or through proxy sales. Laws need to be enforced.
- Research and evaluation to develop more effective approaches: in particular, in relation to disadvantage, gender and ethnicity.

Doctors and smoking cessation

Helping smokers to quit is one of the most cost-effective interventions that doctors can take. For example, using statins (cholesterol-lowering drugs) to prevent heart disease costs nearly £25,000 per life-year gained, whereas NHS smoking cessation support costs less than £1000 per life-year gained (ASH Scotland,

2011). There are national evidence-based guidelines for doctors and other health professionals on how they can help patients quit (NHS Health Scotland et al., 2010). Combining pharmacotherapy with behavioural support increases long-term quit rates to 15% to 20% – four times the unaided success rate. The UK is the only country to provide comprehensive local specialist cessation services nationwide, used by more than 800,000 smokers in 2012–2013.

Helpful websites include ASH (www.ash.org.uk); ASH Scotland (www.ashscotland.org.uk); Tobacco Tactics (www.tobaccotactics.org); treatobacco.net (www.treatobacco.net).

Stop and think

- Around half of British teenagers will try at least one cigarette, but fewer than half of these will become regular smokers. Thinking about yourself, what were the factors that influenced you whether or not (1) to try your first cigarette and (2) to continue to smoke?

Smoking, tobacco control and doctors

- Global deaths from tobacco are increasing rapidly and young people continue to take up smoking.
- Smoking in the UK is highly associated with disadvantage and is a major cause of inequalities in health.
- The tobacco industry needs to keep recruiting young people to replace smokers who quit or are killed by tobacco.
- Reducing the harm caused by tobacco requires comprehensive action to increase prices, ban tobacco promotion, reduce access to young people, increase health education, provide cessation support and reduce SHS exposure.
- Doctors have an important role to play in supporting both patients to quit smoking and comprehensive action by the government and other agencies.

42 | Eating, body shape and health

For the first time in recorded human history, more people are overweight or obese than are malnourished, an 'obesity epidemic' stemming from an imbalance between energy consumed and expended (see pp. 106–107). For many people the system responsible for appetite regulation is unable to cope adequately with these pressures. Obesity has well-documented health risks, including heart disease (see pp. 104–105), diabetes (see pp. 124–125), high blood pressure and stroke. Of particular concern is the increase in childhood obesity, resulting in a range of health-related complications. Obesity also has psychological effects, with increased depression, feelings of ugliness and low self-esteem. These psychological impacts of weight gain are exacerbated by unrealistic ideals about body shape. Consequently many individuals attempt to diet. However, disorders of eating associated with attempts to diet are also increasing, and the modern clinician is faced with the conundrum of how to promote healthy eating amongst people who are underweight through excessive dieting and how to help overweight individuals lose weight (see Case study).

Assessing weight status

The body mass index (BMI; Table 42.1) assesses weight status and helps identify people who are outside the normal weight range. BMI figures are not definitive measures of health. The BMI of many elite athletes is above the 'normal' range, but their excess is muscle rather than fat. In general, however, BMI remains a good approximation of weight status.

The perfect body

The ideal body shape portrayed in magazines has changed markedly over time, and anyone looking at pictures of women used as models in art across the ages will see remarkable changes in physique. Today the figure portrayed as ideal is excessively thin and athletic but often with enhanced breast size. This is unattainable for the vast majority of women. The most extreme example is the use of 'size zero' fashion models in advertisements aimed at women. Even the dolls idolized by young girls have BMIs in the anorexic range (Fig. 42.1), coupled with a bust size that could only be obtained through surgery. Whilst the ideal has got thinner, the average body size has increased, so the disparity between ideal and actual body shapes has grown. The result is widespread dissatisfaction with body shape in women, which contributes to the association between obesity and depression. Men, too, are increasingly concerned about body shape, although eating disorders for men tend to be concentrated in professions where weight is an issue (e.g. ballet dancing, jockeys and some athletes) and in homosexual men, who appear more sensitive to societal pressures (Peplau et al., 2009).

Dangers of undereating

The idea that healthy, often academically gifted and likeable girls should refuse to consume sufficient food to maintain a normal body weight has baffled clinicians since anorexia nervosa was formally defined in 1873. Descriptions of the disorder predate that time, challenging the common view that anorexia nervosa is the modern dieting disease. Anorexia is associated with excessive dieting and a morbid preoccupation with body shape, to the point where the sufferer refuses to consume adequate food to sustain a normal body size. It remains a rare disorder, affecting 1 in 1000 even in the most at-risk groups (high-achieving middle-class girls aged 12–16 years). Claims that anorexia has become more frequent are hard to verify because of changes to diagnostic criteria, the most obvious is the relaxation of diagnostic criteria between *Diagnostic and Statistical Manual of Mental Disorders*, 4th Edition (DSM-IV) and DSM-V. Many psychologists see the full disorder as the tip of an iceberg of women (and increasingly men) whose lives are controlled by attempts to diet. Although traditionally interpreted as a socio-cultural disorder, there is increasing evidence of a genetic component that predisposes some individuals to develop anorexia (Trace et al., 2013) and of comorbidities with other conditions such as obsessive-compulsive disorder. Mortality is high, and the disorder is very hard to treat.

Dangers of dieting

Guides to dieting feature heavily in the media and few people in Western societies have not at some time tried to restrict their eating. The increased prevalence of obesity indicates that these attempts rarely work, even though many diets result in initial rapid weight loss. One consequence of frequent failed attempts to diet is the phenomenon of weight cycling, where a *positive energy balance*, defined as energy intake in excess of expenditure, results in weight gain, which leads to short-term dieting and consequent

Table 42.1 **Body mass index (BMI) calculation and classification***	
BMI	**Classification**
<18.5	Underweight
18.5–24.9	Normal
25.0–29.9	Overweight
30.0–34.9	Mildly obese
35.0–39.9	Moderately obese
40.0 +	Severely obese

*BMI = weight (kg)/(height (m))^2.

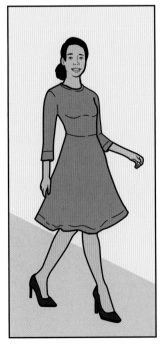

Fig. 42.1 A woman with a figure the same as that of a popular doll would have a body mass index of 16.6.

weight loss, only for weight to be regained and the cycle continued. Research suggests that this pattern itself has adverse effects on health, particularly on the cardiovascular system. Health professionals recommend people who are not obese to maintain a stable weight to minimize these risks.

Binge eating: cause or consequence of dieting?

The defining feature of binge eating is the consumption of a much larger amount of food in a given time than is normal. Binge eating can be associated with obesity and a subtype of anorexia nervosa but is best known in the specific disorder bulimia nervosa (Table 42.2). Here the sufferer has a regular behaviour pattern of dieting followed by periods of excessive eating. Bingeing is followed by attempts to counteract the anticipated consequences of the binge on body weight by self-induced vomiting, use of purgatives or excessive exercise and dieting. The classic psychological model of binge eating was to see it as a secondary consequence of dieting. Accordingly, binge eating was characterized as compensation for the lack of food intake during dieting by overeating when the ability to maintain dieting broke down. The corollary of this is that binge eating should be seen only in people who are currently attempting to restrict their intake. However, sufferers from binge-eating disorder present the behavioural manifestations of binge eating but score low on measures of dieting (Dingemans et al., 2002). This suggests that the tendency to binge eat may be a characteristic of certain individuals, but since unrestricted binge eating will lead to weight gain, binge eating itself may lead to attempts to diet. Dieting may then exacerbate the tendency to binge, and so lead progressively to bulimic behaviour. Thus binging and dieting are interrelated, but one may not inevitably lead to the other.

Promoting a healthy lifestyle

The increase in obesity and eating disorders in Western societies has occurred during a period when other aspects of eating have altered. Most notable has been the increase in use of 'fast foods' and pre-prepared meals at the expense of fresh produce. These types of food often have high energy density and high fat and salt content. Increased energy density does not lead to equivalent increases in satiety and so promotes passive overconsumption. Likewise variety, palatability and larger portion size all promote overeating. With obesity and eating disorders both increasing in incidence, and dieting itself having potential harmful effects on health, how should society tackle these issues? Some see dieting as a necessary evil, since lack of dietary restraint in the face of plentiful high-energy food and low levels of exercise leads to obesity. Most health care professionals concur that promotion of a healthy lifestyle, including healthy eating together with increased energy expenditure, is preferable. Indeed, many clinicians now

routinely prescribe exercise as a component of their treatment for obesity but poor adherence (see pp. 92–93) can render such interventions ineffective. Nonetheless, a lifelong commitment to exercise programmes is recognized as the most effective alternative to drug-based therapy for obesity. However, excessive exercise and dieting together are also features of anorexia, so it is important to monitor effects of prescribed dieting with exercise to ensure that this does not lead to a secondary eating disorder.

Case study

A family (parents in their early 30s, daughter aged 14 years) were seen by their GP during a routine 'well-family' surgery. The daughter was in perfect health, but both parents were overweight and so were advised to increase their levels of exercise and reduce their fat intake. One year later, both parents were still overweight, but the daughter had lost considerable weight as a consequence of excessive dieting and was now diagnosed as having anorexia nervosa.

The GP had no intention of drawing the girl's attention to her weight. However, adolescent girls have a heightened awareness of issues relating to body shape, and awareness of this sensitivity is crucial when communicating health advice.

Eating, body shape and health

- Being obese has serious consequences for physical and mental health.
- Anorexia nervosa has a high mortality rate.
- Repeatedly gaining and losing weight (weight cycling) has more health risks than remaining mildly overweight.
- The ideal body shape depicted by society is unattainable for most people.
- Binge eating can be found in obesity, anorexia nervosa and bulimia nervosa.

Many obese individuals falsely attribute their problems to genetic influences associated with disturbed metabolism and/or appetite, whereas less than 4% of morbid obesity can be traced to a specific genetic disorder. This means for nearly all people reducing their obesity level lies in changing individual eating and exercise behaviour and public health measures to make the healthier option the easier one (see spread 38, pp. 76–77 and spread 53 obesity, pp. 106–107).

Useful websites include those of the National Institute of Diabetes and Digestive and Kidney Diseases' (NIDDK) site on weight loss and control (http:// https://www.niddk.nih.gov/ health-information/diet-nutrition); and the American Obesity Association (http://www.obesity.org/).

Table 42.2 **Clinical diagnoses associated with binge eating**	
Characteristics	**Clinical diagnosis**
Binge eating with no dieting	Binge-eating disorder, often leading to obesity
Binge eating with dieting, excessive exercise, self-induced vomiting or use of purgatives, but no excessive loss of weight	Bulimia nervosa

---

Stop and think

What are the consequences for health and psychological well-being of the following?
- Being constantly overweight
- Cycling between overweight and normal weight
- Being underweight
- Alternately binge-eating and dieting

43 | Deciding to consult

Understanding why people with symptoms do or do not consult a doctor can help improve health services. It is also important because some doctors feel frustrated and angry about 'inappropriate or trivial' consultations, whilst some patients feel frustrated and angry about doctors whom they perceive as uninterested in their problems. Both sets of feelings influence subsequent consulting behaviour, medical treatment, adherence and well-being. Delay may seriously affect a patient's risk of disease progression and the development of complications.

Understanding why people consult or delay consulting is also important because changes in access to doctors and other health professionals (particularly nurses and pharmacists) may significantly affect workload and quality of patient care.

The symptom iceberg

Estimates of the proportion of people who experience symptoms of ill health vary from survey to survey, although the recent Scottish and English health surveys generally reveal similar prevalence rates. Box 43.1 summarizes some results of the 2013 Scottish Health Survey.

Fig. 43.1 is easier to remember and, although the proportions are not strictly accurate, the general picture is valid. Over a 2-week period, about 75% of the population will experience one or more symptoms of ill health. About one-third of these people will do nothing about their symptoms. About one-third will self-medicate or seek the advice of an alternative practitioner (see pp. 144–145), and about one-third will consult their GP. How high/low the iceberg sits in the water will reflect access to doctors and other health care professionals (including complementary and alternative medicine), costs to patients and patients' confidence in their self-care abilities. More patients are being offered alternative ways of accessing doctors by using telephone or internet-based

Box 43.1 **Prevalence of ill health in Scottish Health Survey 2013 (4894 adults and 1839 children)**

- 74% of adults reported their health as good or very good
- 95% of children (under 16 years of age) reported their health as good or very good
- Around one in 10 adults had two or more symptoms of depression, indicating moderate to high severity.
- 9% of children (under 16 years of age) reported long-term limiting conditions.
- 5% of adults had attempted suicide at some point in their life: women (6%) and men (3%).

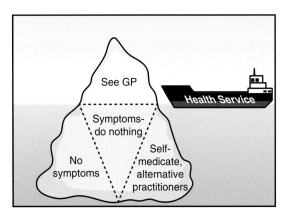

Fig. 43.1 The symptom iceberg.

consultations. In the UK face-to-face consultations with GPs grew by 13% between 2010–2011 and 2014–2015, whilst telephone consultations rose by 63% (Baird et al., 2016). The NHS provides a 24-hour information service (by phone and online), and a nurse-led advice service uses nurses to triage the nature and urgency of the caller's problem and directs the caller to the most appropriate health professional. It appears that improved access to health information through telephone triage can actually increase demand (so-called supply-induced demand), rather than encourage people to look after themselves better (Baird et al., 2016).

It has long been known that the proportion of people with significant medical symptoms who do not consult a doctor is higher than the proportion of people with minor medical symptoms who do consult a doctor, 26% and 11% respectively (Hannay, 1979). More recently, Fielding et al. (2015) suggested that 13% of GP consultations were for minor ailments. Morris et al. (2003) have found that 40% of 240 patients they interviewed indicated that they were consulting about a minor ailment but that, in approximately half of these cases, their GPs thought that the patient was right to consult. Women, preschool children and adults aged 65+ years are most likely to consult a GP over a year.

Differences in symptom perception

Three features of symptoms are important for people's perceptions of their seriousness: (1) the intensity or severity of the symptom; (2) the familiarity of the symptom; and (3) the duration and frequency of the symptom. For example, a severe headache may cause a person who has rarely had a headache to go to the doctor, whereas a person who has experienced migraine for some years is unlikely to consult. This person may consult, however, if the symptoms are unusual in some way or if the headache persists for longer than usual or recurs more frequently than usual.

Differential explanation

At the same time as they perceive their symptoms, people try to make sense of them and to explain them within the context of their lives. They do this using their own lay knowledge and experience and the knowledge and experience of their family and friends (see pp. 98–99). Lydeard and Jones (1989) investigated the health concerns of a sample of consulters with symptoms of dyspepsia and a sample of non-consulters with similar symptoms and found that consulters were significantly more likely to be worried that their symptoms indicated a serious or fatal condition, particularly heart disease or cancer. People with a family history of stomach cancer were also more likely to consult, seeing themselves as 'more vulnerable'.

Differential evaluation

People weigh up for themselves what the relative costs and benefits will be of going (and of not going) to the doctor or other health practitioner (see pp. 36–37). People often decide that other things in their lives are more important than dealing with symptoms of ill health; indeed, doctors themselves are classic examples of people who battle on at work because they perceive themselves as indispensable. Many patients temporalize: they wait, possibly take some medication that they already have with them and see if the symptoms go away over time and only decide to consult if they do not.

People also weigh up what they think the doctor will think of them and what the doctor or other health worker can actually do for them and their symptoms. Research with people with breathing difficulties has shown that people who perceive their symptoms to be serious may delay going to see their doctor if they believe that they will not be able to communicate the seriousness to the doctor (see Asthma and chronic obstructive pulmonary disease, pp. 128–129).

It is also common for people to consult their doctor with symptoms that appear minor to the doctor but the decision to consult reflects anxiety that things might be serious, and they are consulting to confirm that they have reached the right explanation and to reassure themselves that there is nothing seriously wrong. In a qualitative study of parents' concerns when their preschool children became acutely ill, Kai (1996) found that parents felt particularly anxious when their self-care management failed to control their child's symptoms and the threat that these symptoms could imply.

Mothers are also very aware of the moral dilemma they face every time they perceive their child not to be well: do they consult with what might be trivia and risk being seen as 'bad' consulters, or do they delay and risk being labelled as 'bad' parents?

Stop and think

Studies of patient information leaflets or apps designed to reduce GP consultations by patients with symptoms of minor illness have found no change in consultation rates.

- Does this surprise you?
- Why do you think they had no effect?

Access

People experiencing symptoms are less likely to visit their doctor if they live further away from the clinic/surgery, affecting rural patients in particular (see Health: a rural perspective, pp. 158–159). Access to childcare arrangements or the provision of a sitting service for a dependent relative, the availability of a telephone to make an appointment, the availability of a suitable appointment slot and the approachability and friendliness of the doctor and the practice staff are also important factors affecting accessibility.

In many countries, but less so in the UK where most medical care is free at the point of use, the financial cost of payment may act as a deterrent to consulting a doctor (see Organizing and funding health care, pp. 148–149).

Influence of family and friends

According to some studies, up to 50% of symptoms are taken to a doctor on the advice of family or friends. It appears that family members are more likely than friends to recommend a visit to the doctor, possibly because they have the responsibility for caring for the individual.

Research with pregnant women has found that social class IV and V women with extensive and strong lay support and advice, sometimes referred to as *people's lay referral network*, are less likely to attend hospital antenatal classes compared with women from social classes I and II with less lay support. It has been suggested that both the relative number of lay advisers and the degree of congruence in culture between the woman and the doctor will affect the woman's decision whether or not to consult.

People who move to a new area away from their friends and family have been found to make more visits to a doctor in their first year after moving. This raised consultation rate may reflect not only the absence of social support but also the increased risk of ill health arising from the stress of moving house.

Triggers

Several studies have shown that it is not always the experience of symptoms that brings a person to see the doctor. A symptom or an anxiety may have been present for some time, but something else in the person's life triggers the person to consult. A relative may become concerned about a continuing problem and suggest a visit to the doctor; a change at work or in one's personal life may make the symptom more noticeable or incapacitating than before, precipitating a consultation. Media coverage of particular health issues and scares can increase consultation or reduce, for example, the uptake of vaccinations (see Media and Health, pp. 52–53).

Delaying

A good example of the problems associated with patients who delay when they experience symptoms relates to the symptoms of having a heart attack. Such delay in receiving medical care is often associated with higher mortality, which might have been avoided had treatment (defibrillation and/or thrombolytic therapy) been instituted earlier.

Ruston et al. (1998) found that people who did not delay seeking medical care had a better knowledge than 'delayers' of a wider range of symptoms of a heart attack and were more likely to consider themselves at risk. Delayers were more likely to be taking medicines for other conditions such as dyspepsia and would take these medicines and temporalize. Similarly, Horne et al. (2000) identified a mismatch between symptoms expected of a heart attack and symptoms actually experienced, leading to delay.

Case study

In a study of people experiencing angina (chest pain on exertion), Richards et al. (2002) found that compared with residents living in an affluent area of Glasgow, residents from a deprived area reported greater vulnerability to heart disease but that this was not associated with higher reported use of a GP. Instead they interpreted their symptoms as 'normal' and did not present to their doctor for fear that they would be reprimanded by the GP for bothering them with trivia.

Deciding to consult

- The decision to consult a doctor is a complex interplay of physical, psychological and social factors.
- Many people go with relatively minor symptoms because they are anxious that something serious may be indicated.
- People may delay with serious symptoms because of anxiety, lack of knowledge, mismatch of knowledge, use of substitute medication and the relative greater importance of other things in their lives.
- There is often a mismatch between what doctors and patients perceive as appropriate reasons for consulting.
- The perception of what the doctor can do for them and how they will treat them is a significant factor in individuals' decision to consult.
- A change in a person's social setting or relationships may trigger a consultation even when there has been no change in the symptoms.

Every weekday in the UK, almost one million people consult their GP. The consultation between patient and doctor is at the core of all medical practice, be it with a GP or hospital doctor, and be it in the UK or elsewhere. Although an intensely personal and private meeting, usually conducted behind closed doors or curtains, there are rituals and social norms (expected ways of behaving) that provide structure and coherence to what happens in a particular culture.

Doctor–patient relationship

Four models of the doctor–patient relationship have been identified: (1) paternalistic; (2) mutual; (3) consumerist; and (4) default.

Paternalistic

The paternalistic relationship or *disease-centred* approach has, until the late 20th century, been the most commonly observed type of relationship. The doctor, a medical expert, makes a systematic enquiry with the patient answering relatively specific and closed questions, carries out appropriate tests and reaches a diagnosis or a range of possible diagnoses. The doctor then decides on the appropriate treatment, which the patient (the lay person) is expected to follow without question. The process is relatively technical and specific to the symptoms/problem that the patient presents.

In the 1980s, studies of doctor–patient relationships demonstrated that patients, particularly those with chronic illnesses, were also 'experts' in what the symptoms/problem meant to them and their families (Tuckett et al., 1985). This and other research suggested that patients sometimes held different ideas from their doctors about their illnesses, why they were ill or what they wanted to do about it.

Mutual

The mutual relationship is now becoming more common, partly as a result of greater patient knowledge, particularly about chronic disease and partly because of a general cultural shift for individuals not to be passive followers of authority but autonomous agents in their own right. It is characterized by the doctor recognizing both this patient autonomy and the importance of the patient's own beliefs and knowledge of health and illness, as well as the social context in which the illness is dealt with. This model involves the doctor working with a *patient-centred* approach and is discussed in more detail later.

Consumerist

The consumerist relationship is becoming more common in the UK as a result of the extension of private health insurance, the introduction of patient charters, the increasing emphasis on extending patient choice and initiatives to provide quicker access to a doctor. It is characterized by patients 'shopping around' for their preferred care and is accompanied (as exemplified in the USA) by relatively high levels of investigation and treatment and by litigation.

Default

The fourth model, sometimes labelled *default*, is characterized by low levels of engagement between doctor and patient. It can be observed when the doctor can find nothing organically wrong to explain the patient's symptoms and where the patient is labelled

as *somatizing*. There are very particular problems associated with the way patients and doctors respond to such situations, and there is a considerable risk that patients will become trapped in a cycle of over-investigation and treatment.

The patient-centred approach

In its recommendations for undergraduate education in the UK, the General Medical Council (2009) emphasized the importance of learning the patient-centred approach. Box 44.1 highlights five key features of the approach.

Stewart (2001) contrasts the patient-centred approach with 'what it is not – technology-centred, doctor-centred, hospital-centred and disease-centred' (see The biopsychosocial model, pp. 2–3). This is unfortunate as there are good reasons for hospital doctors to use the patient-centred approach, particularly as many inpatients and outpatients are in hospital with acute episodes of illness often associated with, or complicated by, chronic illness. They have important information needs and have their own perspectives on what is happening to them (see spread Deciding to consult, pp. 86–87).

The skilled doctor, whether in hospital or in the community, should be able to move easily between dealing quickly and effectively with acute, life-threatening symptoms by using a disease-centred approach to taking a more patient-centred approach as soon as the threat to life has diminished (see pp. 94–95). Furthermore the acute, disease-centred approach does not have to be at the expense of treating the patient with dignity, respect and humanity. Rather than being seen as two separate and incompatible styles, it is better to think of them as two approaches working in parallel so that the doctor is skilled in both approaches. The importance of being able to work with both approaches is well illustrated by Kinmonth et al. (1998), who reported evidence of poorer disease management of people with type 2 diabetes by doctors who had received extra training in the patient-centred approach (see pp. 124–125).

The research evidence for the practice of patient-centred care is complicated by different definitions and methods of measuring patient-centred care. Similarly definitions of and methods of measuring the outcome of care are not precise. Not all studies have reported a positive association between the practice of patient-centred care and the outcome of that care (Mead et al., 2002), but the weight of the evidence is that patients are more satisfied when they receive patient-centred care.

This judgement is confirmed by a review of longer consultations (Freeman et al., 2002). Patient-centred consultations generally

---

Box 44.1 **Patient-centred care**

- Explores the patient's main reason for the visit, concerns and need for information
- Seeks an integrated understanding of the patient's world – that is, the patient as a whole person, his or her emotional needs and life issues
- Finds common ground on what the problem is and mutually agrees on management
- Enhances prevention and health promotion
- Enhances the continuing relationship between the patient and the doctor

Adapted from Stewart, 2001.

Table 44.1 **Negotiation strategies**	
Patients	**Doctors**
Disclose	Physical setting of room
Suggest	Language
Demand	Technical/non-technical
Leading question	Open/closed questions
Non-verbal behaviour	Tone of voice
Hesitation/silence	Clarifying/functional uncertainty
Delaying tactics	Listening/interrupting
'Whilst I'm here…'	Picking up/ignoring cues
See a different doctor	Non-verbal behaviour
	Interest/disinterest
	Calm/haste
	Prescription

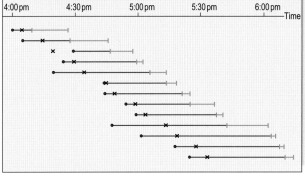

Fig. 44.1 Afternoon surgery with appointments booked every 7.5 minutes. X indicates appointment time. *Red line* indicates waiting time and *green line* the actual visit.

take more time (Howie et al., 1992), and the review reported that longer consultations were associated with:

- Less prescribing (judged as desirable)
- More advice on lifestyle and health-promoting activities
- Better recognition and handling of psychosocial problems
- Better patient enablement (Howie et al., 1998)
- Better clinical care of some chronic illnesses
- Higher patient satisfaction

A patient-centred consultation still involves taking a systematic history of the patient's presenting and underlying problems, but it differs from the more traditional paternalistic relationship by integrating it with an enquiry into the patient's ideas, knowledge, beliefs, concerns and expectations (see pp. 36–37). In their study of doctor–patient relationships, Tuckett et al. (1985) showed that consultations were most likely to break down and patients were most likely to be dissatisfied and non-compliant (see pp. 92–93) when doctors failed to elicit and respond empathetically to patients' beliefs and expectations. Of course, patients will sometimes hold unrealistic or inappropriate expectations. In such cases it is important that the doctor and patient are clear what the patient's expectations and beliefs are and that the doctor explains in a manner that does not make the patient feel stupid or defensive why the belief or expectation is inappropriate. In some cases this will involve negotiation. Some of the strategies that patients and doctors use to control consultations are summarized in Table 44.1. Working-class people may sometimes express themselves rather directly, which doctors may interpret as a demand for a particular test or treatment (see Social class and health, pp. 42–43). On occasion no resolution may be found, and both patient and doctor are likely to feel dissatisfied with the consultation.

It is also important to remember that a single consultation between a patient and a doctor does not occur in isolation, particularly in general practice. A 5- or 10-minute consultation may be but one of a series of consultations during which patient and doctor may negotiate the diagnostic and treatment possibilities, and the implications for the patient's general well-being. Continuity of care is important for many patients.

Lack of time may frequently constrain a doctor from being properly person-centred, and this puts pressure on the doctor and on the patient. Fig. 44.1 illustrates a patient-centred doctor who has a personal commitment; the surgery is due to end at 6.10 p.m. She uses the first hour to see three patients but, despite trying to

catch up, she reaches 5.45 p.m., with only 15 minutes available for three patients, each having waited almost an hour past their appointment times.

Patients themselves are very conscious, not only of their responsibility not to consult for trivia (see pp. 86–87), but also of their responsibility not to take up too much of the doctor's precious time. Patients often feel intimidated by doctors and are reluctant to ask questions, mention anxieties or voice other things (agendas) they want to raise. Barry et al. (2000) described a qualitative study of 35 patients who had revealed in pre-consultation interviews that they had a total of 188 agendas they wished to raise. Only four voiced all their agendas, and, in total, 73 agendas were never mentioned. Agenda items that were not mentioned were associated with negative outcomes, particularly major misunderstandings.

Given that people frequently have anxieties that relatively minor symptoms may mask something more serious, and given their reluctance to present with mental health problems (see pp. 86–87), it should not be surprising that they often feel unable to mention their worries lest the doctor should think that they are wasting the GP's time with trivia or taking more than their 'fair share'.

Stop and think

- Not all studies have found that patients prefer patient-centred care. Why might this be?
- Will the consumerist model become the dominant type of patient–doctor relationship, and if so, how will this affect the patient-centred approach?

Seeing the doctor

- Doctors and patients have different knowledge, beliefs, wants and expectations, and consultations often involve negotiation.
- The process and outcome of care differ not just between patients but also between doctors, especially due to differences in doctors' styles.
- Doctors with a patient-centred approach to care are more likely than those with a disease-centred approach to identify patients' psychosocial problems and to deal with their patients' anxieties.
- Patients are often reluctant to voice their ideas and anxieties in case they are thought of as inappropriate, stupid or time-wasting.

45 | Placebo and nocebo effects

A placebo is often thought of as something that looks (and tastes) like the real medicine but does not (or should not) have any direct action on the condition or symptoms. The placebo effect (from the Latin 'I will please') is important to understand because it can have a great effect on treatment. Placebos are used and abused, but often little understood.

The emergence of placebo effects

Until the 20th century no neat distinction could be made between drugs whose mode of action for a specific disorder was known and understood and any other drug (Fig. 45.1). With the development of scientific medicine, people then began to identify active ingredients and to become more suspicious of drugs whose action was not understood. This introduced the notion that there were drugs that would treat a particular condition by a particular route and other substances that might be placebos.

However, placebos have been shown to bring about clinical improvement in many branches of medicine: surgery, the treatment of cancer, dentistry, psychiatry, paediatrics and numerous others. They can produce the same phenomena observed with other drugs:

- Habituation (a tendency to increase the dose over time)
- Withdrawal symptoms
- Dependence (an inability to stop taking them without psychiatric help)
- Inverse relationship between severity of symptom and efficacy of placebo

The nocebo phenomenon

It is also possible for a drug or procedure to produce adverse effects that are not the result of any known pharmacological mechanism. These are called *nocebo effects*, from the Latin 'I will harm'. Nocebo has been defined in different ways, most commonly as the clinical effects on patients when verbal suggestions suggest clinical worsening (Olshansky, 2007). Others have used the term to refer to adverse events that occur after an inert substance is administered (Data-Franco and Berk, 2013); in this case, negative psychological expectancies are assumed to be responsible. Although effects can be severe, reported nocebo symptoms are more usually generalized and diffuse: for example, drowsiness, nausea, fatigue and insomnia. In clinical trials these nocebo effects can be severe enough to lead to non-adherence, discontinuation and drop-out (see pp. 92–93).

A recent systematic review of 89 studies of nocebo effects (including 70 experiments) found that the largest predictors of nocebo effects were higher perceived dose, explicit suggestions of an adverse effect, high expectations of symptoms and seeing others experiencing symptoms from the exposure (Webster, Weinman and Rubin, 2016).

Placebos and clinical trials

To demonstrate the efficacy of any new treatment, many clinical trials include a placebo for comparison so that such effects can be separated from the effects of the experimental compound. These are often double-blind trials: i.e. neither the patient nor the member of staff who gives it knows which one is the experimental drug and which one the placebo. This ensures that nothing can influence a patient's expectations about the drug and, therefore, the response. Although placebo effects are most commonly thought of in relation to pharmaceuticals, a recent systematic review and meta-analysis has shown that they also make a large contribution in trials of minimally invasive surgical procedures (Holtedahl, Brox and Tjomsland, 2015).

Types of placebo

- Pure placebo: thought to contain no active ingredient, for example, a sugar pill
- Impure placebo: contains an active ingredient, but one that is not known to have any effect on the condition being treated, e.g. a vitamin C tablet being given for headache
- Placebo procedure: a procedure, for instance, taking blood pressure, which is not known to produce any clinical change

What makes one susceptible?

The literature on personality traits as a way of predicting who will and will not experience placebo or nocebo effects has failed to show any reliable predictors. Interpersonal factors such as the therapeutic relationship with the carer appear to be more important. However, circumstances and presentation appear to be the most influential (see also pp. 22–23). For example, people's perception of pain depends on the situation: people injured in combat appear to tolerate pain better than those with similar injuries in hospital (see also pp. 146–147). In war an injury means evacuation to safety and thus brings great relief; this is not the same in civilian life. With placebos, experiments have demonstrated a number of factors that produce a response, for instance:

- The physical appearance of the placebo: for example, green tranquillizers reduce anxiety more than yellow or red ones (Schapira et al., 1970).
- Branding: products that have been marketed or are branded rather than generic will produce greater effects than unbranded products or placebos.
- The reputation of the setting: e.g. a university research unit will enhance treatment more compared with a back-street clinic.
- The patient's perception of staff attitudes affects response: for example, where doctors are judged as more interested and enthusiastic, the results are more positive.

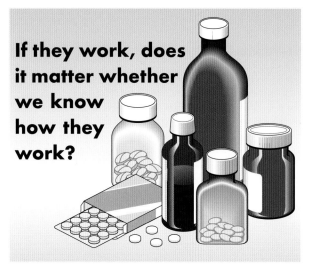

If they work, does it matter whether we know how they work?

Fig. 45.1 Drugs and modes of action.

The nocebo phenomenon has been found to be more common in women than in men, and although cultural and ethnic factors are thought to be important, there is little empirical evidence (Barsky et al., 2002). A recent scoping review of nocebo effects (Symon et al., 2015) found that they are more likely to be found in:

- People who expect to experience side-effects
- Patients who have been previously conditioned to experience side-effects
- Patients with certain psychological characteristics such as anxiety, depression or neuroticism

How do they work?

The placebo and nocebo effects are simply a part of a wider field linking social and meaningful processes with human biological processes. This has been termed *sociomatics* (Kleinman, 1986). Consequently there are various possible contributory mechanisms:

- Social influence – doctors are perceived as people in authority and, therefore, their direction and expectations are followed (see pp. 164–165).
- Role expectation – the doctor's role is to organize treatment, and the patient's role is to get better, so he or she plays that role.
- Classical conditioning – for a patient, past experiences of taking drugs led to improvement, so the administration of a new drug is more likely to produce the same response (see pp. 20–21).
- Operant conditioning – the doctor rewards the patient who shows any sign of improvement, thus increasing the probability that the patient will continue to report improvement (see pp. 22–23).
- Cognitive influence – the patient has firm beliefs about medical treatment: for example, 'modern medicine is based on scientific evidence, therefore this drug will be effective'. Of course, the opposite would also be true: if the patient believes modern medicine to be harmful, he or she may be less likely to respond and may, in fact, experience adverse effects (see Biopsychosocial model pp. 2–3).

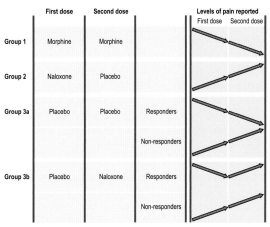

Fig. 45.2 Levels of pain reported in a double-blind trial of naloxone/placebo *(from Levine et al., 1978, pp. 654–657, with permission).*

What are doctors' attitudes to placebo effects?

Many doctors have strong feelings about the use of placebos in medicine: some are positive, but many are negative, perhaps because the placebo effect is similar to faith-healing, when many doctors prefer to see medicine as a science. Although most health professionals are aware of the therapeutic aspect of placebo, fewer are aware of the nocebo phenomenon. Views about placebo effects can range widely:

- Placebo effects are a nuisance that interfere with the understanding and practice of medicine.
- Placebo effects are powerful, but to use placebos in practice is a betrayal of trust between doctor and patient.
- Placebo effects are powerful and should be usefully incorporated to enhance treatment.

Case study

Levine et al. (1978) hypothesized that placebo effects that relieve pain are mediated by endorphin release. If that were the case, then naloxone (an opiate antagonist) would block them. They gave medication to patients after surgery in a double-blind trial (Fig. 45.2). The patients all had wisdom teeth removed. Group 1 was given morphine, group 2 had naloxone and group 3 got a placebo. Of those initially given a placebo (group 3), half were given another placebo 1 hour later (group 3a), and half were given naloxone 1 hour later (group 3b). Our interest lies in these two groups of patients. When they were initially given the placebo, 39% reported a significant decrease in pain, but if they were in group 3b, those given naloxone, the pain increased again. For those who had not responded to the placebo, the naloxone made no difference. So it appeared that some patients obtained significant pain relief from a placebo, but this was reversed by an opiate antagonist. The experiments concluded that endorphin release must have occurred with the placebo.

Placebo and nocebo effects

- Placebo effects have been demonstrated in many branches of medicine.
- Nocebo phenomena are usually generalized and diffuse adverse symptoms.
- Placebo effects ought to be controlled in experimental trials of medical procedures.
- There are no established personal characteristics that will predict a therapeutic response to a placebo.
- Nocebo phenomena are more likely among people who expect to experience adverse effects or have been previously conditioned to experience adverse effects.
- Effects are influenced by context: culture, expectations and beliefs.
- There are ethical issues involved in the clinical use of placebos.

Stop and think

Many people in prison are vulnerable and have in the past been dependent on drugs or alcohol. They feel the need to continue to take something 'to help with nerves'. Part of this dependence is psychological rather than chemical, and they frequently come to the medical officer asking for medication.

- Should a health professional prescribe a placebo in this case 'to keep the patient happy, to persuade the prescriber that he is doing something positive or useful or both'?

Compliance, adherence and concordance are related but subtly different terms. All three imply the type of doctor–patient relationship occurring. Compliance refers to the extent to which someone complies with advice provided by a doctor, suggesting that a paternalistic, doctor-centred, relationship is occurring, with the patient being a passive recipient. Adherence refers to the extent to which an individual adheres to *agreed* advice, suggesting a less doctor-centred relationship where a patient could decide to not agree with the physician's advice. Concordance describes the outcome of a process whereby a doctor and patient come to a *mutually agreeable* route of action, which is more in line with a patient-centred relationship. Concordance around medical advice therefore would be the gold standard for health professionals to aspire to. However, most research examines patient adherence to medical advice and is, therefore, the focus of this chapter.

Do patients adhere to health professional advice?

Medical advice can pertain to various tasks such as changing behaviours, completing physiotherapy exercises or taking medication as recommended and usually contains information regarding how to follow the advice to ensure the most efficacious outcome for the patient. Methods of assessing adherence behaviour are varied, with examples including self-report behaviour or pill counts (correct amount of pills been taken on time?), amongst others. But how accurate are these assessments of adherence? Medication may require to be taken at specific times of day to be of most benefit and pill counts may not tell you this has been achieved. The measurement of adherence behaviour should not be confused with measuring the clinical outcome: for example, if a doctor advises an individual on behaviour changes aimed at controlling blood sugar levels, you might expect their

blood sugar levels to remain fairly constant and low. So could adherence be assessed by monitoring their blood sugar levels, rather than their behaviour? Interestingly the match between adherent behaviour and clinical outcomes, such as blood sugar levels is not always perfect, and so this type of indirect measure of adherence may not be useful.

Around 25% of patients are non-adherent to health professional recommendations. Nonadherence can be costly to both the patient and the health service. For example, adherence in patients with coronary artery disease significantly improved health outcomes, including reductions in hospitalizations, likelihood of recurrent myocardial infarction and mortality rates. Further, when patients were adherent to advice, there was a 10% to 18% reduction in health care costs per patient compared with non-adherent patients. Understanding the reasons why patients may not adhere to advice and how health professionals can try to improve such adherence may improve outcomes.

How can health professionals improve adherence?

The reasons for non-adherence to advice may be intentional or unintentional. Adherence to medication has been linked to patient socio-economic, health care system, condition, therapy and patient-related factors (Box 46.1). The communication within consultations is included within health care system factors (see Clinical communication skills, pp. 94–95). Patients who have a physician who communicates well adhere over two times better than when a physician is a poor communicator. Similarly when a physician is trained in clinical communication, the likelihood of a patient adherence is 1.6 times greater.

So what communication behaviours can doctors utilize to help patients adhere to medical advice? Here it is helpful to introduce the Information-Motivation-Strategy (IMS) model, which was

Box 46.1 Determinants of patient adherence

Socio-economic	Health care system	Condition	Therapy	Patient
Family support	Barriers to health care (e.g. language)	Presence of symptoms	Adverse effects	Age
Other carer factors	Drug supply	Disease severity	Patient friendliness of regimen	Gender
Social support	Prescription by specialist	Clinical improvement	Drug effectiveness	Marital status
Stigma	Information about drug administration	Psychiatric condition	Duration of treatment	Education
Costs of treatment	Patient–health professional communication and relationship	Specific diagnosis/ indication	Drug type	Ethnicity
Prescription coverage	Follow-up	Disease duration	Well-organized treatment	Housing
Socio-economic status				Cognitive function
Employment status				Forgetfulness and reminders
				Knowledge
				Health beliefs
				Psychological profile
				Co-morbidities
				Alcohol or substance abuse
				Transportation difficulties

Source: Kardas, Lewek and Matyjaszczyk, 2013 with permission.

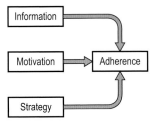

Fig. 46.1 Information-Motivation-Strategy model *(based on Martin, Haskard-Zolnierek and DiMatteo, 2010).*

designed to assist health professionals (Martin, Haskard-Zolnierek and DiMatteo, 2010) (Fig. 46.1).

The first domain of the IMS is *information*. This addresses situations where patients are non-adherent because they do not understand what they are supposed to do. Lack of understanding can relate to many aspects of the illness itself and to treatment options, or it may be because of the cognitive capacity of the patient. Allowing patients to tell their illness stories in their own words provides an environment in which patients are not fearful of showing they do not understand, making it more likely they will ask questions. People ask questions about points they are interested in or that concern them, ensuring concerns are voiced and there is an opportunity to address them. Information should be provided in a clear and specific manner so that people are more likely to remember specific directions such as 'take these tablets 30 minutes before each meal'. The provision of information alone does not mean that a patient will understand that information or remember it. Checking patients understanding and recall of information will help here. A final point regarding information is that patients require adequate understanding if they are to take an active role in decision-making.

The second domain of the IMS is *motivation*. Lack of motivation to follow advice may stem from the health beliefs of patients towards their illness or the treatment suggestions, coping strategies, co-morbidities and mental well-being, or it may relate to aspects of the illness itself (Kardas et al., 2013). An understanding of patients' beliefs towards their illness or treatment options is vital to a patient-centred approach, meaning that concordance between patient and doctor is more likely. Cultural, peer and family beliefs are often taken into account by patients when making decisions about health care, as are beliefs regarding the efficacy of the treatment suggestions being made. Individuals are less motivated to attempt something they believe they cannot successfully achieve, so patient self-efficacy should also be a topic for discussion. An additional approach to boost the motivation of patients to adhere, is to ensure they are aware of the implications of non-adherence (DiMatteo et al., 2011).

The final dimension of IMS is *strategy*. Sometimes treatment plans are just not practical for patients, making adherence difficult. Low income and the high costs of some drugs may mean difficulties in affording appropriate care; likewise poor access to services or treatments mean patients are unable to act upon medical advice. Complicated drug regimens may also contribute to non-adherence. Finally, aspects of the illness itself may be limiting: for example, if a patient is in severe pain, he or she may be unable to carry out physiotherapy exercises aimed at improving his or her condition (Kardas et al., 2013). Initiating a

patient-centred conversation should actively involve the patient in the identification of barriers and the development of solutions to overcome them. This conversation should include discussion of the support available to patients in terms of the financial cost or assistance from friends or family or groups who could remind patients to take medication or assist them to change behaviours.

The IMS model as a whole embodies health professional communication behaviour within a patient-centred consultation style. Patient-centred communication should assist in achieving concordance with a patient regarding medical advice, which should improve adherent behaviour.

Case study

Keiran is a 20-year-old student diagnosed with type 1 diabetes 6 weeks ago. He collapsed at university and ended up in hospital for 3 days, where he was diagnosed. A diabetes nurse explained how to measure his blood sugar levels and inject himself with insulin. The nurse also gave Keiran some advice about diet changes, but he was so worried at the time about injecting himself that he did not take it in, although he vaguely remembered something about eating sweets if his blood sugar levels got too low and avoiding alcohol.

After 3 weeks Keiran was feeling fine and started to wonder what all the fuss was about. He felt perfectly normal and perceived that he was managing his blood sugar levels appropriately. He always carried a bag of sweets around with him 'just in case' and started to notice he was putting on weight. Up until then he had avoided alcohol but started thinking that it was a waste of time as he did not feel ill in the slightest. So at the next party he had a few drinks and felt absolutely okay. Monitoring his blood sugar levels just before he went to bed was tricky to say the least, so he had given himself a few extra units of insulin, just to be sure.

After that experience Keiran decided to continue using this strategy of carrying on as normal and giving himself some extra insulin if he thought he needed it as he continued to feel well. As far as he was concerned, he was managing his diabetes appropriately.

Stop and think

- Keiran has come for a routine check-up for his diabetes (see Case study) with his doctor. How do you approach the subject of adherence during that consultation?

Patient adherence

- Around 25% of patients are non-adherent to medical advice.
- Non-adherence can be as a result of socio-economic, health service, illness, treatment-related or individual reasons.
- Health professionals should aim to achieve concordance with a patient when discussing advice.
- The IMS is a useful model to consider when communicating with patients about adherence to health professional advice.
- Clear and specific information provision along with checking patient understanding can result in greater adherence.
- Taking a patient-centred approach, which explores psychosocial aspects of patients' lives, including health beliefs, and actively encouraging them to identify problems and solutions can improve adherence.

47 | Clinical communication skills

Clinical communication skills are essential for all health professionals. A clinician must integrate four components to achieve a successful patient-centred consultation: clinical knowledge, communication, examination and clinical reasoning skills. Excellent factual knowledge is limited if you cannot identify the reason why your patients attended; help them understand the management options, if appropriate; and achieve shared decision-making.

Clinicians who have poorly developed or maintained clinical communication skills may encounter difficulties in their clinical practice with patients and colleagues. A doctor who is poor at doctor–patient communication, increases the risk of:

- Poor adherence to medication because patients do not understand what medications they take and why adherence is important for their health (see Chapter on Adherence, pp. 92–93)
- A gap between what patients want and what the doctor thinks a patient wants (e.g. Mulley, Trimble and Elywn, 2014)
- Patient complaints

For doctors, the importance of communication skills in clinical practice is recognized by the General Medical Council (GMC; the organization that registers doctors in the UK and ensures proper standards in the practice of medicine) as described in *Good Medical Practice* (Good Medical Practice, 2013). For example, GMP states that all doctors must listen to patients, take account of their views, respond honestly to their questions and give them the information they want or need to know in a way they can understand. The GMC also recognizes the importance of showing respect for patients and (doctors) not expressing their personal beliefs to patients in ways that exploit their vulnerability or are likely to cause them distress. Doctors whose performance is seriously deficient in communication skills can have their registration removed or restricted.

A consultation involves several key communication tasks, summarized in the Calgary Cambridge framework (Silverman, Kurtz and Draper, 2013) as:

- Building a relationship with the patient (rapport)
- Gathering information (history-taking)
- Explanation and planning (e.g. test results)
- Carrying out these tasks in a coherent, logical way

Building rapport

Building rapport depends on two things: preparation and planning, and non-verbal communication (NVC).

Preparation and planning

- Have the right information ready before you see the patient (read the notes).
- Seating: remove barriers such as tables and desks. Sit at 45 degree angle rather than directly facing the patient, and ensure that you are sitting at the same level as the patient.
- Privacy: unless patients know they will not be overheard, they are unlikely to talk freely.
- Noise and interruptions: try to make sure you will not be disturbed, particularly if talking about a sensitive subject or breaking bad news.

Non-verbal communication

- First impressions do count: does your greeting convey warmth and caring or that you are time pressured? Think about body language and how you are dressed.

- Proximity: sitting a comfortable distance from a patient assists communication. Being too distant makes the doctor seem aloof, whilst being too close may feel threatening. Remember that different cultures have different boundaries for personal space.
- Posture: sitting upright but relaxed, with arms and legs uncrossed and leaning slightly toward the patient, conveys attentiveness.
- Eye contact: this is very powerful for initiating, maintaining and ending communication. The clinician's gaze should be in the direction of the patient without staring.
- Computers are used in many clinical settings: it is important to balance eye contact with looking at the screen.
- Facial expression: you can show interest, compassion and concern through your facial expression. If you look uncertain, patients may lack confidence in what you are saying.
- Head nods convey understanding and encouragement to say more: however, do not overdo it; vigorous nodding may be interpreted as impatience.
- Touch can be facilitative (e.g. establish a friendly relationship with patient by shaking hands on meeting), functional (e.g. physical examination) or therapeutic (e.g. touching a distressed patient on the hand to console), but bear in mind cultural norms.
- Paralinguistic features: this refers to aspects of verbal messages that serve to modulate their meaning such as tone, pitch and volume. Paralinguistics can determine whether the same words (e.g. 'you took all the tablets') are expressed as a statement, surprise or question.
- Silence: allow the patient time to respond, or think how to answer a question, without jumping in with another question too quickly.

Used skilfully, non-verbal behaviours offer powerful tools with which to encourage a patient to talk and to demonstrate interest in and understanding of the patient's predicament.

Gathering information

Gathering information is not just a matter of discovering the biomedical facts but also an opportunity to assess patients' perspective of their illness as well as relevant social and economic factors. The latter is essential and should not be neglected, even if appointment time is limited.

> **Stop and think**
>
> Patients often complain that doctors do not ask about their feelings or emotional responses, but some doctors argue that their job is just to treat disease, not deal with how people cope with it.
> - What's your view of such medical practice?

There are three important aspects to gathering information. Clinicians need to ask appropriate questions to establish a diagnosis or elicit a patient's problems (described as the content of verbal communication). The way in which you ask questions is important, referred to as *process skills*. The third aspect is to simultaneously analyze the information received and use this to reason through the clinical scenario. Language is critical to getting and giving information effectively. Different aspects of verbal clinical communication can be identified.

Questioning

There are different questioning styles, often a combination of these approaches is required:

- Opening questions or conversation starters encourage patients to tell you why they presented today. It is important not to interrupt the patient early on so that you can grasp the problem.
- Open questions are useful early on for encouraging patients to describe fully their problems.
- Closed questions limit the patient to one- or two-word answers. They are useful for obtaining or clarifying details and allowing functional enquiry.

Typically a consultation will start with open questions and then narrow to closed ones to gather specific information. It is also important to avoid asking more than one question at once as this can be confusing to the patient and to avoid leading questions.

Reflecting

Where you think patients have more to tell you, often about their worries, reflecting means encouraging them to continue by repeating back to them part of what they have said.

Summarizing

When you think patients have told you all they are going to tell you and you have gathered all the information you need, a summary draws together the significant aspects of what has been said. Summaries are very useful for showing the patient you have been listening, to clarify any misinterpretations or to remind patients that there is something else they want to tell you.

Explanations and planning

The second part of a consultation takes place when a working or definite diagnosis has been made. At this stage the emphasis changes from gathering information to explaining, exploring options, if appropriate, and involving the patient in decision-making. Patients are partners in care and should, if they wish, be involved in a management plan, that is, 'shared decision-making'.

Remember that patients now have greater access to medical information than ever before. Moreover media coverage of incidences of poor patient care and abuses of trust by individual doctors are believed to have adversely influenced the public regard for doctors. This part of the consultation is where most clinicians could improve their communication skills (e.g. Joseph-Williams, Elwyn and Edwards, 2014).

The necessary communication skills for this second part of the consultation include delivering lucid, coherent explanations *that the patient understands*.

When giving an explanation, it helps:

- Check what the patient knows already – so you can gauge how much information you need to give and identify any misunderstandings you need to correct
- Ask how much the patient wants to know
- Tell the patient what you are going to do
- Use a series of logical points and give the patient time to ask questions after each piece of information
- Avoid or explain any jargon
- Repeat and emphasize key points
- Use examples and diagrams and write key points down for the patient to take away

- Use web resources and consultation recordings
- Give specific, rather than vague, advice
- Ask for feedback on understanding
- Documentation – for communication with colleagues and patient access to notes

---

Case study

Peter was a 26-year-old physiology PhD student with a recent history of passing blood after mild exercise. At a busy outpatient clinic he had just undergone an intravenous pyelography of his kidneys and was called to see the consultant, Mr Brown. How successful is rapport and information exchange between doctor and patient in each example? Which would you prefer if you were the patient, and why?

Mr Brown (looking at computer): I can find nothing wrong with your kidneys. I think you have a touch of long-march haematuria … happens sometimes to people who exercise a lot.

Peter (hesitating): Oh? … I've read a bit about that condition, and I don't think it fits with what happens to me.

Response 1

Mr Brown (irritated turns to Peter): Oh, you don't! (pause) Well, if you want to be sure that there is not something else going on, we can book you in for a cystoscopy. (Walks off briskly)

Peter (now anxious): Oh dear. Thanks.

Response 2

Mr Brown (surprised but expressing an interest): What makes you say that?

Peter: Well, the blood I pass is bright red. In long-march haematuria I believe it's usually a dark brown.

Mr Brown: I see! That's possibly significant. (pause) Well, we could do a cystoscopy to have a look in your bladder. That would mean passing a fine optic fibre camera up through your penis. How would you feel about us doing that?

Peter (apprehensive): Well …, if you think it will help find out what's wrong.

Structured approach to consultation

This section has been based on the Calgary Cambridge framework, as taught in many medical schools. This is one of a number of consultation models used in clinical practice, each of which has strengths and weaknesses.

Clinical communication skills

- Clinician–patient communication is central to effective medical practice and can affect quality of care.
- Effective rapport, information gathering and giving and carrying out a structured consultation are key tasks in patient-centred consulting.
- Factors that influence doctor–patient communication include:
  - Preparation and planning
  - Non-verbal communication
  - Verbal communication
- Effective clinical communication requires the ability to use consultation skills flexibly in response to different patients.
- Good resources include:
  - www.skillscascade.com
  - http://www.ukccc.org.uk/

48 | Breaking bad news

Bad news has been defined as 'any news that drastically and negatively alters the person's view of her or his future' (Buckman, 1992). Bad news may be giving a terminal or life-changing prognosis (e.g. metastatic cancer or multiple sclerosis), but it could also be news of sudden loss (e.g. telling a young wife that her husband has died after a massive heart attack or parents that their teenage son has been killed in a motorbike accident). It may also be about something seemingly much less dramatic for patients, but no less distressing (e.g. telling a young man keen to be a pilot that he has diabetes). The impact of the news will have not only medical consequences but also physical, social, emotional and occupational consequences, which health professionals often fail to appreciate.

Why is it difficult?

There are several reasons why breaking bad news is an especially difficult task for doctors, irrespective of their age, speciality or professional experience (Box 48.1). In addition it may be made more difficult if family members want to protect the person from bad news and distress. Under these circumstances the doctor may be asked to collude with the relatives to maintain a conspiracy of silence. This situation often puts strain on a previously healthy relationship both with the doctor and within the family and can lead to feelings of mistrust and isolation on the part of the patient.

Although traditionally doctors withheld bad news from patients, believing this to be in patients' best interests, studies now show that most people want the truth about their diagnosis, but the depth of information sought will vary according to individual needs. Despite these findings, truth-telling, particularly with cancer patients, is still not universally practised, and doctors still frequently censor the amount of information they give to patients about prognosis on the grounds that 'what someone does not know cannot harm them'. Research has also shown that doctors

---

Box 48.1 **Difficulties involved in breaking bad news**

Personal
- Fear of own illness/death
- Fear of expressing own emotions (e.g. crying)
- Recent bereavement
- Identification with own experience (e.g. victim may be the same age)
- Embarrassment/distress/discomfort

Social
- Removal of death from home to institution makes death unacceptable and taboo
- Sickness stigmatized

Professional
- Lack of experience or training
- Fear of eliciting a difficult response (e.g. anger)
- Fear of being blamed by person or superiors
- Failure to provide cure
- Fear of causing pain/emotional damage
- Fear of destroying hope

Political
- Fear of litigation

Data from Buckman, R. 1992. How to Break Bad News: A Guide for Health Care Professionals. John Hopkins University Press, Baltimore, MD.

---

find the breaking of bad news so stressful that they adopt a variety of strategies to make the task easier for themselves (see Clinical Communication Skills, pp. 94–95). These strategies, in turn, can affect the amount and type of information doctors give to patients, i.e. their policy of disclosure. For example, some use medical jargon and statistics to explain a prognosis and focus on survival rates, whilst others explain the diagnosis with complex euphemisms to soften the blow.

Reactions to bad news

People react to bad news differently. The impact will depend partly on the gap between what the person hopes for and the medical reality (Buckman, 1992). Reactions may also be dictated by the person's past experiences, personality and coping strategies. The reactions may be unrelated to the type or stage of the disease. Reactions may vary from calm or resigned acceptance to acute distress, anxiety, anger, shock and denial (see Anxiety, pp. 112–113). However, the way a doctor breaks news can also affect how patients later adjust to and cope with their illness as well as influence their treatment choices (see Coping with illness and disability, pp. 140–141). This knowledge, as well as studies of patients' preferences, has led to the development of numerous guidelines to giving bad news. These models usually follow a step-by-step approach from preparation to next steps (Buckman, 1992; Narayanan et al, 2010; www.breakingbadnews.org).

Preparation

Check person's physical ability to take in news

Before attempting to give any information of this kind, it is important to make sure that the patient or relative is physically and mentally able to understand. In the case of a serious diagnosis such as cancer, patients may already be experiencing symptoms that are preventing them from thinking clearly, such as confusion or drowsiness. It is necessary, therefore, to treat any condition that will prevent the person from comprehending the news, before attempting to impart the news.

Check own appearance and readiness

How doctors present themselves during consultations can also help patients accept the news more easily. Making sure that you appear comfortable, relaxed and not rushed will communicate to patients that you have the time to spend with them and feel at ease with the task. Appearing in a blood-stained coat and/or looking tense and harassed will only serve to heighten patients' stress. Doctors should also have familiarized themselves with patients' notes and made a rough plan of what they want to communicate.

Setting the scene

The context of where the news will be broken is as important as how it is broken. The most appropriate place will be a quiet side room on the ward to ensure the person's privacy and concentration. Bleeps and phones should be switched off to minimize the possibility of interruption. People will absorb the news better if they feel as relaxed and comfortable as possible. Most doctors find it helpful to be accompanied by another member of staff, e.g. a nurse, social worker or chaplain, as well as allowing the patient to be joined by a relative or a friend. The presence of other people can often help clarify information that was given by the doctor after the interview, as well as providing emotional support when the news is broken.

Breaking the news

Step 1: It is essential before breaking the news to find out what patients already know and understand about their illness. This will inform the doctor of the degree of insight and provide a baseline on which to build. Sometimes a patient will indicate that he or she already suspects that something is seriously wrong. This may be especially true of people who have been experiencing difficult symptoms or have known a relative or friend who has had the same illness.

Step 2: Before continuing, the doctor should find out what the person wants to know about his or her illness. This can be done by asking the person directly and should leave the doctor in no doubt about how much information to give. For example, some people will only want to know about their treatment without wishing to speak about their diagnosis or prognosis. Others will require much more detail.

Step 3: The news should be broken simply and clearly but avoiding bluntness and euphemisms. To begin with, some information should be given by the doctor to warn the person that the news is not good: for example, 'the results of the tests are more serious than we thought'.

Step 4: Leave silence and allow time for news to sink in. Seek the patient's permission to continue.

Step 5: You can keep giving information as long as the person is asking for it and understands what is being said. Diagrams or drawings can sometimes help patients to understand more clearly. Check if the person wants more information before continuing or stopping.

Step 6: Encourage patients to express their concerns and feelings. This will show that you empathize with them and increase their satisfaction with the consultation.

Step 7: Plan the treatment programme or the next set of actions with the patient or relatives (e.g. with bereaved relatives, this may be viewing the body). Asking them to summarize the main points of the consultation will inform the doctor about how much of the news they have understood. It is also vital that the doctor arranges to see the patient at a follow-up interview to help clarify any misunderstandings or anxieties the person may have about the news. Follow-up plans should be documented in the patient's notes and shared with colleagues.

No news is bad news

An important part of communicating news to patients is conveying the results of tests. It can be difficult to reassure patients who have been anticipating bad news that the news is good. Studies show that patients who are experiencing symptoms but have negative test results may remain anxious long after the consultation and continue to experience the same symptoms, often leading them to consult again. Reasons for this anxiety may be a misunderstanding of what the doctor said or disbelief. Doubt may also be fuelled by conflicting evidence from an individual's personal circumstances – for example, knowing someone with the same symptoms who had died or who had had a false-negative result. In these circumstances direct discussion of the patient's concerns is advocated, rather than referring the patient on for further tests.

Sudden bad news

In cases of trauma, the task of breaking bad news may be even more difficult because of the suddenness and unexpectedness of the death, illness or accident. In addition, there will usually have been no time to establish a relationship with the person beforehand or warn him or her that the news is serious. The situation can be complicated by the fact that the victim may be young, the next of kin may be difficult to contact or the environment cannot be controlled in a busy accident and emergency department or intensive care unit (McLauchlan, 1990). In these situations the police may be a useful source of help in contacting and supporting relatives.

Conclusions

Giving sad and bad news in medicine will always remain a part of the doctor's role. Good communication skills, good training and guidelines can help doctors do this better (Fallowfield and Jenkins, 2004).

Stop and think

- How would you have broken the news to John?
- What factors might have caused John to react the way he did?
- If you were the ward sister, what would you do to help John now?

Case study

John is a 34-year-old man getting married next year. For the past 2 years he has periodically experienced pins and needles in his arms and legs. Although his fiancée and family urged him to go to the doctor, he had shrugged the symptoms off. In the last few weeks, however, an episode of blurred vision and a temporary loss of power in his right leg precipitated his referral to a neurologist by his GP. A series of tests confirmed a diagnosis of multiple sclerosis. Unfortunately the neurologist was unable to give the news himself because of a prior commitment. He, therefore, asked a junior colleague to break the bad news in his place. This worried the colleague because he had never had to do this before. To minimize his anxiety, he decided he would do it whilst taking blood from John. This would give them both something to concentrate on. On hearing the news, John was devastated. He began to cry and then became angry with the doctor. He demanded to see the consultant. Not knowing how to respond to this reaction, the doctor left to find the ward sister.

Breaking bad news

- Ensure the person is physically able to take in the news.
- Find a quiet room where the news can be broken in privacy and without disturbance.
- Allow the person to be accompanied by a friend, relative or staff member.
- Check what the person already knows, understands and requires to know further.
- Give warning to alert the person that the news is serious.
- Continue giving information if the person is understanding and responding positively.
- Monitor the person's reaction and respond.
- Plan next course of action with the person and always arrange follow-up.

49 | Self-care

People experiencing physical discomfort or emotional distress do not always turn to a doctor for advice and treatment. In all societies there is a range of ways in which people either care for themselves or seek help from others. Kleinman (1985) has suggested that health care systems are composed of different sectors or arenas – popular, folk and professional – although these partly overlap (Fig. 49.1). In Western industrialized societies, doctors certainly do not see all the illness and disease that occurs in a community. Indeed, they only see what has been called the tip of the iceberg (see pp. 86–87). This means that there is a considerable amount of unmet need (see pp. 150–151) in families and in the wider community, where people may be experiencing health issues that might respond to medical treatment.

There are different approaches (and philosophies) to care in the professional sector but most are based on a biomedical model (see pp. 2–3). Many people are dealing with a range of both self-limiting and chronic illness themselves by using self-care (the popular sector) or complementary treatments (the folk sector – also see pp. 144–145) based on a range of different philosophical beliefs. We can begin to understand self-care in more detail by looking at the popular sector.

The popular sector

The popular sector is where ill health is first recognized and defined by people themselves. It is also where much ill health is treated and where various health maintenance activities take place (e.g. taking exercise, ensuring a healthy diet or taking vitamin supplements). It includes all the therapeutic options that people use without consulting either medical or folk/complementary practitioners (see pp. 144–145). Three components of the popular sector are important: (1) the lay referral system, (2) self-care and (3) self-help groups.

The lay referral system

Most people discuss their symptoms with someone else, whether this is a friend or relative. Some people in the community have an important place in these lay networks (e.g. those with experience of an illness, raising children and/or those who are or were health professionals). This system of lay referral may influence health and illness behaviours. For instance, if the network or subculture is incongruent with doctors, in terms of beliefs and situation,

there may be a low rate of uptake of medical services (McKinlay, 1973; Freidson, 1975). Alternatively friends and family may encourage attendance at a health professional's surgery or hospital.

Self-care

How people deal with illness themselves will depend on their beliefs, attitudes, resources and access to formal health care. It is estimated that around 80% of care is self-care. Self-care, and specifically self-medication, is a large and important part of the popular sector. It can include both over-the-counter medicines and home remedies. Recent evidence suggests that people want to be more active self-carers and would welcome more guidance from professionals or peers to increase their confidence in self-care. The Self-Care Forum (www.selfcareforum.org), set up in 2010, provides advice to health professionals wishing to support self-care.

Case study *Self-care forum – supporting self-care*

1. Recognize that self-care is one of the few effective strategies for the management of demand.
2. Agree the advice health professionals will give when asked about common self-limiting illnesses (e.g. chickenpox, head lice, vaginal itch etc.)
3. Involve local pharmacists and community nurses in giving the same advice and support for self-care.
4. Involve all doctors and nurses in reviewing policy related to prescribing antibiotics to ensure consistency, best practice and fairness – always consider NICE guidance.
5. Review policy on psychologically active drugs and 'talking therapies' too ensure consistency, best practice and fairness.
6. Use reviews of long-term conditions to inform and educate patients, carers and their families on the aims of, and choices to make in, managing their condition, including relapses.
7. Involve patient participation groups and other users of services to design, plan and gain feedback on your self-care initiatives.
8. Use websites, emails and display areas to offer high quality self-care information.
9. Consider using self-management courses such as the Expert Patient programme to empower some of your patients with long–term conditions.
10. Encourage health professionals to learn how to assess a patient's self-care status and to identify when they are most receptive to self-care information.

NICE, National Institute for Health and Clinical Excellence.

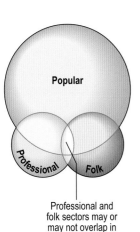

Fig. 49.1 Three sectors of health care. *(From Kleinman, 1985, with permission).*

Popular

Professional Folk

Professional and folk sectors may or may not overlap in particular local settings

There is growing evidence that supporting self-care leads to improved health and quality of life, increases in patient satisfaction and fewer consultations (see spread Quality of life, pp. 50–51).

Stop and think

People may well be experts about their own illnesses, and they certainly may well have self-treated before contacting a GP about symptoms.

• Why is it important for a GP to ask a patient: 'What have you done so far?' or 'What matters to you?'

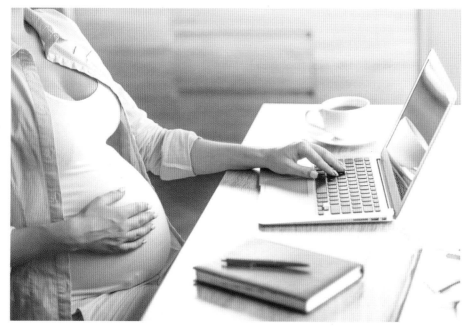

Fig. 49.2 Women helping themselves: searching online for advice on health pregnancy and childbirth. *iStock.com/vadimguzhva*

Self-help groups

A third component of the popular sector is self-help (see pp. 154–155). Self-help groups in relation to health have grown in recent years, often providing an alternative to formal medical care. Self-help groups can often be divided into two broad categories – those with a primary campaigning 'outer' focus and those whose 'inner' focus is to help members (Katz and Bender, 1976). In the health field they cover almost every chronic (e.g. Ileostomy Support Group), lifelong (e.g. Cystic Fibrosis Trust) or mental health (e.g. MIND) condition. Other groups exist for those experiencing traumatic life events, including bereavement (e.g. Compassionate Friends or SANDS, a charity for the support of families with miscarriage, stillbirth and new born deaths).

Self-help groups include mutual support and help. Members have a common experience of the problem, and there is no distinction made between helper and helped. Reciprocity and the sharing of problems is an important part of self-help, as is learning from those who have learned to live with the particular condition. Groups may provide important information or advice to members and may help people overcome stigma or feelings of being different. This type of self-help group should foster the empowerment of its members. Some self-help groups don't even meet in in the physical world as they are solely internet-based. For example, the online group for pregnant women and new mothers called 'Netmums' (https://www.netmums.com/). Netmums advertises itself as the UK's "biggest parenting website offering local info, expert parenting advice, chat, competitions, recipes and friendly support (Fig. 49.2)." The internet offers many opportunities for self-help groups to flourish and can be particularly helpful for those with rare conditions or mobility problems or living in rural areas (see pp. 158–159).

Practical application

Recognition of the vast amount of health care that takes place in the popular sector is important both for doctors working in the community and for those planning health care services. When self-care represents appropriate treatment, doctors should respect this expertise if someone does eventually consult them. Reassurance that the initial response to symptoms is appropriate is one way of doing this; and education about other options helps develop a patient's own resources for care is another. It is also important for doctors to recognize the value of self-help groups in their area and to alert patients to them. This may be particularly important for people living with a chronic illness, although other problems and conditions are also relevant.

Self-care

- Most illness does not come to the attention of doctors but is dealt with by people through self-care.
- Doctors can do more to support patients wishing to self-care. The community pharmacist is an important figure in self-care strategies.
- There are a multitude of self-help groups, based on mutual aid and support.
- With more self-helps groups available online people with rarer conditions, those with mobility problems and those living in remote areas are more likely to access support to continue their self care.

50 | Patient experience

The patient experience may be defined as 'the range of interactions that patients have with the health care system, including their care from health plans, and from doctors, nurses and staff in hospitals, … and other health care facilities' (see www.ahrq.gov). The major features of what a patient is likely to experience when they consult professional health care givers are vital for a doctor to understand. With an appreciation of the probable 'journey' that your patient may have travelled through the health care system, it is more likely you will identify the myriad of issues that are raised for the patient from their perspective. The typical stages of care are outlined (Box 50.1). These many aspects identified from the patient experience are dealt with in some detail in other areas of this book and will be referred to. The aim is to alert you to the use of behavioural sciences in identifying these key issues from the patient's viewpoint.

Link between patient experience and health outcome

Why focus on the 'patient experience'? The answer is that patients who report a good experience of their health intervention tend to show better outcomes. This link has been recently acknowledged by research bodies and auditors who have stated that the assessment of quality health care should note carefully the patient experience. The association has been challenged, however, to such an extent that the criticisms of relying on patient's accounts of their experience has been classified under three main points. Each of the criticisms includes a short rejoinder:

1. Patient lack medical training. *This is refuted as patient satisfaction measures are linked to adherence to clinical guidelines.*
2. Patients base their rating of experience on their health status. That is, patients with poorer health status would report poorer experiences of their care. *There is very limited empirical support for this statement.*
3. Patients report dissatisfaction if they do not get the treatment they expected. *The data, however, are contrary to this statement as patients who report better satisfaction is unrelated to the number of treatments provided.* (Manary et al., 2013)

Living with chronic disease

The experiences of patients, as listed in Box 50.1, will vary enormously according to whether their condition develops from an acute phase to a chronic phase. The expectations of the patient will require substantial change when contemplating a time-limited disease process to one where their condition is not resolvable in the short term. Patients with a chronic illness will experience

Box 50.1 **Patient journey**	
1	Sensations
2	Symptoms
3	Seek advice
4	Have tests
5	Told diagnosis
6	Receive treatment
7	Recover
8	Rehabilitate

health care that is designed principally to assist the management of living with the illness, coping with symptoms such as pain and adjusting to changes of life circumstances (relationship, family and work situations).

Reaction to life-changing diagnosis

The experience of patients with their doctors when given a life-threatening or life changing diagnosis is critical for the subsequent engagement with the health services. (see section Breaking bad news, pages 96–97). Briefly, the patient experiences a combination of shock, disbelief and poor retention of the facts and supporting information (see Cases). The careful attention by the health team members to their communication with the patient is vital (see section Clinical communication skills, pages 94–95). Hence the call by many practitioners to develop a strong patient-centred approach (see section Seeing the doctor, pages 88–89). Patients vary in their information requirements. Some value as much detail as possible, whereas others prefer to limit these to bare essentials. The doctor is recommended to ask the patient about their preference. Likewise similar variations in patient wishes are found with their interest to share decisions on their care, and this will have a strong impact on the experience of care (see section Setting priorities and rationing, pages 152–153).

When patients experience symptoms, they tap into previous experiences of illness of themselves or friends and relatives. These take the form of illness representations that have been outlined in the Common Sense Model (CSM) of illness by Leventhal (Leventhal et al., 2016). The illness representations reflect a knowledge base (consisting of correct facts and also inaccuracies) and also an emotional response (e.g. anxiety, disgust, sorrow, anger or frustration). These representations form an integral part of the patient experience and trigger a number of typical coping responses, including denial, avoidance of the symptom and its meaning or acceptance and agreement to follow advice on management or treatment of the symptoms. After attempts to cope with the changed perception of health as experienced by the patient, a further stage results. This forms an appraisal process where patients assess their coping responses and decide if they have succeeded or otherwise. This cycle of symptom experience, developing illness representations, coping and appraisal are cornerstones to Leventhal's CSM (Fig. 50.1). The understanding by the health care team of these processes experienced by the patient can improve communication and development of advice and treatment planning.

Medically unexplained symptoms

Patients with no organic indication of their complaint are defined as patients with medically unexplained symptoms (MUS). Health care use by patients with MUS accessing primary care patients has been estimated to be significantly greater. This places a large burden on health services. It is known that common complaints tend to resolve themselves with 50% of all outpatient visits triggered by common symptoms such as cough, dizziness, fatigue and pain. Approximately 75% patients presenting with these complaints report improvements in 2 weeks, no matter what their symptom, and at least a fifth of all symptoms are medically unexplained. It is critical for the patient experience to be listened to by the health care team and all symptoms taken seriously. However, sensitive approaches will need to be utilized by the

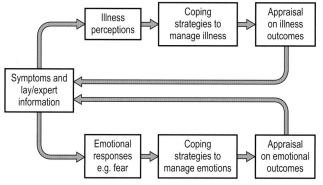

Fig. 50.1 Schematic diagram of Leventhal's Common Sense Model.

Behaviour	Survey responses (preferred)	Video observations (actual)
Pt names		
First (e.g. Jane)	50%	14%
Last (e.g. Ms Smith)	17%	33%
Both (e.g. Jane Smith)	24%	3%
DK	9%	0
Not mentioned by Dr	0	50%

Table 50.1 Preferences of patients on how they wished to be greeted and the actual behaviour shown by doctors

DK, Don't know; Dr, doctor; Pt, patient.

From Makoul, G et al., 2007 with permission.

doctor to assuage real concerns as experienced by patients and, in many cases, their families and relatives.

Doctor's behaviour

There are some clear findings that have shown that the way doctors behave with their patients has a long-lasting and important bearing on the patient experience. The system of care and its quality and management has shown some poor linkages with assessments of the patient experience. This was shown in one of the largest studies examining these relationships (Groene et al., 2015) The importance of communication skills is paramount, and the sensitive use of some key elements of social behaviour that have been modified into the clinical setting can have far-reaching effects on patient satisfaction and on being understood and treated medically competently (Street, 2013). Hence careful attention paid to the patient experience through the elaborate use of communication skills will increase the probability of good outcomes. There are attempts to make recommendations to doctors of good practice through the publication of professionally inspired and created guidelines. The observance of these widely publicised guidelines is a matter of professional audit and debate. However, some relatively simple observations such as the use of greetings with patients in practice serve as an interesting example to illustrate the discrepancy between the perceived and actual behaviours of doctors. The starting point of the doctor–patient interaction might be a suitable point for detailed inspection of an aspect of the patient experience.

Stop and think

- In your contact with patients during community or hospital placements, how do you refer to your patients? By forename, last name or full name and with or without title? How would you determine which approach the patient prefers?

Greetings in medical encounters

The first contact with patients is a vital start in the process of health care, and the evidence base is not advanced to recommend how to greet new patients. In a study that compared patient

preferences (n ≡ 415) to actual events studied from video of interactions (n ≡ 123) between doctors and patients, it was clear that patients tended to prefer (56%) being called by first and last names. It was found that 50% of doctors did not use either of the patients' names (Table 50.1). For safety and preference purposes it is advisable to call the patient by both names. Approximately three-quarters of patients preferred to shake hands with their doctor, and the video confirmation of around 80% was shown. Doctors would be performing well if they did shake their patient's hand, although with the proviso that they watch for non-verbal signals that indicate that this would not be appreciated by the patient (Makoul et al., 2007).

Case study *Reactions to diagnosis*

Woman with breast cancer (approximately 50 years of age): 'I've always heard that people seeing a doctor can switch off from bad news. I actually didn't realise I'd done it, but I'd had one sentence came out of him, and I completely blanked.'

Man with prostate cancer (approximately 65 years of age): 'I was absolutely devastated. There was no real information at all. I was basically told, 'You've got prostate cancer, and it's at an advanced stage. I only wish somebody would have sat down with me initially and gone through all that with me.'

Patient experience

- The patient experience is a crucial aspect of health care delivery and outcome assessment.
- Care provided for acute and chronic conditions brings very different elements of the patient experience.
- Patients report symptoms and have their own illness representations based on facts and an elaborate set of beliefs. The CSM presents a helpful framework of how patients experience illness, cope and appraise their attempts to manage their illness.
- Many symptoms are not the result of organic changes, and are classified as MUS; however, patients experience them as very real sensations that need to be managed by doctors.
- Good communication skills are essential to assist with doctor–patient interactions and relate positively to the patient experience.
- Doctors' behaviour is implicitly linked to the patient experience and requires close attention.

Psychological preparation for surgery is important because it has been shown to reduce anxiety and to improve recovery in the post-operative period (e.g. reduce pain and time to return to normal activities).

Anxiety

Anxiety is an unpleasant emotion associated with threatening situations or thinking about threat. People differ in the degree to which they experience anxiety when facing challenges such as surgery. High anxiety makes it more difficult for the patient to understand information and to cooperate fully with instructions and can interfere with psychological and physiological recovery processes, including wound healing (see stress spread, pp. 125–126).

Anxiety in surgical patients

Patients are anxious before surgery for a number of reasons: they have an illness requiring surgery; they have to undergo the surgical procedure; and there may be uncertainty about the outcome and the likely speed of recovery. In addition, patients worry about being away from home and how their family is coping, as well as continuing to worry about their usual preoccupations such as money and relationships. For some patients, anxiety persists after surgery, and it may be that worries such as how they will cope with being discharged home have a part to play (Carr et al., 2005).

Anxiety before surgery has been found to relate to many post-operative outcomes, including distress, pain, use of analgesics, physiological functioning, return to normal activities and length of hospital stay. Therefore methods of reducing anxiety are likely to improve patient outcomes.

Methods of psychological preparation

A variety of methods of preparing people for surgery have been developed. Some methods are aimed directly at reducing anxiety, whilst other methods guide what the patient does. They are typically administered on the day before surgery, although some have been used in outpatient visits prior to admission. Some of these methods can be delivered to groups of patients, and others incorporate the use of booklets, audio and video tapes/DVDs. Methods used are discussed below.

Information giving
Procedural information

Patients are informed about the procedures they will undergo, when they will happen and where they will be: e.g. they might be told about waking in the recovery room and the possibility of having a drip or catheter.

Sensation information

Patients are informed about the sensations they are likely to experience: e.g. they might be told that pre-medication will not necessarily make them feel drowsy or that after major abdominal operations, they may experience pain caused by wind.

Behavioural instruction

Behavioural instruction involves telling patients about things they can do to facilitate the procedure or their post-procedure recovery.

For example, they may be taught how to cough without pulling on the wound incision or how to turn over in bed without causing unnecessary pain.

Cognitive interventions

Cognitive interventions aim to change how the patient thinks. Based on the assumption that patients' thoughts about what is happening may either raise or reduce their anxiety, interventions aim to encourage more adaptive cognitions. For example, patients may be trained to re-interpret events in a more positive manner: e.g. a patient thinking that a doctor passing the end of her bed is a sign that her condition is giving rise to concern may, after training, propose that this is a sign that she is making progress. Or she may be trained to use techniques that have been useful in other situations: e.g. if the patient reports that distraction has been useful in previous anxiety-provoking situations, she may be advised on how to use such a technique before and after surgery.

Relaxation/hypnosis

Patients can practise a variety of general relaxation procedures and hypnotic techniques before surgery, even when in bed, sometimes using audio-recorded instructions.

Emotion-focussed/psychotherapeutic discussion

Patients are invited to discuss their worries, either one to one with a therapist or in groups including other patients. There are no clearly specified instructions for this type of intervention, but they generally aim to help patients manage their feelings, for example, by putting them into context of past experiences or by helping patients to understand their emotions and give them meaning.

Modelling

This method, which is most commonly used with children, involves showing the patient a film of a similar-aged patient going through various stages of the surgical procedures. The method communicates a considerable amount of procedural information and may demonstrate use of any of the other methods.

Results of psychological preparation

The first properly controlled trial of presurgery anxiety reduction randomly allocated 97 patients to special preparation or normal care (Egbert et al., 1964). The specially prepared group had less pain and used fewer analgesics post-operatively, and their hospital stay was, on average, 2.7 days shorter than that for patients in the control group.

The results of studies involving comparison of groups randomly allocated to psychological preparation versus normal care have been aggregated using meta-analysis and clear benefits for patients have been demonstrated (Johnston and Vögele, 1993). Fig. 51.1 shows the mean difference between the psychologically prepared and control groups, expressed in units of standard deviations (with 95% confidence intervals) for each outcome.

The group receiving psychological preparation showed statistically significant benefits where the mean difference is greater than zero and where the confidence interval does not pass through zero. Thus there is evidence of benefit on measures of

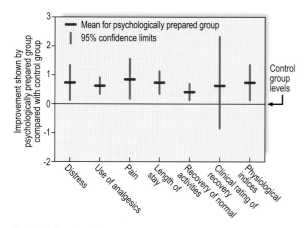

Fig. 51.1 Benefits of psychological preparation for surgery. This is a summary of 40 clinical trials *(diagram based on data from Johnston and Vögele, 1993)*.

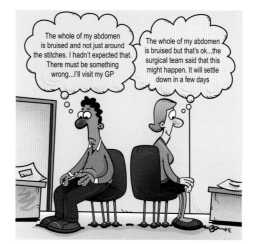

Fig. 51.2 Preparation for post-discharge recovery: Impact of worry on health-service use and the benefits of sensory information.

distress; pain; use of analgesics; physiological indices, such as heart rate and blood pressure; behavioural indices, including resumption of normal activities; and length of hospital stay. Clinical ratings of recovery did not show a reliable difference. One might have expected to find improved patient satisfaction, but too few studies have examined this variable to draw conclusions.

Since this 1993 meta-analysis was conducted, many more studies have been conducted, and surgical and hospital procedures have evolved. A more recent systematic review and meta-analysis found that psychological preparation was associated with lower post-operative pain, length of stay and negative emotion, but many studies were poorly reported (Powell et al., 2016). An example of a study included in the review is by Yang et al. (2012). The authors demonstrated that an intervention that included a high level of procedural information (e.g. explaining procedures that occur in the intensive care unit) and sensory information (e.g. about possible throat irritation caused by the trachea tube) resulted in lower post-operative anxiety than for control participants who received the standard preparation that included less detailed procedural information.

Preparation for the post-discharge period

It is important that information covers not only the immediate surgical procedure but also the postsurgery recovery process. Many surgical procedures (e.g. elective inguinal hernia repair surgery) are now carried out with a minimal stay in hospital for the patient – some even undergo such procedures as day-case patients. This means that many patients are discharged very quickly to their home environment where they do not have immediate access to professional medical support. Some post-surgical experiences such as swelling and extensive bruising may be seen as part of the normal recovery process by medical professionals, but if the patient is not aware that such symptoms are normal, further concern is likely to result and further medical help sought (Powell et al. 2009; Fig. 51.2). Thus, providing patients with a good understanding of what is to be expected after surgery can minimize anxiety and conserve health care resources (see Patient Experience spread, pp. 100–101).

Case study

Mr Jones was admitted to a surgical ward for abdominal surgery. He was anxious about the procedure and particularly concerned about undergoing anaesthesia. On the morning of surgery, he could not contain his anxiety and discharged himself. He returned to his general practitioner (GP) as a patient who required surgery but could not tolerate the procedures.

The GP referred Mr Jones to a psychologist who used psychological preparation procedures involving relaxation training and cognitive techniques. Mr Jones was trained to use relaxation as a distraction technique, especially when experiencing worrying thoughts. He was taught to recognize negative thoughts such as 'What if I die during surgery?' and to deal with them by thinking of counteracting thoughts such as 'I've never heard of that happening to anyone I know – why should it happen to me?'

Mr Jones was able to return to the surgeon and to proceed with treatment without further interruption.

Stop and think

- Although the benefits of psychological methods of preparing patients for surgery have been known for at least 20 years, they have not been widely implemented. Why might this be?

The limitations in implementing these techniques may be due to lack of appropriately trained staff. Alternatively some staff may be trained in how to prepare patients for surgery but feel they do not have the time to spend with a patient. The development of booklets, audio-recorded instructions or internet-based resources may facilitate the use of these techniques but such approaches need to be fully evaluated.

Psychological preparation for surgery

- Patients are anxious before and after surgery.
- High pre-operative anxiety is predictive of poor post-operative outcome.
- A variety of methods has been developed for preparing patients for surgery (e.g. information-giving, behavioural instruction, cognitive coping, relaxation, emotion-focussed discussion and modelling).
- These methods have been shown to improve post-operative outcomes in well-controlled clinical trials.

Coronary heart disease (CHD), sometimes called ischaemic heart disease (IHD) or coronary artery disease (CAD), is a disease in which plaque builds up in the coronary arteries (atherosclerosis). Specific conditions within CHD include (unstable) angina pectoris and myocardial infarction (MI). Angina pectoris refers to a sensation of tightness or chest pain caused by a brief obstruction or constriction of a coronary artery, but this pain is relieved during rest. In unstable angina the pain does not go away, even during rest. MI refers to death of heart muscle (myocardium) as a result of blockage of a coronary artery that prevents oxygen reaching the myocardium.

The main medical interventions are (1) pharmacological (medications to reduce blood pressure, prevent clotting and reduce serum (blood) cholesterol); (2) revascularization: percutaneous coronary interventions (PCI), coronary artery bypass grafts (CABG); (3) cardiac rehabilitation; and (4) life style interventions.

Causation and prevention

CHD is the leading cause of death worldwide and a major cause of morbidity and loss of quality of life (see Health: a global perspective, pp. 156–157). Major well-established risk factors are smoking, hypertension and high serum cholesterol. Additional lifestyle risk factors include poor diet, overweight/obesity (see pp. 106–107) and psychological factors such as hostility, stress and distress (see pp. 112–113).

The Systematic COronary Risk Evaluation (SCORE), developed by the European Society of Cardiology, is a useful tool for estimating cardiovascular risk. The risk estimation (10-year risk of CVD) is based on a number of risk factors: age, gender, smoking status, systolic blood pressure and total cholesterol. Separate risk charts are available for countries categorised as low and high risk (https://www.escardio.org/static_file/Escardio/Subspecialty/EACPR/Documents/score-charts.pdf).

The type A behaviour pattern (competitive, time-urgent and hostile) was identified in the 1960s as typical of the coronary-prone individual. Subsequent research has indicated that high hostility alone is the factor most associated with greater risk of CHD (see Personality and health, pp. 18–19 and What is stress?, pp. 126–127). In surveys, patients and healthy populations believe stress to be the commonest cause of MI (see pp. 126–127). The challenge for health professionals is to also educate the population about the importance of behaviours such as smoking in heart disease (see Changing cognitions and behaviour, pp. 72–73 and Smoking, tobacco control and doctors, pp. 82–83).

CHD is related to socio-economic disadvantage (see pp. 42–43). This may be due, in part, to patterns of smoking, diet and stressful work experience, as lower socio-economic groups smoke more, have a poorer diet and are more likely to have jobs where they have little control and high demands compared with those in the higher socio-economic groups. CHD is also the major cause of death for both women and men in Western countries (see pp. 156–157). Whilst awareness of CHD (once considered a male disease) has increased among women in recent years, a challenge is they may present with different symptoms of heart disease compared with men. Similarly, symptoms that doctors attribute to cardiac conditions in men are sometimes attributed to other conditions when presented by female patients (see Gender and health, pp. 44–45). This effect is more common when doctors are working in stressful, time-pressured settings (see Life as a trainee doctor, pp. 162–163).

CHD mortality has been declining in many Western countries in recent years. This can be attributed to both treatments (medication and interventions) and lifestyle changes. However, in recent years the importance of looking at CHD mortality by age has been emphasized because reductions in the mortality rate in some age groups may obscure less positive trends in other age groups. These differences may reflect higher levels of obesity (see pp. 106–107), lower levels of physical activity, an increase in type 2 diabetes in younger adults and smoking levels amongst younger adults. Some researchers have cautioned that these negative trends could begin to slow the previously observed decline in mortality rates within younger age groups.

Stop and think

As a doctor, what differences in stress levels and/or psychological well-being might you expect in a patient of 80 with a MI compared to patients younger than 40?

Response to symptoms and myocardial infarction

Individuals may often misinterpret symptoms. A large number of patients referred to cardiology departments present with non-cardiac chest pain, probably resulting from anxiety about physical symptoms. Equally, many patients experiencing an MI do not recognize the symptoms and delay seeking help, even when they have experienced MI before (see Deciding to consult, pp. 86–87). Given the importance of early revascularization, such delays may critically determine the patient's treatment and survival (see Case study). A rapid response ensures more effective treatment and, therefore, better outcomes.

MI is a sudden life-threatening event, and many patients experience high levels of anxiety and depression after MI. Close family members may be even more distressed than the patient in the early period whilst the patient is in hospital. These high levels of distress are unrelated to the severity of the MI and may persist for months or years. Both anxiety and depression are associated with increased risk of further MI and mortality post-discharge, with depression (see pp. 114–115) conferring higher risk than anxiety symptoms. This increased risk is independent of severity of MI or other CHD risk factors (Pogosova et al., 2015). Despite the fact that 20% of post-MI patients would have major depression, identification of depression in these settings is poor. However, two brief screening questions can help:

1. "During the past month, have you often been bothered by feeling down, depressed, or hopeless?"
2. "During the past month, have you often been bothered by little interest or pleasure in doing things?"

If a patient answers 'no' to both, you can be confident that they are not depressed. However, a 'yes' response requires further investigation (see also Health screening, pp. 66–67).

Cardiac rehabilitation

Cardiac rehabilitation programmes have been shown to:

- Reduce psychological distress for patients and their families
- Improve cardiovascular fitness

- Reduce mortality and hospital readmissions (by 13%–31%) (Heran et al., 2011)
- Increase rate of return to paid employment
- Reduce health service costs

Benefits from such programmes persist for years. Programmes may involve education, exercise, dietary and vocational counselling and psychological components such as stress management. The addition of psychological components to exercise- and education-based programmes results in greater patient benefit (see Helping people to act on their intentions, pp. 74–75).

Patients and their families are often anxious about resuming physical activity after a cardiac event or intervention. Routine testing and rehabilitation classes can promote patient self-efficacy (i.e. belief in their own ability to complete behaviours successfully). For instance, a study where spouses were allowed to observe routine treadmill testing to assess cardiovascular fitness increased both patient and spouse self-efficacy in the patient's ability to engage in energetic activities (see Adherence, pp. 92–93). Assessed at follow-up, those with higher self-efficacy (and not necessarily those who did best on the exercise text) were more physically active, in line with doctors' advice, in the weeks after the test (see Self-care, pp. 98–99).

Stop and think

- Psychological factors are involved in many aspects of CHD. How might a psychologist contribute to the work of a cardiology department?

Response to stressful medical procedures

Medical procedures may be stressful as a result of the discomfort or pain experienced as well as the uncertainty about the outcomes. Psychological preparation can reduce the stressfulness of procedures and improve outcomes (see Psychological preparation for surgery, pp. 102–103, and Cognitive-behavioural therapy, pp. 138–139). These principles can be applied in coronary care settings when patients are being prepared for CABG surgery and PCI. Research has also shown that patients can provide important role models for other patients in ways that can speed recovery. Pre-operative cardiac surgery patients randomized to share a double room with a post-operative patient having the same surgery were found to be less anxious before the surgery and to recover more quickly after the procedure. They also became more active more rapidly post-operatively and were discharged earlier than control patients (Kulik et al., 1996).

Case study *Delay to treatment for symptoms of a myocardial infarction*

On the way home from restaurant, Mrs MacDonald feels pressure in her chest. She thinks it unlikely to be anything more serious than indigestion at her age (51 years). She does not like to mention it, as it would spoil the evening. Going upstairs to bed the pain intensifies, and she comes out in a cold sweat, so she lies down to see if she feels better. Her husband worries that it is a heart attack, but Mrs MacDonald says: 'I don't think so – women don't have heart attacks. It's more likely to be the menopause!' After some hours of increasing symptoms, she calls an ambulance. Unfortunately, by the time she gets to hospital, she has already had substantial damage to her myocardial (heart) muscle and so will not benefit as much from available cardiac interventions as she might have by presenting earlier.

Heart disease

- CHD may be prevented or delayed by changes in behaviour and lifestyles.
- Socio-economic disadvantage and stress are associated with higher incidences of CHD.
- Patients may fail to recognize the symptoms of MI, with resulting delays in seeking medical treatment.
- Anxiety and depression are common responses to MI of both patients and their partners and family.
- Depression and anxiety after MI are an independent predictors of mortality.
- Cardiac rehabilitation, including psychological components, enhances patient outcomes and survival.
- Psychological preparation for medical procedures reduces their stressfulness and improves post-operative recovery.

Malnutrition, as in malfunctioning, means incorrect/inappropriate nutrition. The term covers both consuming too much and too little food. Although many use the term 'malnutrition' to refer specifically to under-nutrition. In low-income countries, many would immediately think of starving children with hunger oedema, but a far greater problem is the chronic under-nutrition suffered by many more people. In terms of overnutrition, it is no understatement to say that obesity is the greatest public health problem of our time in high-income countries such as the UK and the USA. Whether someone is under- or over-nourished is not simply an issue of weight. We generally use weight categories that are measured by BMI (body mass index). BMI is weight in kilograms (kg) divided by height in meters squared (m²). This classification has five categories (Box 53.1), although sometimes six (see spread Eating, body shape and health, pp. 84–85).

Ordinary people find it hard to work out their BMI. Even if you know how to do the calculation many people over-estimate their height and under-estimate their weight. Upper arm circumference, clothes size, or waist line, might be easier to understand, but each of these ways of classifying healthy versus unhealthy body sizes has its own disadvantage as a measurement.

The BMI for children is calculated the same way as for adults, but there are no agreed BMI cut-off points defining overweight and obesity. Instead, overweight and obesity in children can be classified into percentiles (Box 53.2).

Undernutrition

People are undernourished if their diet does not provide adequate calories and protein for growth and maintenance or if they are unable to absorb the food as a result of illness that they would normally take in. Under-nutrition can affect every system of the body such as the muscular system (resulting in fatigue, lethargy and decreased peripheral and respiratory muscle strength), the immune system (predisposing to poor recovery from infection) and psycho-social function, including anxiety and depression (Schenker, 2003). Under-nutrition is an important factor in morbidity and mortality in low-income countries (see Health: a global perspective, pp. 156–157). In addition, it is a problem in rich countries, in specific patients' groups, e.g. older adults in hospitals; people living with specific conditions are at a greater risk, including people with learning difficulties or those living with HIV or anorexia. It has been suggested that 70% of undernutrition in the UK goes unrecognised and therefore untreated (Schenker, 2003). As a doctor it is important to recognize that certain diseases can reduce patients' appetite or change their taste, smell and preferences for particular foods.

Obesity

Obesity is body fat deposition simply resulting from having a greater calorie intake than expansion. In brief, people are using less energy through physical activity than they take in through eating. Obesity at a population level is a public health problem. Underlying causes include the increasing availability of cheap calories in fast food restaurants and convenience delivery companies, processed food and increased portion sizes (affected by marketing) and energy density. At the same time many people experience an increasingly sedentary lifestyle, both at work and at home. Fewer people have a physically demanding job; many of us have office jobs and use labour-saving machinery in the home and workplace. Moreover, in our leisure time we spend more hours playing computer games and/or watching television. Many have gotten used to driving cars over relatively short distances. Calories are too cheap, and calorie-rich food with low nutritional status is often too easily available.

Obesity is a medical problem in itself, as it is an illness, especially morbid obesity. Moreover, obesity is also a risk factor for a range of other medical conditions such as cardio-vascular disease (see pp. 104–105), chronic obstructive pulmonary disease (see pp.128–129), diabetes (see pp. 124–125) or cancer (see pp. 110–111). In addition, obesity can also have a highly detrimental effect on people's general well-being. Some question whether obesity is a psychological disorder. Obesity is associated with several common disabilities such as arthritis, mental illness, learning disabilities and lower back pain. At the same time being overweight might be protective against fractures in women in later life, and there is some evidence that fit fat men live longer than unfit slim men.

Obesity is also a social cost, hospitals are required to invest in special operating theatres, ambulances and so on, which can take the physical bulk and weight of severely obese patients. Obese people are more likely to die in a car crash than people in similar accidents who have a lower range of BMI.

Dealing with obesity

Obesity is not only a physiological issue, it is often also a psychological one. The former would suggest medical solutions that may include bariatric surgery, gastric bands, stomach stapling, appetite suppressing drugs and so on.

Psychological interventions used in weight management include cognitive therapy, psychotherapy, relaxation therapy, hypnosis and behaviour therapy. The key aim of many psychological interventions is to increase the individual's self-esteem and self-worth, reduce anxiety and increase self-efficacy. The last includes the person's confidence in their own ability to reduce snacks and calorific intake and to manage relapses such as the occasional binge-eating episodes. Psychological theories and the

Box 53.1 Body mass index (BMI) categories (adults)

BMI	Category
Lower than 18.5	Underweight
18.5–24.9	Ideal
25–29.9	Overweight
30–39.9	Obese
40 and higher	Very obese

Box 53.2 Body mass index (BMI) categories (children)

BMI percentile cut-off	Category
At or below 2nd percentile	At risk of underweight
Above 2nd percentile and below 85th percentile	Healthy weight
At or above 85th percentile and below 95th percentile	At risk of overweight
At or above 95th percentile and below 98th percentile	At risk of obesity

From http://www.gov.scot/Resource/0046/00464858.pdf.

behaviour they promote appear to be useful when combined with dietary and exercise strategies.

What we really need is to encourage lifestyle changes with the aim of the general public health message – to make the healthy option the easy option. The National Institute for Health and Clinical Excellence (NICE) points out that even small reductions in weight, especially delivered by relatively inexpensive interventions can be cost effective if this weight loss is maintained. The solution to the obesity problem is prevention and weight management. Both prevention and weight management should be addressed at an individual level or at a societal level. The key strategies of obesity prevention are simple, dietary change and increased physical activity, or a combination of both. At an even more basic level the strategy would be to take in fewer calories or use up more calories, or a combination of both. The public health messages for this approach are fairly easy to understand, so why is it so difficult to change behaviour (see Helping people to act on their intentions, pp. 74–75)? One barrier to healthy eating might be low income. Poor people spent a greater proportion of their income on food compared with rich people. Therefore poorer people are more 'price sensitive' to the cost of certain food items. As the prices of healthy fresh fruit and vegetables are higher than those of processed equivalents, poorer people are 'forced' to choose the unhealthier foods.

Obesity as a social issue

Obesity is not just an individual issue, that is, a burden to the person involved, it is a societal issue, as it is a cost to the NHS and society (see Organizing and funding health care, pp. 148–149). The Foresight Report (2007) predicted that 60% of men, 50% of women and 25% of children in the UK will be obese by 2050. Such costs include more expensive hospital beds, ambulances and crematoria to accommodate the increased size of patients. In short the costs of obesity to both the health system in particular and society in general are considerable, and money spent on treating obesity cannot be spent on anything else (see Setting priorities and rationing, pp. 152–153). A scientific review of the evidence base surrounding obesity concluded that the large rise in the numbers of people affected was an outcome of multiple factors arising largely from exposure to the UK's obeseogenic environment (Butland et al., 2007). The review mentions factors such as our economic, psychosocial and cultural milieu as well as our behavioural responses that arise in response. Yet interventions designed to tackle obesity have overwhelmingly focussed on the role of individual behaviour and our so-called lifestyle choices. Perhaps as a society we need to think more about interventions such as the so-called sugar tax (Fig. 53.1). In 2018 the UK joined a small number of countries which have introduced a tax on sugary drinks to help reduce obesity.

Weight management

Differences between men and women, children, in epidemiological trends and possible solutions (HTA). Adult men and women in the Health Survey for England 2015 were equally likely to be obese (27%), but men were more likely to be overweight (41%) compared to women (31%). Men are less likely to join weight management interventions, but they are more likely to stay and to succeed. As fewer men join such interventions, they

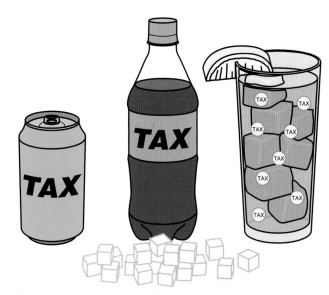

Fig. 53.1 Sugar tax makes unhealthier drinks with loads of sugar more expensive.

are different from the women who have a less engaged population in terms of motivation and staying power. There are online interventions and apps to help people manage their weight through the measurement of food intake, calories and level of exercise (see spread Gender, pp. 44–45). As health professionals it is important to find out why people might want to lose weight. Some may be interested in improving their body image and others in improving their fitness or the chance of seeing grandchildren (see Health beliefs, motivation and behaviour, pp. 70–71). Each of these different factors could be a starting point in a discussion about weight management with a different patient.

How do we define success in weight management? Typically public health interventions run for a couple of years, and participants' weight levels are measured up to a year after the end of the intervention. Several studies have suggested this follow-up period is too short. The reason for this seems to be that the majority of weight management participants return to their pre-intervention BMI within 1 to 5 years (Dansinger et al., 2007; Kraschnewski et al., 2010; Wing et al., 2006).

Stop and think

- What would you do to encourage poorer people to choose healthier diets?
- Why do people eat more than they need to?

Malnutrition and obesity

- Malnutrition refers to both under- and overnutrition
- Obesity is a growing public health issue
- Doctors can help individual patients with and/or refer for weight management.
- Behavioural change techniques can help motivate people to make lifestyle changes
- We need both individual interventions and societal ones to reduce obesity.

Human immunodeficiency virus (HIV) appeared at a time when it was widely believed that science had brought infectious diseases under control, and it seemed that all of a sudden a new incurable disease presented itself. Until recently it was only possible to treat some of the secondary effects of HIV and acquired immune deficiency syndrome (AIDS – the disease stage of most infected people), and since the infection is currently not curable, the main remedy still lies in prevention. Since the virus can be transmitted in different ways (Box 54.1), prevention requires targeting different types of behaviours.

Although HIV is widespread – worldwide 37 million people were living with HIV by late 2016 – it is clear that the infection is not equally spread amongst members of society or between societies. Even within the UK there are regional differences in the proportion of people infected through sexual intercourse between men and intravenous drug use (IDU). The figure for women as a percentage of the total number of people living with HIV, for example, differs from region to region and the proportion of IDU among the people diagnosed with HIV/AIDS in Scotland is higher than in the UK as a whole. Thus certain groups of people have a far higher infection rate than others, depending on different parts of the country.

The disease has distinct social aspects. Firstly, at the social level it involves several taboos such as sex, drugs, and death and dying; consequently it is heavily stigmatized. Secondly, at the personal level, the acceptance of being diagnosed as HIV-positive can be very difficult. People can feel isolated, shocked, frightened, panicked and/or guilty; profess denial; and become depressed, but some also display a sense of coming to terms with themselves and even acceptance. Such emotions are understandable, as people have to accept that they have a long-term illness (in high- and middle-income countries) and/or become more aware of their own mortality (in many low-income countries). Treatment using anti-retroviral drugs is expensive. It was estimated that only 21 million people out the 37 million living with HIV were receiving anti-retroviral treatment by mid-2017, which is particularly a problem in sub-Saharan Africa (see pp. 156–157).

Double stigma

HIV has what is called a double stigma attached. *Stigma* refers to the identification and recognition of a bad or negative characteristic in a person or group of people and the treatment of them with less respect or worth than they deserve as a result of this characteristic (see Labelling and stigma, pp. 60–61). *Double stigma* refers to terminal illness *and* sexually transmitted infection. Stigma is also applicable to cancer and other terminal diseases. Double stigma refers to stigma attached to 'deviant', 'unnatural' or socially undesirable activities such as men having sex with men (MSM), injecting drug use or prostitution. Alonzo and Reynolds (1995) explained that stigma is the 'identification of some sort of moral contamination that causes others to reject the person bearing it'. Thus people living with HIV are regarded as

'dangerous, dirty, foolish and worthless' in comparison with descriptions of patients with cancer or stroke.

Experiencing stigma (stigmatization) may lead to low self-esteem in the infected person, reduced willingness to seek medical and social help and increased difficulty in sharing worries with friends, relatives and neighbours. At the societal level in some countries, fear of HIV/AIDS still exists despite the fact that it has been scientifically demonstrated that AIDS is not communicable by day-to-day social contact. This fear and stigmatization can easily be translated into discrimination and victimization of people with HIV. HIV/AIDS is branded a plague, which implies that people living with HIV are threatening and dangerous, rather than threatened, because they carry the potential to contaminate the healthy through transmission of a contagious disease. This has led to some dentists and doctors refusing treatment in the past, even when safe procedures were available.

Society also often makes a distinction between 'innocent' and 'guilty' victims. It is believed that the people with HIV bring it on themselves through their own doing, and they are blamed for their disease and as a result are branded as 'guilty' victims. In contrast, 'innocent' victims are infected through mistakes by the medical profession or through infected blood. Babies of HIV-infected mothers are included as innocent, whereas their mothers may be seen as guilty.

The use of the phrase 'risk group' reinforces the idea that HIV infection can only happen in certain people. The idea of stressing risky behaviour is far more meaningful both in terms of reducing the stigma attached to being HIV-positive and in terms of preventing the spread of the infection. It is not what people are that puts them at a higher risk, but what people do.

HIV and the media

The media are a major source of information for people, as well as influential in forming or at least confirming people's opinions (see Media and health, pp. 52–53). Many people in industrialized countries will not personally know anyone who is infected with HIV; consequently the perception of the disease is likely to be mediated or even formed by mass media. This includes 'facts' reported and comments made in newspapers, television news and social media and 'fiction' in soap operas and movies.

In an interview with *The Independent* newspaper (3 November 1993, p. 23), Suzanna Dawson, who played the role of the wife of a character who had AIDS in a soap opera, said:

> I've had some terrible experiences of the kind of prejudice HIV-positive people face … I've been slapped and spat at in the street, booed off the field in a charity match … it makes you feel so alone, so scared … I've picked up the phone at 2 a.m. to hear some guy screaming: 'You're a dirty bitch, spreading disease throughout the world'.

The actress (Dawson) suffered this level of abuse even though she was only an actress playing a fictional role.

Psychological issues

One key set of psychological issues centres on the question: 'Who do you tell?' Being diagnosed HIV-positive may involve having to adapt one's behaviour and outlook on life. Telling a partner or family could mean having to admit to injecting drugs, having sex with another man or being sexually unfaithful. Telling your employer might mean losing a job, not necessarily because the

---

Box 54.1 Routes of transmission of HIV

- Unprotected penetrative sex (vaginal, oral or anal)
- Unsterilized needle/syringe previously used by someone infected with HIV
- Mother to child during pregnancy, childbirth and breast-feeding
- Infected blood or tissue transfer
- Receiving semen from an infected man for artificial insemination

employer wants to get rid of you but because your colleagues do not want to work with you any longer. Bringing up the issue of using safer sex methods can also be problematic. It is a difficult enough issue for most, especially at the time of the first sexual intercourse. However, people with HIV might find suggesting the use of condoms with prospective sexual partners difficult because of the fear of being rejected, both emotionally and physically (see pp. 62–63).

Health promotion and HIV

The Joint United Nations Programme on HIV/AIDS (UNAIDS) launched its 'Fast-Track' strategy in 2014 with the '90-90-90 target' to be achieved by 2020, meaning that 90% of people living with HIV know their HIV status; 90% who know their HIV-positive status are on treatment; and, 90% of people on treatment have a suppressed viral load. Box 54.2 lists the current Public Health England advice on HIV testing. The first 90%, that is, of those living with HIV being diagnosed, has not yet been achieved in Scotland in 2016, although the country was not far off, with a testing rate of approximately 85%. It is unlikely that the proportion of people infected being diagnosed is reached in countries with far less organized health care systems. Meanwhile the health promotion message has to be aimed at all men and women who are sexually active, not just the high-risk groups, since (1) people with HIV are generally not recognizable until the end-stages of the disease; and (2) the virus has a long incubation time. Recently, HIV pre-exposure prophylaxis (PrEP) became available through the NHS in Scotland in July 2017.

Fig. 54.1 shows one of the advertisements with a safer sex message targeting the general population. The message is clearly aimed at men, unlike previous health promotion activities for condoms, when condoms were 'only' contraceptives and often seen as a woman's responsibility (see spread Gender, pp. 44–45).

Case study

George (age 21 years) is a third-year medical student. He took an HIV test with his new partner when they started a sexual relationship. He felt it was a waste of time and only went along to please his partner. Although he was counselled at the time, he was very shocked to be told that he tested HIV-positive. His thoughts jumped back and forth between his partner and what would happen to the relationship, his study and career. He wondered: 'Who gave me the virus?' and 'Which private habits do I have to disclose and to whom? Will I die young or be on medication all my life?'

Stop and think

- What other issues might the medical student in the Case study face after his recent diagnosis?
- Why is society's reaction to people with HIV generally negative?

Despite all health promotion messages over the past 3 decades, talking about condom use and sexual desires still proves to be difficult for many people. Moreover there is growing evidence that young people in the UK are less aware of the risk of HIV.

HIV/AIDS in low-income countries

The majority of people with HIV live in developing countries (see pp. 156–157). In Africa HIV is mainly transmitted through heterosexual contact; MSM is still a leading factor in Europe and the USA, although heterosexual transmission is increasing. Many areas of Africa do not have the resources to screen blood consistently, which means that HIV is still being transmitted

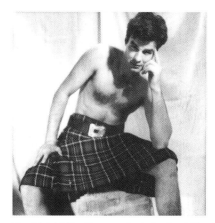

Fig. 54.1 HIV health promotion in Scotland. The slogan reads: 'What should a real Scotsman wear under his kilt?' Answer: 'A condom!' *(Courtesy of Scottish AIDS Monitor and Lothian Health).*

through blood transfusions, and very few medicines or social services are available for people living with HIV/AIDS. It is worth remembering that for some African nations hit hardest by AIDS, the entire national health budget is only equal to that of one large hospital in the USA. Consequently many developing countries cannot afford to offer the kind of treatment that has made long-term survival of HIV patients common in industrialized countries.

People living with HIV/AIDS in developing countries can also experience discrimination and stigma, leaving them isolated and deprived of social care and support. The death of parents in several countries, especially in sub-Saharan Africa, has led to a large number of so-called AIDS orphans, whose life chances are drastically reduced compared with children with a living parent.

HIV/AIDS

- People living with HIV/AIDS often suffer from a double stigma.
- Mass media have played an important role in influencing public perception of the disease.
- We should move away from thinking in terms of risk groups to risk behaviour. It is not important who you are, but what you do is.
- The majority of people with HIV live in the developing world, where much less funding is available for prevention and (often expensive) care (www.unaids.org/hivaidsinfo/index.html).
- Prevention is the main, or even the only, approach to stop the spread of HIV/AIDS.

Despite differences in the progress of different cancers and the increasing effectiveness of medical treatments, cancer continues to be the most widely feared group of diseases. It creates greater anxiety than coronary heart disease, which has approximately doubled the fatality rate. Psychological and social factors are involved in the aetiology and response to the disease and its treatment.

Aetiology and progression

In a review of the preventable causes of cancer, behavioural factors were implicated in the majority of cancers (Doll and Peto, 1981): smoking (involved in 30% of cancers); diet (35%); reproductive and sexual behaviour (7%); and alcohol use (3%). Thirty-five percent of the seven million global deaths from cancer in 2001 have been attributed to nine behavioural or environmental risk factors. The lead risk factors were smoking (596,000 deaths), alcohol use (88,000), overweight and obesity (69,000), low fruit and vegetable intake (64,000) and physical inactivity (51,000 deaths) (Danaei et al., 2005). There is also accumulating evidence that risk factors such as stress, depression and social isolation have relationships with processes of cancer progression, including immune response, angiogenesis (the development of blood vessels) and the ability of cancer cells to avoid anoikis (a form of programmed cell death) (Lutgendorf and Sood, 2011). However, the extent to which such associations affect patient survival is still unclear.

Communication about cancer

Cancer is associated with many social and clinical taboos. In popular language and in medical settings, euphemisms such as 'growth', 'tumour', 'lump', 'shadow' and 'the Big C' are used to avoid the word 'cancer' (see spread Breaking bad news, pp. 96–97). These communications may arise from the fears and misconceptions surrounding cancer, but, in turn, they also give rise to such fears. Thus patients with benign disease sometimes suspect that they have malignant disease but that their doctor is withholding the information. On the other hand, such language may lead a patient who does have a malignant cancer to misunderstand the full implications of their condition.

Communications about cancer are fraught with problems due to negative attitudes of patients, their families, health professionals (including doctors and nurses), other hospital personnel and the wider lay community (see Labelling and stigma, pp. 60–61). Doctors' ratings of the quality of life of cancer patients are significantly worse than the patients' own ratings. Health care staff members sometimes worry that giving patients with cancer information about their condition or treatment may increase anxiety. However, a systematic review of interventions to improve information given to patients with advanced cancer found positive results (e.g. improved satisfaction with communication) in six of eight trials. The other two trials showed no effect of the intervention (Gaston and Mitchell, 2005).

Members of the general public are much more likely to say that they want to be informed of a terminal diagnosis than doctors estimated they would (Jenkins et al., 2001) and want to be told personally, rather than have other people (such as a relative) told first. Not only do patients appreciate being informed about their illness, but many people with cancer also prefer to actively participate in decision-making about their illness (see Breaking bad news, pp. 96–97). Providing patients with information enables them to decide whether or not they would like to participate in decision-making (rather than leaving the decision-making to medical professionals) and, if they wish to be involved in decision-making, helps them to arrive at the optimal decision for their personal situation (see Helping people to act on their intentions, pp. 74–75).

Delay

People may not seek medical help when they experience potential cancer symptoms (see Deciding to consult, pp. 86–87) and may not choose to participate in cancer screening programmes. Screening for the detection of pre-cancerous cells or for the early diagnosis of treatable cancers has often had poor uptake rates (see spread Health screening, pp. 66–67).

Patient delay in seeking help when a symptom is noticed has four components: (1) appraisal delay (deciding the symptom indicates an illness); (2) illness delay (deciding that the illness merits a consultation with a doctor); (3) behavioural delay (making the appointment); and (4) scheduling delay (time between making appointment and actually seeing the doctor) (Andersen et al., 1995; Fig. 55.1). Appraisal delay can form a major part of the delay time. For example, a person with a cough might initially ignore or not notice the cough, until it becomes clear that it is persistent. Even so, if the person was a smoker, they might attribute the cough to 'smoker's cough' rather than an illness and therefore not realize that it could be a symptom of a serious condition such as lung cancer early enough to obtain the most effective treatment.

Response to diagnosis

Even when the term 'cancer' is used in giving the diagnosis, patients may subsequently report that they have never received

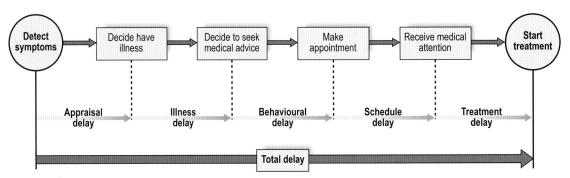

Fig. 55.1 Stages of delay in obtaining treatment *(adapted from Andersen et al., 1995).*

such a diagnosis. To ensure that patients can recall the full description of their condition and the potentially reassuring communication about treatment and prognosis, some clinicians have provided patients with an audio-recording of the diagnostic consultation (see Clinical communication skills, pp. 94–95). Evidence suggests that many patients find such recordings useful both for aiding their recall of the consultation and for helping them to communicate information about their condition and its treatment to their families.

Patients have varied ways of coping with a cancer diagnosis. Kübler-Ross (1969) proposed a sequence of staging of the response to a poor prognosis ranging from shock and denial, through anger, depression and, finally, to acceptance. Whilst there is considerable doubt about the actual sequence of stages, this range of response is commonly observed in patients with cancer. Researchers have investigated whether some coping methods may result in better adjustment. In general, coping strategies that focus on emotional aspects of the response are associated with poorer emotional adjustment. By contrast, patients whose strategies focus on thinking about the issue in a different way, e.g. on reaching acceptance of the condition or on seeking solutions to problems, show better subsequent adjustment (e.g. Carver et al., 1993).

Early research suggested that coping strategies, e.g. 'fighting spirit', influence prognosis and survival (Greer, 1979; Spiegel et al., 1989), but this has not been consistently supported (Petticrew et al., 2002; Coyne et al., 2007). This work has emphasised the role of psychological factors in morbidity and quality of life rather than mortality.

Response to treatment

Where two medical treatments are thought to have a similar prognosis, patients may be offered a choice of treatment. For instance, in patients with advanced prostate cancer, orchidectomy (surgical removal of testicle) or bi-monthly hormonal injections (synthetic luteinizing hormone) with minimum side-effects have similar survival rates. Yet when given the choice of treatment, a large proportion – 23 out of 50 men – opted for the mutilating surgery rather than the minimally invasive injections. It may be that people have more confidence in a surgical procedure that allows them to feel that the cancerous tissue has been physically removed.

Two studies of patients receiving chemotherapy examined the impact of side-effects on participants (Nerenz et al., 1982; Love et al., 1989). Some side-effects (e.g. vomiting and tiredness) were associated with distress and disruption, others were not. For example, hair loss was not, by itself, associated with emotional distress, perhaps because it is less debilitating than other side-effects that affect how patients physically feel and what they are able to do, or because they understood hair loss to be caused by the treatment while other side-effects might be interpreted as a result of the cancer itself (Fig. 55.2). People who had more side-effects or felt they had failed to cope with side-effects were more distressed.

Many patients experience anticipatory nausea and vomiting as chemotherapy progresses. For the initial treatments, nausea is experienced during and after the treatment. With later treatments, the nausea can occur before treatment, on arrival at the hospital or even on the journey to the hospital. This effect has been explained in terms of classical conditioning [see spread Understanding learning, pp. 20–21] – the patient learns to associate the visit to hospital with the administration of chemotherapy and therefore responds as if to chemotherapy, with nausea and vomiting. Considerable success has been achieved in training patients in relaxation techniques that they can then use in anticipation of and during chemotherapy (see Luebbert et al., 2001 for a meta-analysis aggregating the data of 10 controlled studies). Reducing nausea using such psychological techniques means increased comfort for the patient and reduced need for anti-emetic drugs.

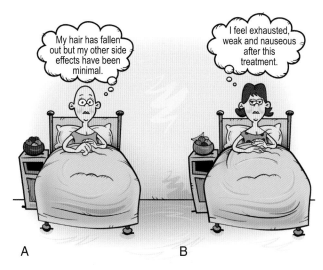

Fig. 55.2 Which patient is likely to be more depressed – A or B? Which patient is the observer likely to think is more depressed?

Case study *Providing test results in an oncology clinic*

Doctor: The tests on your breast lump are negative …

Alison: So there's nothing you can do …

Doctor: Oh yes. Don't worry; we don't leave things like this. We'll be proceeding with local excision of the necessary tissue.

Alison: That means I'll have to have the operation after all. What's the point?

Doctor: That's how these lumps are always managed. Everything will be fine. Try not to get upset. We'll fix a date for doing this as soon as possible. What about Wednesday next, coming in on Tuesday evening. OK?

- What did the doctor understand by the word 'negative'?
- What did Alison understand?
- What is Alison likely to think when she comes into hospital for surgery?

Stop and think

Patients with lung cancer in the UK have poor survival rates compared with those in other developed countries.

- Why do you think this might be the case?
- How much do you think this is caused by patient behaviour and how much by doctor behaviour?

Cancer

- Cancer is the most widely feared of all diseases.
- Behavioural factors are important in the aetiology of cancer and, therefore, offer opportunities for prevention.
- Communication about cancer may be limited by social taboos, concern to avoid upsetting patients and undue pessimism about the impact of the disease.
- Delay in reaching treatment can negatively affect prognosis, and there are a number of stages where this can be addressed.
- Patients' coping strategies can affect subsequent adjustment.
- Patients' choice of, and response to, treatment may be unexpected from a medical point of view but may be psychologically meaningful.

Feeling anxious can create a range of mild to severe levels of fear and anxiety in people and can be characterized by lifelong debilitation and periods of relapse and remission (Rynn and Brawman-Mintzer, 2004). Anxiety can either be a temporary state and an adaptive way of dealing with a situation (e.g. exam revision) or longer lasting, which can be more intrusive into everyday life. Anxiety disorders can start at an early infancy (see Development in early infancy. pp. 8–9) with one in six young people having experienced an anxiety related episode at some point (www.anxietyuk.org.uk). Anxiety disorders can be linked to childhood experiences (e.g. child abuse), age, socio-economic issues, long-term conditions and lifestyle choices (e.g. diet, drug misuse). Hence it is important for health care professionals to have an understanding of anxiety, the types of anxiety disorders, how these can present and treatment options available.

What is anxiety?

Anxiety is a commonly occurring problem that produces a response out of proportion to the actual threat. The disorder is recognised as having four components:

Physical – symptoms and sensations, for example, increased heart rate, chest tightness, shortness of breath, dizziness, faint feeling, headaches and nausea.

Cognitive – thoughts and worries associated with anxiety can create 'what if?' questions in relation to the anxiety provoking situation (e.g. 'what if I fail?', 'what if I embarrass myself?').

Behaviour – changes in behaviour can reduce anxiety. Actively avoiding an anxiety provoking situation can be one type of behaviour as are lifestyle choices (e.g. alcohol consumption or drug misuse). These behaviours, unfortunately, are maladaptive coping strategies to decrease high anxiety levels.

Emotional – anxiety can produce emotions such as fear, dread, panic, frustration, anger, sadness and depression (pp.114–115). This shift in emotions not only affect the individual experiencing them, but also relationships with family and friends.

The Case study illustrates how these four components combined with an individual's environment, can interact to create and maintain anxiety and contribute to avoidance.

Types of anxiety disorders

What should we look out for as signs of the disorder? It has been recommended that 'people with a suspected anxiety disorder receive an assessment that identifies whether they have a specific anxiety disorder, and look at specific symptom severity and functional impairment, so that tailored treatment can be delivered' (NICE, 2014). Several different types of anxiety disorder exist. People may suffer from more than one. These include:

Panic disorder – involves sudden waves of intense anxiety that seem to come out of the blue without any apparent cue. People may be overwhelmed by feelings of loss of control and concerned about having repeated, unexpected panic attacks. They occur in public places and involve feelings of being trapped (agoraphobia) and associated with fear of shopping, crowds or travelling.

Obsessive compulsive disorder (OCD) – people with OCD suffer from obsessional ruminations, which are intrusive and recurrent, with distressing thoughts or images (e.g. about contamination or harming others). They may also experience compulsions to perform certain repetitive behaviours such as checking and re-checking and lengthy cleaning rituals.

Post-traumatic stress disorder (PTSD) – this is a response to an extreme stressor (e.g. experience of accident, environmental disaster or war). Its symptoms involve the individual frequently re-experiencing the traumatic event, becoming distressed and unable to avoid or forget the trauma (see pp. 112–123). This disorder can contribute to poor sleep and concentration.

Body dysmorphic disorder – in this instance an individual can experience excessive worry about their appearance and have a distorted view of how they look and are seen by others. This can be severely debilitating for the individual and affect self-esteem, confidence and social interaction.

Social anxiety disorder (social phobia) – is an intense fear and avoidance of social interactions that can involve being scrutinized or focus of attention. This can significantly affect everyday life, self-esteem and self-confidence. It is common in adolescents where situations that cause embarrassment are avoided.

Phobia – a fear that is posed by a particular object or situation creating excessive symptoms and behaviours. Common specific phobias are to blood and injections, enclosed places such as being in a lift, animals and aspects of the natural environment (e.g. storms and water). Physical reactions to phobias can be characterised in some instances by decrease (or increase) in heart rate and fainting. The individual, if often treated through graded exposure, as shown in Fig. 56.1, and demonstrates that a feared object can become unthreatening.

General anxiety disorder (GAD) – is a commonly occurring condition, characterized by excessive worry or anxiety about everyday events (e.g. work, school) to the point at which the individual experiences considerable distress and difficulty in performing day to day tasks. Often the individual experiences uncontrollable worry not linked to any specific situation, causing restlessness and somatic complaints.

How can health care professionals address anxiety?

Anxiety can be screened for using self-report questionnaires, and for a diagnosis of anxiety to be made, the symptoms need to have been present for at least 6 months, have impacted on functioning and are seen to have produced heightened reactions (Diagnostic and Statistical Manual of Mental Disorders, 5th edition (DSM-V)) (American Psychiatric Association, 2013). Identification of anxiety disorders has been found to be poor especially within primary care, this results in very few individuals suffering from this disorder receiving appropriate treatment. People with an anxiety disorder, and their significant others/carers, require patient-centred care tailored to the nature of the disorder and its symptoms. The National Institute for Health and Clinical Excellence (NICE, 2014) provides recommendations for health professionals in diagnosing and treating the specific needs of the variety of anxiety-related disorders.

Psychological therapies

Psychological interventions (or 'talking treatments') can be effective treatments for anxiety disorders and are recommended first-line treatments in preference to pharmacological treatment (see Cognitive-behavioural therapy, pp.138–139). Health care professionals should usually offer or refer for the least intrusive,

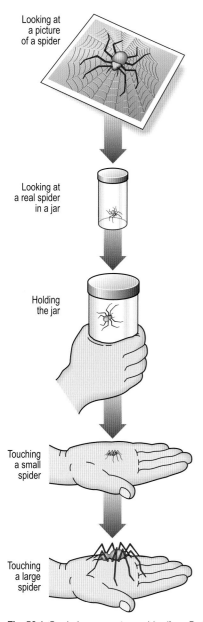

Looking at
a picture
of a spider

Looking at
a real spider
in a jar

Holding
the jar

Touching
a small
spider

Touching
a large
spider

Fig. 56.1 Graded exposure to a spider *(from Puri et al., 1996).*

most effective intervention first. Treatment can vary depending on age, needs, requirements and informed choice made by the individual and could involve either low- or high-intensity interventions.

Cognitive behavioural therapy (CBT) is a goal-orientated, skills-based treatment, commonly used to treat anxiety disorders. It is delivered in a supportive environment and assists through identification of its cause, how the individual behaves and feels in relation to the situation and then works towards changing these responses. Internet-based treatments (e-interventions) have grown rapidly in helping people with anxiety disorders.

Mindfulness-based therapy is growing in popularity and is another effective approach for treating anxiety disorders. It encourages an individual to focus on what they are experiencing in the present moment and has been shown in practice to reduce anxiety.

Anxiety

- One in nine people worldwide has suffered an anxiety disorder in past year.
- Untreated anxiety disorders can become chronic.
- Women are more susceptible to anxiety than men.
- Persistent anxiety, associated physical symptoms and maladaptive behaviour can severely impact on engagement with daily life.
- Identification of anxiety, especially within General Practice, has been reported as poor.

57 | Depression

The World Health Organization ranks depression as the leading cause of disability globally. One in 20 individuals suffer from a significant depressive disorder, and about 17% of the population will suffer from a major depressive disorder at some point throughout their life (Hammen and Watkins, 2007). Depression can be disabling, and patients may be unable to function effectively for several months. Suicidal thoughts and attempts are the most disturbing features of depression, as 4% of patients hospitalized for an affective disorder eventually die of their own volition. The highest suicide rate is among men aged 40–44. In the UK, three times more men than women commit suicide. It is now recognized that children and adolescents can suffer from depression and that this is often not diagnosed or treated.

Definition

The key features of depression are low mood and anhedonia (loss of interest and enjoyment of activities). Box 57.1 shows the diagnostic criteria from the International Classification of Diseases, version 10 (ICD-10), and symptoms must be present for a minimum of 2 weeks for a diagnosis. Low mood may show diurnal variation (more pronounced in the morning than in evening) and largely unaffected by daily events. Typically patients have a systematically biased negative view of themselves, their world and future (Beck's cognitive triad). Depression can be a chronic or recurring condition.

Classification

Depression can be classified by severity – as mild, moderate or severe – based on the number, type and severity of symptoms encountered and level of difficulty in completing daily activities (Box 57.1). Mild depressive episodes are commonly managed in the primary care setting whereas severe episodes may require admission to a psychiatric inpatient ward. In general practice the Patient Health Questionnaire (PHQ-9) is a useful self-report instrument for screening, measuring and monitoring depression severity.

In many cases of depression, interlinking risk factors play a role. These include physiological, gender, genetic, individual and environmental factors. The pathophysiology of depression is poorly understood, but the role of neurotransmitters, in particular serotonin, noradrenaline and dopamine, is suggested by the efficacy of medications. Studies report approximately a 2 : 1 rate of depression for women compared to men (Hammen and Watkins, 2007). However, this may partially reflect a greater readiness of women to admit distress and to seek help. Men may present their distress in a disguised manner, e.g. through somatic complaints such as pain. Men may be more prone to self-medicate in response to depression, e.g. by alcohol abuse.

Some types of depression tend to run in families. McGuffin et al. (1996) reported concordance for lifetime major depression in 46% for monozygotic twins compared with 20% in dizygotic twins, with both rates being higher than lifetime depression in the general population. This suggests a genetic contribution to the development of major depression.

Individual factors such as stressful life events, including divorce, bereavement, challenges in the workplace, physical illness and pain and traumatic early life experiences, can increase susceptibility to depression. Beck's cognitive theory of depression suggests that an individual's pre-existing negative pattern of thinking (schema) act as a vulnerability factor for depression e.g. when faced with stressful life events.

A crucial environmental factor is the availability of good-quality support from friends and family. This seems to offer protection in helping individuals deal with stressors that may otherwise precipitate a depressive episode. The lack of an intimate or confiding relationship is a good example of increasing the risk for depression.

Differential diagnosis (i.e. competing conditions with similar features to depression): schizophrenia; mood disorder; grief reaction; adjustment disorder; dementia; substance-induced mood disorder (both prescription and illegal drugs); endocrine disturbance (e.g. hypothyroidism); and sleep disorders (e.g. sleep apnoea).

Treatment

A particular problem with depression is that many patients are reluctant to seek treatment. They may worry about the stigma (see pp. 60–61) of being labelled with a psychiatric disorder. Some patients do not recognize themselves as being depressed but rather believe that they are lazy, wicked or simply undeserving of treatment. For those who do seek treatment (often after persuasion by friends and family), treatment options include psychotherapy, medication and, if indicated, electrical convulsive therapy. The National Institute for Health and Care Excellence (NICE) recommends a stepped care model (Table 57.1). NICE advocates not prescribing anti-depressants to treat mild depression because the risk–benefit ratio is poor. Instead they recommend starting with brief psychological interventions such as guided self-help.

Psychological treatments

Cognitive-behavioural therapy (CBT) (see pp. 138–139) and interpersonal psychotherapy (IPT) are structured,

---

Box 57.1 International classification of diseases – 10 depression diagnostic criteria

Diagnostic criteria for depression ICD-10 uses an agreed list of ten depressive symptoms

Key symptoms:
- persistent sadness or low mood; and/or
- loss of interests or pleasure
- fatigue or low energy
- at least one of these, most days, most of the time for at least 2 weeks
- if any of above present, ask about associated symptoms:
  - disturbed sleep
  - poor concentration or indecisiveness
  - low self-confidence
  - poor or increased appetite
  - suicidal thoughts or acts
  - agitation or slowing of movements
  - guilt or self-blame
- the 10 symptoms then define the degree of depression and management is based on the particular degree
  - **not depressed** (fewer than four symptoms)
  - **mild depression** (four symptoms)
  - **moderate depression** (five to six symptoms)
  - **severe depression** (seven or more symptoms, with or without psychotic symptoms)
  - symptoms should be present for a month or more and every symptom should be present for most of every day

Table 57.1 **NICE stepped-care model**	
Focus of the intervention	**Nature of the intervention**
STEP 4: Severe and complex depression; risk to life; severe self-neglect	Medication, high-intensity psychological interventions, electroconvulsive therapy, crisis service, combined treatments, multiprofessional and inpatient care
STEP 3: Persistent subthreshold depressive symptoms or mild to moderate depression with inadequate response to initial interventions; moderate and severe depression	Medication, high-intensity psychological interventions, combined treatments, collaborative care and referral for further assessment and interventions
STEP 2: Persistent subthreshold depressive symptoms; mild to moderate depression	Low-intensity psychosocial interventions, psychological interventions, medication and referral for further assessment and interventions
STEP 1: All known and suspected presentations of depression	Assessment, support, psychoeducation, active monitoring and referral for further assessment and interventions

time-limited psychological treatments for depression (Luty et al., 2007). They are useful for patients who do not have psychotic symptoms and are able to engage in the learning process involved. CBT is more expensive than drug treatment, but there is evidence that CBT reduces the risk of future depressive episodes (NICE, 2007). A combination of anti-depressants and psychotherapy may be most helpful (Keller et al., 2000). This may be because the drug treatment provides a boost to increase activity and aid concentration, enabling the patient to take an active part in a psychological intervention, which, in turn, may reduce the risk of future relapse. Other forms of psychotherapy, counselling and alternative treatments are available; however, few have a strong evidence base regarding their efficacy (see www.nice.org.uk/CG023).

Medication

The common anti-depressant medications include tricyclics and selective serotonin reuptake inhibitors (SSRIs). It usually takes time before patients note any benefit, so they need to persist with treatment. Many anti-depressants have side-effects, particularly in the early stages, and this can lead to patients discontinuing treatment. The SSRIs are as effective as the older tricyclic antidepressants and are less likely to be discontinued because of side-effects and are safer from overdose. Many patients may be reluctant to take anti-depressants because of fears regarding dependence and toxicity. Such fears should be elicited and addressed during the consultation.

Electroconvulsive therapy

Electroconvulsive therapy (ECT) is a controversial treatment for severe depression. Electrical stimulation of the brain produces a grand mal seizure. It is the seizure itself, rather than the electricity, which has the therapeutic effect. ECT has been shown to be effective in controlled clinical trials. It should be used only to achieve rapid and short-term improvement of severe symptoms after an adequate trial

of other treatment options has proven ineffective and/or when the condition is considered to be life-threatening in individuals with a severe depressive illness. Patients often complain of memory loss after ECT (Rose et al., 2003).

There is no perfect treatment for depression and many have high drop-out rates. Reasons for patients with depression dropping out include lacking energy and concentration and finding clinic visits difficult and having a pessimistic view of the treatment (e.g. a sense of hopelessness). Moreover treatment takes time to show benefits.

Depression in the general medical setting

Depressive illness is strongly linked with physical disease. Up to one-third of physically ill patients attending hospital have depressive symptoms. Depression is even more common in patients with:

Life-threatening or chronic physical illness
Unpleasant and demanding treatment
Low social support and other adverse social circumstances
Personal or family history of depression or other psychological vulnerability
Alcoholism and substance misuse
Medicines that cause depression as a side-effect, such as anti-hypertensives, corticosteroids and chemotherapy agents (Peveler et al., 2002).

Comorbid depression may also be associated with poor prognosis in medical conditions: e.g. after myocardial infarction, patients who were depressed have significantly increased mortality rates. This may be because they see the future as bleak and pointless and do not have the motivation or energy to engage in cardiac rehabilitation programmes or change unhealthy behaviours (e.g. smoking, exercise, diet) and may not adhere to prescribed medication. Unfortunately many patients do not get their depression diagnosed or treated, yet even in terminal disease states such as metastatic cancer, treating an underlying depressive illness can markedly improve the patients' quality of life.

Health and social policy implications

It is important to consider preventive measures at the individual, family, community and population levels. Increased social support, income support, employment opportunities and housing could all potentially help reduce psychosocial stressors. The provision of health professional resources and training to identify depression may help to reduce the high rate of untreated depression. After the initial treatment of depression, follow-up is crucial. A simple protocol involving telephone follow-up and review by the practice nurse has resulted in markedly improved outcomes in general practice. At 2-year follow-up, 74% of patients treated with this 'enhanced care' approach were in clinical remission versus 41% of those who received 'treatment as usual' (Rost et al., 2002). Depression can be treated in primary care and is largely effective. However, accessible and speedy referral pathways to specialist mental health services are vital, particularly for treatment-resistant, recurrent, atypical and psychotic depression and for patients at significant risk. Greater public awareness can help to remove the stigma around mental illness.

Case study

Jacqueline is a 33-year-old bank clerk, married 12 years with three young children. Recently both her parents died, and she had been promoted at work to a more demanding position. The family moved to a new home recently, and two children had problems settling in at school. For 6 weeks, Jacqueline was wakening at 4 a.m. and was unable to get back to sleep. She worried constantly about moving home, and regrets taking up her new post. She became increasingly convinced that she was failing in her job and as a wife and mother. She could not confide in her husband, lost her appetite and felt constantly exhausted and irritable. She felt joyless and saw the future as bleak. She was convinced that her family would be better off without her. Her husband became increasingly concerned and this made her feel even more guilty for causing concern. Eventually her husband persuaded her to go to her GP, who diagnosed a major depressive episode. She was treated with a combination of anti-depressant (paroxetine) and CBT. Jacqueline reduced her working hours, joined a gym and met new people. Over a 3-month period she gradually improved and was slowly getting back to her 'old self'. The GP recommended that she stay on her medication for a further 6 months.

Inflammatory bowel disease (IBD) illustrates how social and psychological processes have an impact on the response to and the experience of illness, and some of the issues that these processes generate for medical care. Ulcerative colitis (one type of IBD) will be used to demonstrate this (Kelly, 1992).

Clinical features

Ulcerative colitis is a disease of the lining layer of the large bowel. It can occur at any age. Its principal symptoms are chronic unpredictable diarrhoea accompanied by heavy anal bleeding, weight and appetite loss and abdominal pain. Its causes are unknown but an autoimmune process is suspected. There is presently no medical cure. For the moment the mainstays of treatment are rectal and systemic 5-aminosalicylic acid derivatives and corticosteroids, with azathioprine in steroid-dependent or resistant cases (Ghosh et al., 2000). Most recently the use of monoclonal antibodies (adalimumab, golimumab and infliximab) that inhibit the pro-inflammatory cytokine tumour necrosis factor (TNF)-alpha have been recommended where other treatments have failed (NICE, 2013).

The complications of colitis can be severe. There may be perforation of the bowel, and the effects on the overall health of the patient can be extremely serious. Where the disease is present for more than 10 years, there is a very greatly enhanced risk of the development of bowel cancer. At present the best treatment option available in the face of unremitting symptoms and grave deterioration in the patient's health or the development of cancer is the surgical removal of the bowel. This involves either creating an internal pouch to collect the waste matter of digestion with normal anal evacuation or simply redirecting the faeces through the abdominal wall via a stoma, a procedure called *panproctocolectomy and ileostomy*. The operations are major and, in the case of ileostomy, have profound effects on appearance because the small bowel protrudes externally, and although patients are cured of the colitis, they are incontinent of faeces. They will always have to wear a bag to collect the products of digestion.

Onset

When the first symptoms – usually diarrhoea – appear, the typical response by the sufferer is to minimize or ignore them. Diarrhoea is commonplace, so the sufferer typically assumes that the symptoms will remit of their own accord, as diarrhoea usually does. This reaction may continue until such time as blood appears in the motion. This is usually regarded by the patient as very significant and frightening. Whereas diarrhoea is common, anal bleeding is not. Contact with the medical profession is frequently made some time after the appearance of blood, although some patients do seek help for their diarrhoea. When the symptoms of diarrhoea are presented, they are sometimes misdiagnosed.

I was working. I had two children …

I began to feel, y'know, unwell. Went to my GP. Didn't examine me at all, and told me I was suffering from piles, haemorrhoids, and gave me some medication. The piles wouldn't go away, and I was back there. And by this time it was terribly painful. And I started to get really worried because I was losing blood. So I made another appointment with another doctor in the practice, and she took me into the examination room, examined me straight away, and within a week I was up at St George's Hospital (38-year-old teacher) **(Kelly, 1992).**

The important social–psychological concept involved here is help-seeking (see pp. 88–89). Diarrhoea comes well within the range of the normal experience of most people. They generally wait to see whether it passes in a day or two (temporizing behaviour). The observation of blood in their motion signals something out of the ordinary and acts as the trigger for them to consult the doctor. From a medical point of view, rectal bleeding is something requiring investigation. It is, however, quite unlikely to engender the same degree of anxiety as experienced by the patient. As far as colitis is concerned, bleeding does not necessarily indicate an exacerbation of the illness. Thus the patient's estimation of the seriousness of the symptom may not necessarily correspond to the doctor's. However, to manage the patient's symptoms and anxieties successfully the doctor must be aware not only of the physical symptoms but also how they are being interpreted by the patient. The fact that the patient believes a symptom to be grave is what is important in understanding why the patient has gone to the doctor.

Diagnosis and treatment

Confirming the diagnosis will involve inspecting the patient's colon with a colonoscope or a sigmoidoscope (NICE, 2011). Barium enema can provide radiological confirmation. From the patient's perspective, these procedures are undignified, uncomfortable, frequently painful and often highly stressful. One patient described barium enema:

So I got the appointment for the X-ray department, went in, without a care in the world. I came out absolutely devastated … it was terrifying … And you go into this place, which had this revolving table and everything and this room, and they pump all this stuff into you. It was ghastly (33-year-old female school teacher) **(Kelly, 1992).**

Most Radiology departments have little or no time to prepare people for these procedures, and the fear and anxiety that may be generated are considerable because the patient is uncertain as to what is happening. The stressfulness of these kinds of experiences has been shown to be significantly reduced if patients have been well prepared in advance (Fig. 58.1) (see pp. 102–103).

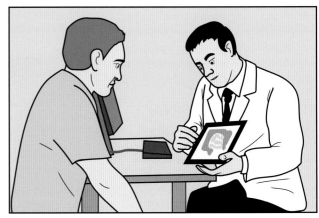

Fig. 58.1 It is important to check a patient's understanding of the disease, and of any procedures before they happen, to manage stress and anxiety *(from http://www.crohnsandcolitis.org.uk/).*

Furthermore, recognizing the indignity of the procedures can also be reassuring for the patient.

Diagnosis is not always straightforward, and determining whether it is colitis or another form of IBD can be difficult. However, having made the diagnosis, the physician faces a dilemma. If the disease can be brought under control, all well and good. However, what the physician also has to convey is that this may offer only temporary respite and that the patient may face a long period of chronic illness of varying degrees of severity. Although the patient is entitled to receive a full description of the likely prognosis and the treatment options available, for many patients this raises more problems and questions than it solves. Discussions of cancer, surgery or long periods of severe ill health may terrify patients and cause them to lose hope and certainly may lead to raised levels of anxiety. And the treatment options are not necessarily clear-cut either. The disease process is uncertain; phases of exacerbation and remission are unpredictable. The long-term risk of cancer and sudden and major acute deterioration must also be borne in mind. From a lay point of view, this is a large amount of unwelcome and irresolvable information with no easy options. Moreover it is usually the case that the patient enters treatment for this disease in the expectation of a cure. Eventually patients will come to realize that they are not going to recover fully.

This is further complicated by the fact that, in spite of all the problems, many patients try to live as normal a life as possible in the face of the illness. If patients are trying to live a normal life, they face a tension between the demands of fulfilling usual social responsibilities and accepting the limitations imposed upon them by the illness.

Although this is not easy, people do manage to cope with their illness in spite of the difficulties it presents. Doctors can help here by encouraging patients to live as normal a life as they can and by helping them to recognize the limitations the illness can produce.

Living with the illness

Many aspects of life are likely to be affected by the illness. The chronic, unpredictable diarrhoea means that things such as travel, shopping, walking, eating and socializing are interrupted as the sufferer has to go off and find a toilet. The nature of the symptoms are such that the patient usually has very little warning (perhaps less than 30 seconds) of the need to evacuate. Sufferers become highly skilled in breaking off from social interaction, arranging journeys and trips so that toilets are always within easy reach and carrying a change of clothes for the occasions when they self-soil.

I didn't enjoy shopping or anything.

I was always wanting to be near a toilet; I, well, always felt nauseated with it.

I didn't have the energy to go shopping like everybody else … we couldn't plan anything … (46-year-old housewife)
(Kelly, 1992).

It is sometimes remarked that patients suffering from colitis exhibit odd behaviours such as obsessive attention to detail and concerns about personal cleanliness. However, it is most likely that these behaviours are adaptive in the struggle with the illness, rather than a cause of it.

Surgery

For some patients with colitis the prospect of surgery has to be confronted. There are two important behavioural issues. Firstly,

patients have to deal with the prospect of major body-altering surgery that, with some operations, will leave them with a stoma. Secondly, the patient now faces a new psychological threat. Although the medical decision may be relatively straightforward, it is not automatically viewed in that way by the patient. Some will refuse surgery, believing that the threats arising from the illness are preferable to the threats arising from the surgery. Helping the patient adapt to surgery is, therefore, a key problem in this procedure. Preparations for surgery should not involve trying to make patients 'accept' their illness or the fact that they need an operation. Helping patients to prepare for surgery should be about allowing them to acknowledge the psychological pain and distress and the associated feelings of loss that this surgery engenders. It should aim to help them work through their feelings of hurt. This is a difficult and traumatic procedure from the patient's perspective and one that requires considerable social and psychological skills on the part of the people caring for that patient (see pp. 102–103).

Stop and think

- To what extent might there be a conflict between the medical and psychological management of colitis? Is the refusal of some patients with colitis to have surgery adaptive or maladaptive?

Case study

Gillian is 52 years old. She was first diagnosed as having colitis when she was 46 years old. She is married with two teenage children. Her doctor has just told her she needs to have a total colectomy and ileostomy. She is completely distraught at the prospect. She always has thought of herself as an attractive woman. She is horrified at the prospect of wearing a bag. Yet she is very ill. She has not had a proper night's sleep for 3 years. She has to get up in the night three or four times to go to the toilet. During the day it is even worse. She usually cannot go for longer than an hour before she has to open her bowels. Her work as a secretary is becoming increasingly difficult. Her boss is very understanding, but the fact that she constantly has to leave the office has made things very awkward. Her appetite is poor, and when she does eat, she sticks to a diet of minced breast of chicken and white bread. She and her husband used to go out a lot, but they stay at home all the time now. Her doctor has told her that the operation would make her better. Gillian, however, is resolute in her refusal to have the operation.

Inflammatory bowel disease

- The process of making decisions about seeking help are governed by social and psychological factors as well as the degree of medical seriousness of the condition.
- Symptoms that are regarded as critical by the patient will not necessarily be the same ones as those identified as medically serious.
- In a disease like colitis, social and psychological symptoms may be evident, but they are usually a consequence rather than a cause of the illness.
- As with many illnesses, the treatments for colitis are frequently viewed as more psychologically threatening by the patient than the illness itself. These threats condition patient behaviour as much as the threats from the disease and its symptoms.
- The surgery performed to cure colitis is often associated with very powerful feelings of distress and loss.

59 | Physical disability

Physical disabilities are limitations in the ability to perform activities and can be the result of such diverse conditions as cerebral palsy, rheumatoid arthritis, stroke, multiple sclerosis or accidental injury. As shown in Fig. 59.1, the commonest disabilities in Western industrialized countries are in locomotion, personal care activities (e.g. dressing, washing, feeding and toileting) and hearing. Approximately 21% of adults and children in the UK report at least one limiting long-standing illness, but this rate varies (see Social aspects of ageing, pp. 14–15). For example, the rate increases to 50% in people aged 75 years or over, 30% in those earning £10,000 or less per year, 28% in heavy smokers and 36% in those who are economically inactive.

Activity limitations can result in social disadvantage. Disability present from birth (e.g. in cerebral palsy or cystic fibrosis) may disadvantage individuals throughout their lifetime and affect school, employment, marital, parenting and other social opportunities. By contrast, an injury suffered as a young adult, a myocardial infarction in middle age or a stroke after retirement will have very different impacts on both the individual and his or her family.

Assessing disability

In research or clinical practice, levels of disability are assessed to ascertain the severity of the condition or to evaluate improvement or deterioration. Clinical assessments may be used to make decisions about medical care, referral to rehabilitation services (especially physio-occupational and speech and language therapists), provision of aids or adaptations to the home or recommendations for absence from work, pensions or welfare benefits.

Disability is typically assessed by measures of activities of daily living (ADLs), which assess the person's ability to perform everyday self-care or mobility activities. These measures assess activities that virtually everyone would wish to perform and, therefore, do not include activities that may be important for particular individuals. For example, the Barthel index includes personal toilet (wash face, comb hair, shave and clean teeth), feeding, using toilet, walking on level surface, transfer from chair to bed, dressing, using stairs and bathing.

There are two main methods of assessment: self-report and observation. The first requires individuals to describe difficulties experienced, and in the second they perform defined activities whilst a trained observer notes successes and failures. Self-report

has the advantage of allowing the assessment of a wide range of activities occurring in home and private situations, covering all times of day and night and over days, weeks or months. Observational methods are restricted to what can be assessed in the limited setting of the hospital or in the limited period available for a home visit; patients who can use the toilet independently in the hospital setting may not be able to do so at home if there is less space to manoeuvre or no support to lean on. They may be even more disabled if they need to go to the toilet during the night if this involves additional flights of stairs. Electronic monitors (e.g. pedometers) can record activity through the day in the individual's normal environment.

Models of disability

Three models of disability have each contributed to a broader understanding: medical, social and psychological.

Medical model

The traditional medical model regarded disability as a direct consequence of an underlying disease or disorder (see The biopsychosocial model, pp. 2–3). From this perspective, reductions in disability can only be achieved through the amelioration of the underlying pathology. However, pathology is a poor predictor of disability: for example, the degree of joint degeneration is a poor predictor of mobility disability in people with osteoarthritis (Dieppe, 2004). This traditional model also engenders stigmatizing language (see pp. 60–61) and does not recognize social and psychological factors. More recent models not only recognize the role of impairment in disability but also incorporate social and environmental factors.

Social model

A social model of disability emphasizes that activity limitations and participation restrictions result from social and environmental constraints. So individuals are limited not only by their medical condition per se but also by the behaviour of other people towards them and by environmental barriers such as the inaccessibility of buildings or poor sound systems. These additional features can make it impossible for them to participate fully. A person may be less disabled when activity is supported than in a protective social environment; there is evidence that compassionate attention to activity limitations can increase levels of disability (Romano et al., 1995). In Fig. 59.2 we see an attempt

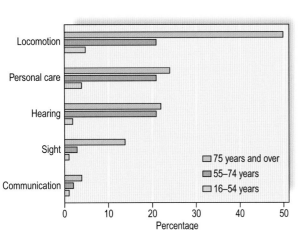

Fig. 59.1 Prevalence of disabilities by age (percentage reporting each disability) *(adapted from Bajekal et al., 2001, with permission).*

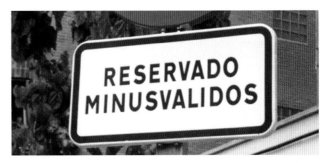

Fig. 59.2 Social values. Would disabled individuals feel valued by a society that offered this 'special' car-parking space ('reservado minusvalidos' means 'reserved for the disabled')? Or would they feel that they were 'minus validity'? English uses similarly stigmatizing vocabulary, e.g. 'invalid' (with two pronunciations) or 'handicap' (derived from 'cap in hand' of the person begging).

to overcome problems of access for individuals with locomotion impairments, but the language used reflects the stigmatizing attitudes that can make participation difficult (see pp. 60–61). The inclusion of a role for contextual factors as well as impairments is necessary to reconcile social and medical models of disability. In addition, it is possible that social participation may affect activity limitations and impairment, e.g. joining a social club may result in increased physical activity, thus reducing joint stiffness.

Psychological model

A psychological model of disability emphasizes that activities performed (or not performed) by someone with a health condition are influenced by the same psychological processes that affect the performance of these behaviours by people without disabilities. So individuals will be motivated to engage in the activity because it results in things they like, because they believe that other people who are important to them would like them to do it and because they believe they can (see Case study). Thus two people with identical medical conditions, living in identical social and environmental situations, may face very different activity limitations because of their cognitions, emotions or coping strategies (see Stop and think box and pp. 36–37). Depressed or anxious people are likely to be more limited because of their associated cognitions. For example, individuals who believe that they can overcome their disability, find the activity more rewarding or see family and friends as being more supportive will be more likely to engage in the activity than someone with different beliefs.

There is ample evidence that psychological factors predict disability outcomes. For example, patients with stroke with a stronger belief that they can influence their recovery are found to do more than patients with less belief in personal control, and this difference persists for at least 3 years after a stroke (Johnston et al., 2005). Interventions that enhance perceived control beliefs have resulted in reduced activity limitations (Fisher and Johnston, 1996).

Integrating across models

These three theoretical approaches have been combined in the World Health Organization's *International Classification of Functioning, Disability and Health* (ICF) model (World Health Organization, 2002b), an integrative model appropriate to the multi-disciplinary management of disability. For example, a stroke patient may require neurologists to address the underlying brain damage; rehabilitation staff deal with activity limitations; psychologists assess cognitive damage, address dysfunctional beliefs and enhance mood; and social services work to adapt patients' living space (e.g. by providing ramp access to their home).

The ICF identifies three components of disability: (1) impairments to body structures and functions; (2) activity limitations; and (3) participation restrictions, each of which is affected by personal and environmental factors (Fig. 59.3). Bodily impairments accommodate the medical model, whilst the inclusion of a role for contextual factors such as the structure of the physical environment and personal beliefs accommodates the social and psychological models. In addition, activity limitations and participation restrictions involve behaviour, which allows for the further integration of psychological models into the ICF (Johnston and Dixon, 2013).

Case study

After a road traffic accident, Miss Lopez did not resume eating and drinking when she was physically capable. She only started eating and drinking normally after a behavioural programme that socially reinforced taking sips of water and enabled her to have the confidence that she could do it.

Stop and think

- Mr Harrison was disabled as the result of a spinal cord injury after falling from a lorry but reported that his quality of life had improved because he was studying for a degree rather than being a manual worker. The clinical team believed that Mr Harrison could learn to walk again but seemed unmotivated. What factors are likely to be influencing Mr Harrison's level of disability? What should the clinical team do?

Stop and think

- Elizabeth Edison uses a wheelchair to get around. What image comes to mind when you picture Elizabeth Edison? Is she elderly and frail in appearance? Or is she a young, fit paralympic basketball champion?
- Social stereotypes can affect how we think about age and disability and how we behave toward people with disabilities. How well are the needs of young people with disabilities accommodated in our society? How valid is the assumption that to be old is to be disabled?

Physical disability

- Disability is assessed by ADL (Activities of Daily Living) measures, using both self-report and observational methods.
- Disability and its impact can be explained in terms of disease and social and psychological factors.
- Disability is influenced by impairment resulting from disease or disorder, the physical environment, the social environment, emotions, cognitions and coping strategies.
- The World Health Organization's ICF provides a comprehensive model.

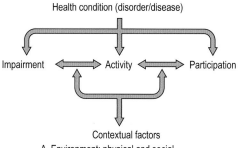

Fig. 59.3 International classification of functions *(adapted from World Health Organization, 2002b).*

60 | Learning disability

The implications of a learning disability for the health of individuals who are affected and their families can be far-reaching, and they may need considerable clinical care and psychological and socio-economic support. 'Learning disability' is the term currently used in UK legislation and policy, although the term *intellectual disability* is becoming increasingly common.

A learning disability is defined by the Department of Health (2001) as a 'significant reduced ability to understand new or complex information, to learn new skills (impaired intelligence), with a reduced ability to cope independently (impaired social functioning), which started before adulthood'.

This means that somebody with a learning disability will have difficulties in understanding, in learning new things and generalizing these to new situations and with social tasks such as communication, self-care and awareness of and responses to danger. It is important to recognize individual strengths and abilities as well as needs, which are likely to vary, depending in part on the severity of the disability. Learning disability fits the social rather than the medical model of disability (see also pp. 2–3); it cannot be cured, nor in any real sense can it be treated, although in some cases it can be avoided by prompt medical intervention or by improved antenatal care, and in many cases its impact can be mitigated by appropriate responses across a range of disciplines. Having a learning disability has been found to have a negative impact on many aspects of quality of life. Children who live in neighbourhoods that are deprived or who live in poorer households have an increased likelihood of having a learning disability.

Prevalence

According to Public Health England (PHE), it is estimated that in 2013 there were 1,068,000 people with learning disabilities. This included:

- 224,930 children
- 900,900 adults (equivalent to 2.1% of the English adult population)

Of these adults, 206,132 (23%) were known to GPs as people with learning disabilities.

Causes

A learning disability occurs whilst the brain is developing. This might be before, during or soon after birth. A number of other conditions are associated with a learning disability, including

Fragile X syndrome (the most common cause of inherited learning disabilities, with almost all boys having at least some degree of learning disability)
Down's syndrome (where all people will have some degree of learning disability)
Autism spectrum conditions/disorders (around 50% of those diagnosed with an autism spectrum condition may also have a learning disability)
Cerebral palsy (although not all people will have a learning disability)

Birth-related disabilities are mostly caused by insufficiencies in the oxygen supply or by prematurity. After birth the most common causes are early childhood illness or physical accident.

The cause of mild learning disability is generally multi-factorial, and the precise mechanisms are not clear.

Health implications of learning disability for the individual

The incidence of ill health in people with learning disabilities is higher than in the general population, much of which is avoidable. Public Health England report that 'these health inequalities often start early in life and result, to an extent, from barriers they face in accessing timely, appropriate and effective health care'. Premature deaths are common, with people with learning disabilities dying, on average, 13 years (men) and 20 years (women) younger compared with the general population. People with profound intellectual (learning) and multiple disabilities are likely to die at an earlier age than those with less severe disabilities.

The most common co-existing health problems are respiratory disease; coronary heart disease; conditions associated with physical impairments (e.g. eating/drinking difficulties); obesity or being underweight; mental health problems (including dementia); epilepsy; or sensory impairments. Of these, complications as a result of eating and drinking difficulties and epilepsy or convulsions were the cause of death reported in 27% of cases. A smaller proportion (5%–15%) of people with learning disabilities displays challenging behaviour. These rates are likely to be higher amongst some groups, e.g. teenagers and young adults and those people who are in hospital settings. People with challenging behaviours can be at particular risk of experiencing both health inequalities and of poor care (including inappropriate use of anti-psychotic medication).

This is a population that is typically denied control over many basic aspects of daily living, is subjected to higher than average experience of bullying and denigration (see pp. 60–61) and has limited opportunity for self-expression or fulfilment – all factors recognized as having an impact on levels of stress, depression and mental illness in the general population (see pp.126–127). Reducing inappropriate prescribing might help to focus attention on factors related to the social conditions of people, rather than on their learning disability.

Access to health care

There are a number of barriers to accessing health services, including difficulties not only in being able to detect, express and seek treatment for health needs but also in being able to access services.

Annual GP health checks were introduced in 2008. After the first 5 years, it was thought that around half of those eligible received a health check, with huge variation across health authorities.

Health implications of learning disability for the family

Although there is now a greater awareness of the importance of how to communicate any diagnosis, it is still the case that many new parents feel inadequately supported when their child is diagnosed as having a learning disability. Nor do they feel well prepared for what this will mean for their family, especially through the early years. Where the disability is not immediately obvious, it can take parents years to achieve a diagnosis and their efforts can have them labelled as anxious, neurotic or worse. Achieving a diagnosis may still leave parents having to fight for effective help or support. This situation tends to worsen when the child makes the transition to adult services. The period around transition (planning for which starts when the child is 14 years of age) can be a time of great anxiety for parents and of renewed battles for support.

Added to the pain of having to let go hopes and ambitions for their child, parents will also have to adjust to a child who will require basic care for a protracted (or indefinite) period, who may have very disturbed sleep patterns and other problem behaviours and who may have co-existing conditions such as epilepsy, cerebral palsy, sensory impairments, eating problems and others.

In such situations, parents are at risk of exhaustion, of neglecting their own health and well-being and of stresses affecting their own relationship and their relationships with other children. There is also good evidence that having a child with a significant disability affects the earning power of a family, thus adding a further stress.

Because learning disability is a lifelong condition and because there is a shortfall in appropriate and acceptable provision, many parents remain carers into their 70s and beyond, and only become known to social services when they become too frail to continue caring. Given the universal coverage of general practice, GPs are well placed to identify earlier these so-called hidden carers (see spread Community care, pp. 154–155).

Implications of learning disability for health services and society

In 1969 there were nearly 60,000 people with learning disabilities living (permanently) in hospital. The last long-stay hospital in England closed in 2009. Policies clearly state (e.g. Valuing people now, 2009) that people with a learning disability should live in their communities. Despite this, in 2015, around 2500 people were receiving inpatient services (including 110 people under the age of 18 years), some of whom have been inpatients for more than 5 years. Out-of-area placements are common, particularly amongst people with challenging behaviour. Once people are moved out of area (which may occur during childhood, e.g.

attending a residential school), research has shown that people often remain out of area.

The social model has prevailed over the medical model. Policy continues to follow the route of individualizing services and transferring control to the person, but disputes over resources and affordability mean service delivery is still far from personalized or user-controlled. Box 60.1 provides some key principles of service delivery.

Case study

John was a 10-year-old boy with severe learning disabilities. He lived in the family home but was mainly restricted to one room. Most furnishings had been progressively damaged and removed. At home, John would not stay clothed, eat at a table or from a plate, use cutlery or use toilet facilities – he resisted bathing, had few settled nights, engaged in little play and frequently hit out and bit. There was little support going into the home and the family resources were exhausted. Transfer to a specialist residential school, out of area, was under active consideration, but the family was not keen.

Intensive partnership working with the family, involving advocacy services, and health, social work, education and housing services working with the support service, saw John and his family carer, 18 months later, in a new home. He still did not have full access to the house, but his bedroom and sitting room were furnished, and he had games, materials and activity equipment indoors and in the garden. Person-centred intervention approaches included active support, positive behaviour support and work to develop his communication. He was experiencing more engagement in activities in and around the home, and at the local parks and beach. He now slept in his bed, with sheets and duvet, bathed twice a day, had settled nights and ate with appropriate equipment at the table. In addition he was using signs and symbols to communicate needs and wants, including the sign for toilet, and indicating choices about food and clothes. The threat of removal to a residential school had receded.

Stop and think

The health care needs of people with learning disabilities are not always looked at well enough in medical education. Nor are wider issues about how doctors should best communicate with them.

- Why is this the case? What can you do to improve your understanding and communication skills?

Box 60.1 Principles of service delivery to people with a learning disability

People with learning disabilities:

- Should be valued. They should be asked and encouraged to contribute to the community they live in. They should not be picked on or treated differently from others.
- Are individual people.
- Should be asked about the services they need and be involved in making choices about what they want.
- Should be helped and supported to do everything they are able to.
- Should be able to use the same local services as everyone else, wherever possible.
- Should benefit from specialist social, health and educational services.
- Should have services that take account of their age, abilities and other needs.

From Scottish Executive, 2000, with permission.
See also the United Nations Convention of the Rights of People with Disabilities (2007).

Learning disability

- Although prevalence of people with learning disability is relatively low, the impact on the individual and the family is likely to be considerable. Carers of people with learning disabilities may experience exhaustion, stress and poor health.
- The social model of disability has made an important contribution to the individualizing of services and to transferring control to the individual.
- The transition from childhood to adulthood can be a time of considerable anxiety to parents and the individual.
- Doctors can be a great support to a family if they listen carefully and work with the individual, the family and other health and social services to obtain the support that the individual and family want and need.

61 | Post-traumatic stress disorder

Post-traumatic stress disorder (PTSD) is a condition where exposure to an intense and frightening emotional experience leads to lasting changes in behaviour, mood and cognition. Often after a life-threatening incident (e.g. a violent assault, rape or wartime experience), the individual re-experiences the event(s), e.g. via intrusive and distressing thoughts, images, flashbacks or nightmares. The individual may also exhibit phobic avoidance and/or physiological reactivity (e.g. increased heart rate) to reminders of the trauma. Increased arousal in terms of sleep disturbance, irritability and exaggerated startle response are common. In addition the individual may exhibit a restricted range of affect and a sense of a foreshortened future and may lose interest in previously rewarding hobbies or activities. The current diagnostic criteria of the International Classification of Diseases (ICD-10) are shown in Box 61.1.

Symptoms of PTSD may occur immediately after the triggering event, or may not develop until weeks, months or years have passed. Many individuals will develop symptoms of an "acute stress reaction" immediately after a traumatic event, experiencing short-term symptoms of PTSD, which resolve as the individual learns to cope. When these symptoms persist, a diagnosis of PTSD can be made.

Effect on memory

As stated previously, PTSD is characterized by intrusive, distressing memories of the traumatic event. Paradoxically it is also often associated with marked impairments in learning and memory for new material (anterograde memory: see pp. 26–27). Patients often complain that they remember what they do not want to, yet cannot remember what they now wish to. Heightened arousal at the time of encoding may result in modulation (strengthening) of the emotional memory trace, possibly via noradrenaline release in the amygdala. Subsequent anterograde memory impairment may be caused by the deleterious effects of prolonged elevated levels of stress hormones (e.g. long-term hypercortisolaemia) on hippocampal functioning. Indeed, some magnetic resonance imaging studies have shown that chronic PTSD is associated with reduction in the volume of the hippocampus, a brain area critically involved in new learning and memory.

Prevalence and risk factors

The estimated lifetime prevalence for PTSD is 6.8%. The most common precipitating traumas are combat for men and rape and sexual molestation for women. It is important to note that (1) most people do *not* develop a disorder after experiencing a stressful life event; and (2) many disorders other than PTSD, in particular phobias, depression, acute stress reaction and adjustment disorders, often develop after adversity.

It is clear that some individuals are more likely than others to develop PTSD after exposure to trauma. Predictive variables that have been identified include trauma severity, dissociation during the trauma, perceived threat and premorbid vulnerability factors, including prior emotional disorder, particularly depression (see pp. 114–115).

Refugees, in particular, may have been exposed to significant traumatic events, and there is accumulating evidence that they may be at 10 times higher risk of developing PTSD compared with the general population. Refugees have often left behind their livelihood, their communities and their possessions. Lack of social support and the challenge of integrating into a new society may further impede recovery. Where culture and language barriers exist, the NICE 2005 guidelines recommend the use of interpreters and bicultural therapists as required to optimize treatment. Trauma-focussed psychological interventions (see in later section) have been shown to be effective.

Debriefing and PTSD

When disaster strikes, there is an understandable desire to try to act quickly to support survivors. With increasing recognition that PTSD can be a debilitating outcome in many individuals who experience trauma, rapid psychological interventions, i.e. single-session critical incident stress debriefing (CISD), became popular during the 1990s. However, systematic reviews of controlled trials in this area failed to find any evidence that CISD reduced general psychological morbidity, depression or anxiety; rather a significantly *increased* risk of PTSD has been observed in those who had received debriefing (NICE, 2005) (Fig. 61.1). This may be because those who did not receive immediate professional treatment instead utilized existing social support mechanisms and gradually came to terms with their traumatic experience over time via discussion with close confidants.

Treatment of PTSD

The most effective treatments for chronic PTSD are trauma-focussed cognitive–behavioural therapy (CBT) and eye movement desensitization and reprocessing (EMDR). In PTSD, symptoms may be maintained via overt and covert avoidance of reminders or thoughts about the event. Exposure-based behaviour treatments have consistently been shown to be effective. These involve patients confronting their fears, either via systematic desensitization (imaginal exposure to feared stimuli whilst in a relaxed state, in a graded, hierarchical fashion) or 'real-life' graded

---

Box 61.1 Diagnostic criteria for post-traumatic stress disorder as defined by the *International Classification of Diseases* (ICD-10)

F43.1 Post-traumatic stress disorder

A. Exposure to a stressful event or situation (either short or long-lasting) of exceptionally threatening or catastrophic nature, which is likely to cause pervasive distress in almost anyone.

B. Persistent remembering or 'reliving' the stressor by having intrusive flash backs, vivid memories, or recurring dreams or by experiencing distress when exposed to circumstances resembling or associated with the stressor.

C. Actual or preferred avoidance of circumstances resembling or associated with the stressor (not present before exposure to the stressor).

D. Either (1) or (2):
   (1) Inability to recall, either partially or completely, some important aspects of the period of exposure to the stressor
   (2) Persistent symptoms of increased psychological sensitivity and arousal (not present before exposure to the stressor) shown by any two of the following:
      a) difficulty in falling or staying asleep
      b) irritability or outbursts of anger
      c) difficulty in concentrating
      d) hyper-vigilance
      e) exaggerated startle response

E. Onset of symptoms within 6 months of the stressor.

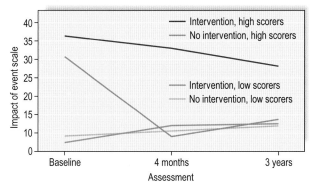

Fig. 61.1 Effects of immediate debriefing on victims of road traffic injury. Those with high initial scores on the impact of events scale (intrusive thoughts and avoidance) had worse outcomes than untreated controls 4 months and 3 years later *(from Mayou and Farmer, 2002, with permission).*

exposure. EMDR is a relatively new technique that consists of imaginal exposure whilst the therapist waves a finger across the patient's visual field with the patient tracking the finger. EMDR is a controversial treatment as initially remarkable claims were made for its efficacy. The effective component of EMDR may be due, in part, to the exposure component.

The evidence base for drug treatments in PTSD is limited and drug treatments for PTSD should not be used as a routine first-line treatment for adults (NICE, 2005). Mirtazapine, amitriptyline and phenelzine have been found to have clinically significant effects in PTSD sufferers (NICE, 2005). The selective serotonin reuptake inhibitor (SSRI) anti-depressant drug paroxetine may also be helpful, and in many cases the traumatized individual may fulfil diagnostic criteria for both PTSD and co-morbid major depression. Where a patient responds well to a drug treatment, it should be continued for a minimum of 12 months before withdrawing it gradually.

PTSD in the general medical setting

A significant number of individuals may be traumatized by their experience of medical events and procedures. This may be particularly so in emergency departments, intensive care units and orthopaedic and plastic surgery clinics. Modern medicine and surgery often employ invasive procedures for which the patient has had little or no preparation (see pp. 102–103). For example, many individuals who previously would have died are now alive because of medical and surgical advances. Although such patients are now discharged as medical 'success stories', some survivors develop PTSD and become markedly disabled. Very often these cases are not identified in the general hospital setting, and appropriate interventions are not offered. Such individuals may subsequently avoid further contact with the medical profession or show poor adherence with treatment regimes (see Adherence pp. 92–93).

Case study

Mrs C, a 30-year-old woman, underwent a tonsillectomy. Whilst in hospital her husband brought their baby to visit her. Mrs C started to hug the baby. Suddenly blood spurted out of her mouth all over the floor. Panic ensued, and she was rushed in a state of hypovolaemic shock to the operating room, where a bleeding artery was ligated. She remembers overhearing a doctor tell her husband that 'she'd had one foot in the grave'. For months after this event, Mrs C lived in a constant state of anxiety. She feared that the pharyngeal scar would open and she would bleed to death. Intrusive thoughts and memories of the event kept her awake at night and disturbed her during the day. She was terrified to make a careless move in case it triggered a further episode of bleeding. She withdrew contact from her baby because of a fear that whilst hugging him blood would again spurt out of her mouth. Treatment involved controlled exposure, involving visiting the surgeon who had operated on her, and receiving accurate information regarding future risk. Gradually she returned to her previous level of functioning.

From Shalev et al., 1993.

Post-traumatic stress disorder

• PTSD is an increasingly recognized, although controversial, disorder.

• PTSD is commonly reported after extreme trauma.

• Most people do not develop a disorder after a traumatic life event.

• Some medical events (e.g. myocardial infarction), treatments (e.g. defibrillation) or settings (e.g. intensive care) can lead to PTSD symptoms.

• Patients with PTSD after medical events are often not identified.

• Refugees are at elevated risk of developing PTSD.

• Sufferers may avoid further medical care and show poor adherence with treatment.

• Improved recognition should lead to appropriate treatment and improved ability to make use of medical care.

• Effective treatments include trauma-focussed CBT and EMDR.

The number of people worldwide with the chronic condition diabetes mellitus has been increasing dramatically in recent years and is expected to go on rising. Over 3 million people in the UK have diabetes, at least another 600,000 are estimated to have undiagnosed diabetes. Without action the total number with diabetes will rise to 5 million in the UK, and represent nearly 10% of the global adult population by 2030. Diabetes consumes almost 10% of the UK National Health Service (NHS) budget, around £10 billion annually (Diabetes UK, 2014). The two main forms of diabetes are type 1 and type 2, with 85% to 95% having type 2 diabetes. Both types result in raised blood glucose, which has adverse short- and long-term consequences. For example, diabetes greatly increases people's risk of developing cardiovascular and kidney diseases, is responsible for over 100 amputations per week and 20,000 early deaths per year in the UK and over 8% of all adult deaths globally (Diabetes UK, 2014).

Type 1 diabetes

Type 1 diabetes is typically diagnosed in childhood or adolescence. As a result of a combination of genetic and environmental factors, which are not well understood, an autoimmune process progressively destroys the cells in the pancreas that produce the hormone insulin. Insulin is necessary to facilitate the uptake of glucose from the blood by body tissue. Without insulin, blood glucose levels rise, leading to characteristic symptoms of frequent urination, thirst, fatigue and weight loss. If untreated, there is a risk of ketoacidosis (build-up of harmful ketones in the body) leading eventually to coma, which can be fatal. Type 1 diabetes is treated by replacing the insulin no longer produced by the body, with insulin delivered by injection or pump. The complex treatment regimen requires patients to monitor blood glucose levels and use the results to balance food consumption, insulin administration and energy expenditure. The aim of treatment is to achieve good glycaemic control: that is, keeping blood glucose levels within the normal range. However, young people with type 1 diabetes in particular often risk experiencing long-term negative health consequences from hyperglycaemia (abnormally high blood glucose levels) to avoid the more salient and upsetting short term symptoms of hypoglycaemia (a "hypo", or abnormally low blood glucose levels), which can result in confusion and loss of consciousness.

Type 2 diabetes

Type 2 diabetes was traditionally a disease of the middle-aged and elderly but is increasingly seen among younger people. This is a result of rising rates of obesity and physical inactivity, as being overweight is estimated to account for 80% to 85% of the overall risk of developing type 2 diabetes (Diabetes UK, 2014). Due to a strong genetic component, having a family history of diabetes also increases people's risk, as does being from a Black or South Asian ethnic background. In type 2 diabetes, blood glucose levels become abnormally high because of both impaired insulin production and insensitivity. The symptoms are similar to type 1, but often less pronounced so that type 2 diabetes can go undiagnosed for years. The management of type 2 diabetes initially involves supporting people to make lifestyle changes to improve their diet, increase their physical activity and lose weight. Tablets for reducing blood glucose levels and/or insulin injections are also usually required in the longer term.

Prevention of diabetes

The development of diabetes is usually preceded by a prolonged period where blood glucose levels are higher than normal but not high enough for a diagnosis of diabetes – this is known as *impaired glucose regulation* or *pre-diabetes*. For many of the 60 million Europeans with pre-diabetes, the onset of diabetes can be delayed or prevented by changes in lifestyle, and especially by moderate weight loss (5% or more of body weight). The Finnish Diabetes Prevention Study and the US Diabetes Prevention Program demonstrated that for people with pre-diabetes, individualized counselling that supported healthier eating and increased physical activity reduced people's risk of developing diabetes by nearly 60% over 3- to 4-year follow up periods in comparison with usual care. The reductions in risk persisted for at least 10 years and the more weight loss, healthy eating and physical activity targets that were met, the greater the reduction in risk (Fig. 62.1).

Guidance on diabetes prevention (e.g. from the UK National Institute for Health and Care Excellence and European Diabetes Prevention Forum) highlights the importance of identifying people at high risk of developing type 2 diabetes. It also provides recommendations for the content and implementation of diabetes prevention programmes to support people in making sustainable lifestyle changes. A recent review has shown that programmes that adhere to these recommendations are more likely to be effective (Dunkley et al., 2014). Currently there are no known interventions to prevent type 1 diabetes, but research on this amongst people with known risk factors is ongoing.

Depression and diabetes

Depression rates are around three times higher in people with type 1 diabetes and twice as high in those with type 2 diabetes

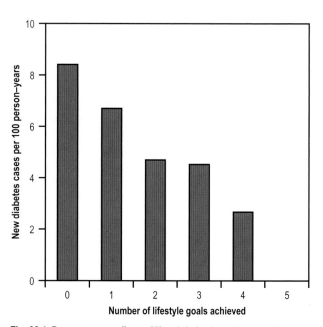

Fig. 62.1 Dose-response effects of lifestyle behaviour change on diabetes incidence (at a median of 7 years of follow-up) in people with pre-diabetes. The goals were (1) no more than 30% of daily energy from fat; (2) no more than 10% of energy from saturated fat; (3) at least 15 g per 1,000 kcal fibre; at (4) least 30 minutes per day of moderate physical activity; and (5) at least 5% weight reduction *(adapted from Tuomilehto et al., 2001, with permission).*

compared with people without diabetes. This relationship is probably bi-directional and results from behavioural and physiological pathways. People who are depressed are more likely to engage in unhealthy behaviours (see spread depression, pp. 114–115), be obese and struggle with self-management of their diabetes. Depression may directly reduce insulin sensitivity and glycaemic control. Moreover the psychosocial impact of having a chronic illness and the demanding self-management regime in diabetes (see later section) is likely to increase the risk of depression. Therefore it is important to assess and treat depression in people with diabetes. However, anti-depressant medications must be used with caution because they can have adverse effects on glycaemic control.

Self-management of diabetes

Good glycaemic control is central to preventing and delaying the onset of complications from diabetes. In both types of diabetes, glycaemic control is largely dependent on the actions taken by the person with diabetes to manage their condition. Diabetes self-management involves performing behaviours related to medical management (blood glucose monitoring; regularly taking tablets, injecting insulin or both), and making and maintaining lifestyle changes to ensure a healthy diet, healthy weight and adequate physical activity. Patients are also expected to take actions to prevent complications (e.g. foot care to prevent problems resulting from reduced blood supply to the feet; attending screening for diabetic retinopathy, which can lead to blindness; and attending regular check-ups). Self-management is particularly challenging in adolescents with type 1 diabetes as physiological and behavioural changes make glycaemic control more difficult, their self-management goals and skills alter over time and there is a shift in the relative influence of family and peers (see Case study).

Supporting diabetes self-management

Despite its importance, few people with diabetes engage in self-management as recommended, often finding the lifestyle changes difficult. Patients can, therefore, benefit from education and support to improve their self-management. Dose Adjustment For Normal Eating (DAFNE) is an example of a programme shown to improve blood glucose control without

adversely affecting quality of life for people with type 1 diabetes. It teaches them how to match their insulin dose to food choices to maximize glycaemic control (DAFNE Study Group, 2002). For the far larger numbers of people with type 2 diabetes, a wide range of interventions focussing on supporting aspects of self-management in one-to-one, group, and technology-based formats, have been developed. The DESMOND and X-PERT programmes are two of the most well known in the UK (Box 62.1). These programmes are highly variable in terms of their aims, approach, delivery, content, contact time and effectiveness but overall have small positive effects on glycaemic control, at least in the short term. Impacts on quality of life and longer-term outcomes, including

complications, are not clear. These programmes, may be improved with increased emphasis on coping with the emotional consequences of diabetes, better use of behaviour change theories and techniques and support to ensure longer-term maintenance of effects. Tailored approaches that focus on motivating and empowering individuals (e.g. motivational interviewing) to address their most pressing self-management problems can be applied. Self-regulation techniques, including goal setting, reviewing progress, managing setbacks, revising goals and engaging social support, appear to be effective (American Association of Diabetes Educators, 2009) (Box 62.1).

Diabetes mellitus

- Diabetes is an increasingly common chronic illness, mainly because of ageing populations in developed countries and the global rise in obesity.

- Type 2 diabetes can largely be prevented by improving diet, increasing physical activity and losing weight.

- The onset of complications in both type 1 and type 2 diabetes can be prevented

or delayed by improved blood glucose control.

- Day-to-day management of diabetes is primarily the responsibility of patients, who need empowering and supporting in their self-management of the condition.

- Interventions to enhance patient self-management are most effective when they are patient-centred and tailored

to individual needs and include elements to address motivation, self-regulation and social support (see Box 62.1).

- Diabetes occurs in all age groups, and is particularly common in certain ethnic groups.

- Different approaches to providing appropriate care and support are needed for these different groups.

Box 62.1 Patient-centred self-management for type 2 diabetes

A patient-centred, group-based self-management programme based on theories of empowerment and discovery learning (the X-PERT diabetes programme) has been evaluated in a randomized controlled trial involving 314 adults with type 2 diabetes. Compared with the control group who received usual care plus brief individual diabetes education via appointments with a dietician, nurse and GP, after 14 months the X-PERT group showed significant improvements in their blood glucose levels, body weight, waist circumference, physical activity levels and other aspects of diabetes self-management (Deakin et al., 2006).

Case study

Part 1: Self-management for a teenager with type 1 diabetes
Tracey is 16 years old and enjoys going clubbing. When Tracey stays out late dancing and drinking with her friends, she misses her evening snack, and the alcohol and physical activity lower her blood glucose levels. Her blood glucose levels continue to drop whilst she is asleep, and she is often hypoglycaemic by the time she wakes up, making her bad-tempered and uncooperative, or worse: Tracey has been rushed to hospital unconscious on several occasions. How can the health workers help Tracey to take better care of herself?

Part 2: How can we help Tracey?
- Encourage Tracey to attend sessions specifically for groups of teenagers with diabetes to discuss how to overcome the lifestyle challenges posed by their self-management.

- Tracey's doctor may be able to suggest an adjustment to her insulin injections on evenings when she is going out.

- The dietician may recommend certain foods Tracey should eat before going out, and snacks or soft drinks that she could have whilst clubbing.

- Tracey or her mother could be advised to leave a favourite snack conveniently by her bed for when she returns home late.

- Tracey's parents should be advised not to relinquish responsibility for Tracey's diabetes too soon.

63 | What is stress?

Although we all know how it feels to be 'stressed', defining what we mean is not easy, precisely because it is a subjective experience. Stimulus-based models indicate that stress means being under a lot of 'pressure'. This idea comes from engineering relating to pressure applied to an object and is applied to individuals with the suggestion that we have a certain tolerance to stress but that if it is too great, we become ill. The response-based model focuses on the physical and psychological experience of 'being stressed' and is seen as an automatic response to an external stressor. This perspective concentrates on investigating the mechanisms linking stress to physical illnesses. Interactional or transactional approaches concentrate on the mismatch between our perception of demands placed on us and our perception of our ability to cope with these demands. This model explains why different individuals find different events stressful and why they differ in their responses to them.

How do we measure stress?

Life events scales are commonly used to measure stress influenced by stimulus-based perspectives. The first scale, Schedule of Recent Experiences (Holmes and Rahe, 1967), only counted the number of actual recent experiences (each event of 43 had the same weight). The subsequent Social Readjustment Rating Scale assigned points to different life events. For instance, death of the spouse is assigned 100, and personal injury or illness is assigned 53 points. Later scales measured everyday events that cause us frustration (Hassles Scale) or make us feel good in our everyday life (Uplifts Scale). The main criticism of such scales is that they do not take into account the individual's own appraisals of these potential stressors.

What influences the experience of stress?

We all find different things stressful, and our reactions to stress and how we cope reflect this individual approach. However, this perspective is not reflected in stimulus- or response-based models. One of the interactional models that have shown usefulness in accounting for individual differences is Lazarus and Folkman's (1984) transactional model of stress and theory of appraisal. This model states that individuals actively appraise an event as stressful rather than passively responding to it. There are two types of appraisal: primary and secondary. When we are faced with a potential stressful event, we first engage in primary appraisal, by which the event can be appraised as irrelevant, benign and positive, harmful and threatening or harmful and challenging. If assessed as threatening or challenging, we engage in secondary appraisal, namely, of our coping abilities. This model suggests that we experience stress when we perceive a discrepancy between our perception of the threat or challenge and our perception of ability to cope with that threat.

What is the relationship between stress and physical illness?

Changes in the immune system can occur as a result of stress. The field that examines the impact of stress on the immune system is known as *psycho-neuro-immunology* (PNI). Research has examined both acute and chronic stress and their consequences for immune function. Chronic stress is associated with some degree of

downregulation of immune systems, as in the case of acute stress, but the findings are less clear-cut; moreover the changes that have been shown are within the normal range of variation for healthy individuals. Research on the common cold shows that stress levels do predict increased susceptibility to catching a cold even after controlling for health behaviours such as smoking and drinking.

Investigations on work-related stress shed light on the psychological mechanisms that might be at work (Fig. 63.1). Two critical constructs in creating job strain appear to be high job demands and low decision latitude (lack of decision-making power over time management). Whitehall II is a prospective cohort study that explores the socio-economic status, stress and cardiovascular disease. This study follows a cohort of 10,308 participants from British Civil Service aged 35 to 55 years (3,413 women and 6,895 men) and collects self-report and clinical data every 2 to 5 years. Kuper and Marmot (2003), using Whitehall II data, found that participants who were at low decision latitude and high demands, i.e. those with job strain, experienced the highest risk for coronary heart disease (see Heart disease, pp. 106–107; Work and health, pp. 56–57).

Stress can have an effect on our health behaviours. When we are stressed, we might engage in a variety of behaviours that are unhealthy. We may skip meals, sleep less or smoke or drink more in an effort to cope.

Stop and think

Many students experience stress before, during and/or after examinations.

- Which thoughts and perceptions increase this stress?

- How could you help a friend who experiences a lot of stress due to a forthcoming exams?

Reducing stress

There are many approaches that can be taken to reduce the experience of stress and/or its impact on our health and quality of life. Ideally we should reduce the stressors in our lives. Thus to

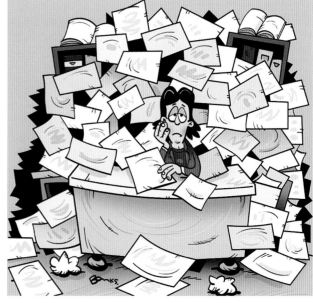

Fig. 63.1 Stress at work: A sense of being overwhelmed and lacking control.

reduce job strain, we should redesign work by reducing psychological demands; giving people more control over their day-to-day jobs, enabling them to have more task variety and providing more leadership opportunities may improve long-term health. Such strategies of getting rid of stressors may not always be within the control of the individual. Since part of the stress response is secondary appraisal of our coping abilities. Therefore it may be helpful to work on our appraisals of our coping abilities. For instance, we may want to remind ourselves how we have coped in similar situations in the past and that actually we do possess the ability to successfully manage the situation. Or we may want to consider working on our primary appraisal and re-evaluate how important the stressor is.

Our relationships with our social networks can have an influence on our health and quality of life. Whilst social relationships can be a source of fun and positive experience, relationships that involve abuse or negative interactions are some of the major stressors we can face. Berkman and Syme (1979) in their landmark study with 6,928 adults found that those lacking social and community ties were more likely to die in the 9-year follow-up period than those with more extensive networks. Although we need to be mindful of what we mean by social support (the size and structure of the network or perceived social support), our networks might be a source of help to cope with stressful events (see also Self-Care, pp. 98–99).

Stress management courses have also been developed to help people. Although Miller and Cohen's (2001) review showed that there was little evidence that stress management interventions alleviated the immune dysregulation associated with stress, van der Klink et al.'s (2001) review of interventions for work-related stress indicated that interventions based on cognitive–behavioural methods had positive impact (See Box 63.1).

Box 63.1 Stress among medical students and health care professionals

Being a health care professional can be a very stressful experience. Consider the context of Graham's experience and what might be going through his mind. How would you help Graham who says he feels very stressed?

Graham started his first month in his new clinical placement at a regional hospital in a major city in an area. He is in local rented accommodation, which is poorly heated and maintained. It is temporary until he can find a better alternative. The job is completely different to expectations, with significant responsibilities, high turnover of patients, hectic schedule and a ward team not sympathetic towards new staff arrivals. His sleep pattern is disrupted, he complains of headaches, his appetite is poor, he is tempted to overuse alcohol in the evenings and he finds himself getting panicky and unable to make quick decisions.

What is stress?

- There are different ways of conceptualising stress and the stress experience: stimulus-based, response-based and interactional/transactional.
- Traditionally stress has been measured by life events scales that count and assign values to significant life events, but these do not take into account individual's own appraisal of the stressor. Physiological measures such as sweating and heart rate can be used as indicators of stress.
- Two appraisal mechanisms affect our experience of stress: primary appraisal (of how stressful the event is) and secondary appraisal (of our coping abilities). Stress arises from discrepancy between how stressful the event is and our perception of our coping abilities.
- Investigations into job strain show that those who lack control over their jobs and face high demands at work experience the highest risk for coronary heart disease.
- Stress can have a negative impact on our health behaviours.
- Stress management techniques that might be suitable for different individuals. Cognitive–behavioural techniques appear to be most successful in reducing work-related stress.

Asthma affects almost 1 in 11 individuals and 1 in 5 households in the UK, occurring from infancy to old age and is genetically based. Chronic obstructive pulmonary disease (COPD) is diagnosed in 2% of the UK population and in 4.5% of those over 40 years of age. In most cases COPD is the consequence of lung damage caused by smoking (<10% is caused by occupational illness). However, this number is growing. Asthma and COPD symptoms have many similarities, such as breathlessness and exacerbations, which can be triggered by infections (for both) or allergens in the case of asthma. For asthma the most important intervention is inhaled corticosteroid, an anti-inflammatory medication. Used regularly, inhaled steroids reduce lung inflammation and prevent asthma symptoms. Higher-dose oral steroids are used in short courses to manage exacerbations. In severe asthma they may be taken in lower doses for regular control.

Broncho-dilating medication is the other main medical intervention. It relaxes airways and relieves symptoms but does not reduce airway inflammation. Patients use this medication when they feel mildly breathless or before exercise.

Quality of life in asthma and COPD

Lung obstruction is, for most, reversible in asthma but not COPD. Breathlessness in asthma is relieved by regular use of inhaled or oral steroids and occasional use of broncho-dilators. With appropriate medication and regular adherence, almost all people with asthma can lead a non-restricted life. For many individuals activities need not be limited, and exacerbations can be reduced to a very low level. However, patients can feel burdened by regular medication and levels of physical activity can still be less than in the general population. For both conditions quality of life can be impaired.

In COPD lung damage is non-reversible and progressive. Moderate-to-severe breathlessness, cough and phlegm production with periods of acute symptoms are characteristic of COPD. Daily activities become limited, sleep is frequently disturbed and severe attacks of breathlessness can lead to hospital admissions and a spiral of inactivity and disability. Pulmonary rehabilitation can help patients cope with constant breathlessness and manage everyday activities.

Adherence in asthma

In mild to moderate asthma, lung inflammation can be controlled by daily use of inhaled corticosteroid, but many patients do not take their inhaled steroid as prescribed. Non-adherence can be unintentional (accidental because of practical barriers) or intentional (purposeful acts based on perceptions). Patients may believe medication is only needed at certain times (pragmatic adherence) or stop to test if symptoms reappear (testing). Some may express steroid phobia. A patient-centred approach to self-management is effective and structured education with personalized action plans and regular review are recommended (British Guideline on the Management of Asthma, 2016).

Self-management in asthma and COPD

Adherence is most likely when patients understand what they are being advised to do, and why (see pp. 92–93). Personalised Asthma Action Plans (PAAP) (Fig. 64.1) aim to encourage individuals to recognize when asthma control is affected (based on symptoms and peak flow) and to identify actions required: for example, making changes to medication regime such as increasing or initiating steroids or seeking help from a health care professional. They should be discussed and agreed upon between the health professional and the patient as part of structured self-management education. Use of PAAP's has been shown to improve outcomes for asthma and quality of life and to reduce emergency health care use and symptoms.

COPD action plans aim to increase recognition of an exacerbation and encourage prompt treatment and can reduce emergency admissions and hospital stays. In recent years, distinct self-management programmes for COPD have been developed with the aim to provide education, psychosocial support and, in some cases, an exercise intervention. These have met with varying success but can reduce health care use and increase exercise performance and knowledge.

Smoking cessation in COPD

Smoking cessation is the main method of controlling further deterioration and early death in COPD (Fig. 64.2). In asthma, it is important for symptom control and reducing the risk of asthma in children (see pp. 82–83)

Family and health professional advice are important influences in encouraging quit attempts. Brief doctor advice increases the likelihood that a smoker will stop by about 2% to 3%, and advice plus nicotine replacement therapy leads to increased cessation of about 10% (Fig. 64.3).

Use it, don't lose it!

Your action plan is a personal guide to help you stay on top of your asthma. Once you have created one with your GP or asthma nurse, it can help you stay as well as possible.

People who use their action plans are four times less likely to end up in hospital because of their asthma.

Your action plan will only work at its best to help keep you healthy if you:

1 **Put it somewhere easy for you and your family to find** – you could try your fridge door, the back of your front door, or your bedside table. Try taking a photo and keeping it on your mobile phone or tablet.

2 **Check in with it regularly** – put a note on your calendar, or a reminder on your mobile to read it through once a month. How are you getting along with your day-to-day asthma medicines? Are you having any asthma symptoms? Are you clear about what to do?

3 **Keep a copy near you** – save a photo on your phone or as your screensaver. Or keep a leaflet in your bag, desk or car glove box.

4 **Give a copy of your action plan or share a photo of it with a key family member or friend** – ask them to read it. Talk to them about your usual asthma symptoms so they can help you notice if they start. Help them know what to do in an emergency.

5 **Take it to every healthcare appointment – including A&E/consultant.** Ask your GP or asthma nurse to update it if any of their advice for you changes. Ask them for tips if you're finding it hard to take your medicines as prescribed.

Fig. 64.1 Personalised Asthma Action Plan (PAAP).

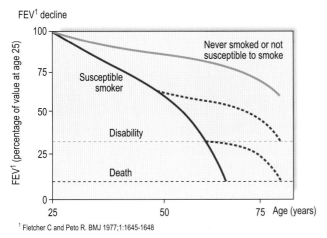

FEV¹ decline

Fig. 64.2 Smoking and lung function decline: Peto graph.

¹ Fletcher C and Peto R. BMJ 1977;1:1645-1648

Stop and think

- Do you or does someone you know have asthma? Does it have a major or minor effect in your life or their life?

What prompted an attempt to stop smpking?

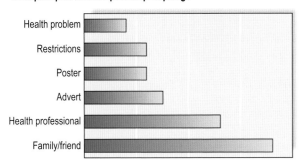

Fig. 64.3 Influence on smoking cessation attempts.

Pulmonary rehabilitation in COPD

Pulmonary rehabilitation includes physical exercise (e.g. walking to improve exercise capacity, and education to support self-management and lifestyle changes); typical topics include disease education, breathlessness management, energy conservation and anxiety management. It is run by a multi-disciplinary team, including physiotherapists and nurses for small groups of patients. Pulmonary rehabilitation has been shown to improve patient quality of life, exercise tolerance, respiratory muscle strength and anxiety and depression, even when objective indicators of lung function do not change.

Psychological issues in asthma and COPD

Asthma deaths are uncommon, but psychiatric morbidity is high among the small group of people (<1%) with a history of severe life-threatening asthma attacks. A summary of psychosocial adverse factors associated with fatal and near-fatal asthma attacks is shown in Box 64.1.

Intensive management programmes, with one-to-one contact and fast access to health professional support, have been a successful approach to reducing life-threatening attacks among

this high-risk group. Molfino et al. (1992) followed up 12 patients who had had near-fatal asthma attacks and who were recommended for closely supervised follow-up. Seven of the 12 agreed and all survived. Five refused; of these, two died within 6 months of hospital discharge. Psycho-educational programmes that target patients with severe asthma have shown short-term gains in self-management and reduced hospital admissions.

Stop and think

- Do you know anyone with COPD? What effect does it have on their life?

Case study

Adolescents and asthma

In a focus group study, 28 teenagers (13–17 years) with asthma talked about their experience with asthma and health care. The teenagers were concerned about adverse effects and medication costs and wanted more information about asthma and its treatment. They considered themselves compliant with therapy but felt that they had had conflicting advice and inappropriate rules from adults about medication use. The group wanted complete responsibility for medication and believed that they did not disobey adults or that peers had a negative influence on them.

In 1997 the National Asthma Campaign carried out a national study of UK teenagers' attitudes towards asthma. This showed that worries about asthma attacks and about use of inhalers was greatest among younger teenagers and lessened as teenagers grew older.

From Slack and Brooks, 1995.

Asthma and COPD

- Regular inhaled steroids reduce risk of exacerbations in asthma, but many patients stop taking preventive medication when symptoms reduce.
- In asthma and COPD, agreement on treatment goals between patient and health professional improves outcomes. It is best achieved through a personalised approach to self-management education.
- Smoking cessation is the most important intervention for slowing the progression of COPD. Pulmonary rehabilitation is recommended to improve function and reduce disability.

65 | Death and dying

The medicalization of dying

Dying and death, like birth, are a normal part of everyday life. Over the past few decades, Western societies have largely removed death and dying to the confines of institutions such as hospitals and hospices. Care of the dying and the dead is still, for the most part, the remit of professionals such as doctors, nurses and undertakers. As a result, death has become marginalized and stigmatized and, some would argue, increasingly medicalized (see pp. 2–3). More recently, media images of death, dying and mourning such as the Princess of Wales' funeral in the UK and the events surrounding 9/11 terrorist attack in the USA have gradually re-introduced this topic to the public arena. Public outpourings of grief on national television have become more acceptable. There is growing recognition that people should be encouraged to talk more openly about death and dying so that their wishes for end-of-life care are identified and fulfilled through advanced care planning (www.dyingmatters.org; Henry and Seymour, 2008).

Place of death

Paradoxically although we know that most people would prefer to die at home, in their own beds and surrounded by family and friends, most do not. Data on place of death in England showed that 53% of all deaths occurred in hospital in the year 2010 (Gomes et al., 2011). A combination of factors such as poorly controlled symptoms, lack of family support, the burden on carers, badly coordinated services and changes in people's preferences as their disease progresses can result in people being admitted to a hospital or a hospice before they die. Thorpe (1993) suggested that improvements in care could enable more people to die at home (Box 65.1). However, not all patients want to die at home, and to help patients die where they want, it is important for doctors to explore patients' thoughts and fears in order to understand the reasons for their choice (Faull and Woof, 2002).

Attitudes to death and dying

Many doctors find caring for those who are dying a stressful but important part of their workload. This may be because doctors feel guilty or frustrated at their failure to achieve a medical cure or because they have difficulty in knowing how to communicate with the dying and their relatives. In addition to these professional concerns, most doctors will face common human fears when contemplating the inevitability and uncontrollability of death (Faull and Woof, 2002). The more anxious health professionals are about death, the more negative may be their attitudes and behaviour towards people at the end of life. Patients and their

---

families may also have their own reasons for avoiding these conversations (www.dyingmatters.org).

Stages of dying

Theoretical models have helped us to understand individual psychological responses to death. In her interviews with terminally ill patients with cancer, Kübler-Ross (1970) described the dying process as a series of stages that the person passes through before finally coming to terms with his or her imminent death. These stages include shock, denial, anger, bargaining, depression and ultimately acceptance. Similar staged theories have been used to describe the bereavement process (see pp. 16–17). However, not everyone passes through these stages in sequence, and individuals may fluctuate between acceptance and denial as they try to maintain hope about their prognosis (Johnston and Abraham, 2000). Carers and health professionals, therefore, need to be prepared for fluctuations in patients' moods and behaviours so that they do not misinterpret them.

Caring for people from different faiths

The way we care for people as they die and prepare the body after the death should be guided by the person's cultural and religious beliefs. Unfortunately such beliefs and associated rituals are often compromised by the organizational and bureaucratic barriers imposed by modern health care or by lack of understanding on the part of health professionals. Yet respecting these beliefs and ensuring prescribed rituals are adhered to can help patients to achieve a peaceful and dignified death and facilitate the bereavement process for carers (Firth, 2001).

Viewing the body after the death

Junior medical staff may often be involved in dealing with the relatives after the death. This may involve breaking the news of the death to the relatives and accompanying them to view the body, either on the ward or in the hospital chapel or mortuary where the body has been taken (see pp. 96–97). Although this may be an uncomfortable duty, it is an important part of the grieving process and allows the relatives to begin to absorb the loss and to say their final goodbyes. It will be especially difficult, however, if the death has been sudden or unexpected.

The good death

Helping patients achieve a good death is an important goal for health professionals who work with the dying. Table 65.1 describes the perceptions of one group of palliative care professionals about factors that constitute a 'good' death or a 'bad' death (Low and Payne, 1996). Good deaths occur when patients accept death and have control over the circumstances of their death, whereas bad deaths occur when patients are unprepared and the dying process is managed badly.

The importance of achieving a good death has led to the publication of guidelines and recommendations to help health professionals improve the standard of care for dying patients. For example, a report by the charity Age Concern identified 12 principles that facilitate a good death (Debate of the Age Health and Care Study Group, 1999) (Box 65.2).

> **Box 65.1 Factors that would allow dying people to remain at home**
>
> - Adequate nursing care
> - Good symptom control
> - Confident and committed general practitioners
> - Financial assistance
> - Access to specialist palliative care
> - Effective coordination of resources
> - Terminal care education

Table 65.1 **Factors constituting a 'good' death and a 'bad' death**	
Good death	**Bad death**
Lack of patient distress	**Negative effects on family**
• Family acceptance	• Unfinished business
• Dying in presence of close people	• Relatives' distress
• At peace	• Not dying with close people around
• Continuing previous interests	• Terrible physical symptoms
• No physical pain	
• No anxiety	
• Dying in place of choice	
Patient control during dying process	**Patient non-acceptance**
• Following appropriate cultural rules	• Non-preparation of relatives
• Dying in place of choice	• Non-acceptance of illness
• Cultural perceptions of good death	• Fighting death to the end
• Patient control	• Badly managed death
• Dying in presence of close people	
Role of staff	**Patient fears**
• Comfortable process	• Psychological distress
• Peaceful death	• Not dying in a place of choice
• No anxiety	• Terrible physical symptoms
• No pain	• Fighting death to the end
	• Not dying with close people around

Box 65.2 **Principles of a good death**

- Knowing when death is coming and understanding what can be expected
- Retaining control of what happens
- Being afforded dignity and privacy
- Control over pain relief and other symptom control
- Choice and control over where death occurs (at home or elsewhere)
- Access to information and expertise of whatever kind is necessary
- Access to any spiritual or emotional support desired
- Access to hospice care in any location, not only in hospital
- Control over who else is present and shares the end
- Being able to issue advance directives that ensure wishes are respected
- Time to say goodbye, and control over other aspects of timing
- Being able to leave when it is time to go and not having life prolonged pointlessly

Social death

The stigmas surrounding death and the difficulties in knowing how to talk to those who are dying can mean that terminally ill people experience a type of 'social death' before their bodies fail. This may occur because family, friends and health professionals find it difficult to talk to people who are dying and therefore withdraw from them or because the dying themselves begin a process of disengaging from people in an attempt to prepare themselves for their death (www.dyingmatters.org). This process may be initiated or exacerbated by physical symptoms that prevent patients from leading a normal life. Its result, however, may be that patients become lonely and isolated. Hospital staff may unwittingly compound this isolation by moving dying patients to side wards or hiding them behind bed screens. Maintaining good communication with patients at the end of life is essential to reassure them that they are still supported and valued as people, that they have a purpose in life and that they will be helped to resolve any unfinished business.

Ethical issues

Core ethical principles can be difficult to apply when dealing with those approaching death (Watson et al., 2006). Dilemmas arise when trying to balance the benefits and burdens of life-sustaining treatment with the goal of enhancing end-of-life care for patients: promoting a good death may mean withdrawing or withholding treatment. Confusion around the various definitions of euthanasia and assisted suicide and the extent to which they should be legalized is a matter of continuing debate and one in which doctors will always have a central role. Whilst it has been argued that the emergence of palliative care has precluded the need for euthanasia and assisted suicide, the discipline's approach to pain and symptom control has sometimes led to criticism and accusations from the public and others who misunderstand the importance of relief of suffering as a clinical goal. Similar problems surround the use of cardiopulomonary resuscitation in patients who are dying, and discussion with the patient and his or her family about whether or not to apply a do-not-resuscitate order can be difficult and distressing for the doctor. In addition, cognitive impairment in patients can mean that decisions have to be made on their behalf by either relatives or doctors. Taking time to explore patients' and relatives' wishes and questioning the efficacy of treatments are important to ensuring that interventions are both ethical and legal (Henry and Seymour, 2008).

Case study

You are a junior doctor on a busy medical ward to which an elderly Muslim man, Mr Ahmed, has been admitted. The patient's condition is terminal, and his prognosis is short. The consultant has informed the patient's wife that allowing him to die at home would not be advisable. The patient has a large family, and all of them are very distressed by the news. They want to visit every day and insist on bringing special food that they want the nurses to prepare. Their behaviour is causing disruption, but there are no single rooms available. On the night of Mr Ahmed's death the nurses ask you to tell the family to go home and come back in the morning. You are uncomfortable about this but do as you are asked. A few hours later Mr Ahmed dies. On hearing of his death, his family members are very angry and say that because they were not present at the death to perform special rituals, his soul will never be at peace.

Stop and think

- What steps could you have taken to ensure that Mr Ahmed had a 'good' death?
- How might you have found out more about the rituals that the family wanted to perform?
- How might this experience affect Mrs Ahmed's bereavement process?

Death and dying

- Our attitudes to death may affect the way we care for dying patients. Most patients want to die at home, but most, however, die in hospital.
- 'Good' deaths can be achieved if people are in control of the way they die. End-of-life care can pose challenging ethical questions for doctors.

66 | Counselling

Case study

A 35-year-old married mother of two attends your practice. Mrs Blue tells you she feels frightened all the time; she is irritable with her daughters, aged 2 and 5 years, and her sleep is more disturbed than usual even with two young children. She wonders what is wrong with her. Is she mentally ill? Is she depressed? Is it early menopause? She does not want tablets.

How do you understand Mrs Blue's complaints? Is she depressed or just stressed? Her notes do not mention her husband. She will not have anti-depressants – what are you going to do?

Research from general practice suggests that many patients like Mrs Blue present with psychological and/or unexplained medical symptoms and/or social problems associated with current life difficulties. The need to provide another management strategy, rather than psychotropic medication, is now recognised as important for patient care. GPs' reliance on psychotropic medication is thought inadvertently to push patients into the so-called mental health sick role, resulting in secondary gains to the illness and causing increased practice visits.

The British Association of Counselling and Psychotherapy (BACP, 2013) has provided evidence suggesting that:

1. Counselling and cognitive–behavioural therapy (CBT) are equally effective in the treatment of depression. Both result in post-treatment health gains, such as improved mental health and relationships with others.
2. Depressed patients are more satisfied with counselling than with psychotropic medication.
3. People with obsessive compulsive disorder (OCD) experienced improved functioning with counselling compared with psychotropic medication.
4. Counselling is more cost-effective than routine GP treatment for conditions such as postnatal depression and bulimia.

The advantages of counselling are (1) reduced psychotropic medication; (2) fewer patients presenting with minor physical complaints; (3) referral pathways to qualified colleagues (BACO, 2017); (4) knowing that a counsellor can spend 50 minutes with a patient compared with 6–12 a GP can offer.

What is counselling, and what is its evidence base?

Counselling is 'a boundaried time for people to explore and solve their own problems. Counselling raises people's self-esteem and helps them develop the skills to resolve their own past and present problems'.

Counselling is not giving instruction, information, solutions or support. It is assisting people to identify their own solutions to their own problems. It is used in a variety of situations, including bereavement, work-related stress, sadness or symptoms of reactive depression, anxiety, current-life difficulties, reduced confidence and sexual identity.

What is needed?

The setting for counselling is a quiet and confidential space in which the patient is in control and encouraged to speak freely. The role of the counsellor is to listen actively to what the patient is saying and especially to what has been omitted. The counsellor assists the patient to overcome their difficulties, or resistances, when speaking of their problems and concerns, which they may feel are embarrassing, childish or critical.

A person-centred approach

Counselling is person-centred with the patient in control. This is an essential component. The patient determines the pace and the course of the counselling. Fig. 66.1 shows the continuum from clinician-centred to person-centred interactions. When the clinician is in control, the patient is passive, being provided with information and advice. This reflects a paternalistic model of the clinician–patient interaction. When the patient is in control, the patient is active; the clinician may appear as passive but is, in fact, an active participant – listening carefully and following where the patient leads. The clinician's role is to provide interpretations and thus enable the patient to understand the source or cause of the presenting symptom. This interaction is the epitome of a mutual-participative model of the clinician–patient relationship.

A mutual-participative counsellor–patient interaction

The interaction is dynamic in nature. This is essential to achieve a mutual-participative interaction between counsellor and patient. It has three features, which change in their quality throughout the course of the counselling. The model is known as the *psychodynamic model* (Greenson, 1965). The first feature is the real relationship. This is a reality-based, adult-to-adult relationship, in which the patient has chosen the counsellor, based on their knowledge of the counsellor's skills.

The second feature is the therapeutic alliance. This is also an adult-to-adult interaction and, like the reality-based relationship, is an interaction between equals. Working together, in a mutual-participative manner, the patient is able to accept the treatment the counsellor is offering:

> 'The reality-focused elements [that] allow the patient to identify with the aims of the [counsellor] … an essential condition for successful treatment'
> **(Sterba, 1934).**

Difficulties, however, exist with the formation of the treatment alliance when the patient is too anxious and/or fears

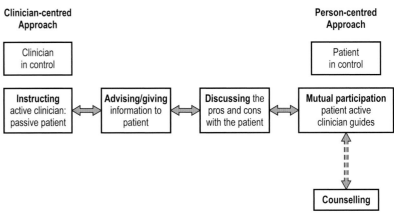

Fig. 66.1 From clinician-centred to person-centred.

the counsellor's criticisms. When this happens the patient's anxiety will destroy the formation and/or maintenance of the treatment alliance. In such situations the counselling will discontinue. It is essential that the counsellor effectively communicates with the patient to create, to nurture and to maintain the treatment alliance. It is, therefore, a special form of the clinician–patient relationship, which is founded upon effective communication (pp. 94–95) and the clinician's/counsellor's ability to contain the patient's fear and anxieties.

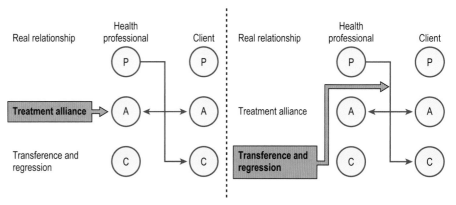

Fig. 66.2 A psychodynamic model for the clinician-patient relationship.

Transference

Transference is a distinctive dimension of the interaction: it is a repetition of the past and where important relationships are played out within the present. The patient does not feel like the adult they are, but starts to feel like the child they were once. Remembering in action rather than in thought, the counsellor is now put in the position of an important other – such as the parent – with all of the emotional reactions that belonged to the parent and not to the counsellor. With the transference the patient will experience a change in the emotional state. They start to experience a shift from more controlled to less controlled emotional states. In other words they will have regressed from being an equivalent and adult participant to feeling like a powerless small child in the interaction with the counsellor. The characteristic of this dimension of the psycho-dynamic model is that of a parent–child interaction (Fig. 66.2).

Two types of counselling

The two strategies most commonly used are (1) CBT and (2) psycho-dynamic counselling.

Cognitive–behavioural therapy

CBT is based on the perception that thoughts, feelings, physical sensations and behaviours are all inter-related. The problem arises when negative thoughts and affects result in being caught in an unbearable cycle, resulting in negative feelings – such as depression and/or anxiety. CBT examines current difficulties, in the here and now, and assists the patient to find practical solutions to solve their problems. Using problem-solving, the counsellor assists the patient to appreciate that their problems are connected to a situation that stirs up unbearable thoughts, which result in difficult behaviours. The patient is assisted to identify thoughts, behavioural patterns, and an action plan to develop the skills to stop the unbearable thoughts,

physical feelings and behaviours. From the action plan, new skills are identified, practised between sessions and are used to replace the unhelpful thoughts. Gradually the patient appreciates how the unhelpful thoughts impinge on their lives and uses the new skills to achieve better psychological functioning.

Case study

How could CBT help Mrs Blue? She is anxious and depressed. Her behaviour with the children and sleep are affected. You ask her when the frightening thoughts occur. She says they happen when she puts her daughters to bed and she sits alone. The dying thoughts start, followed by a dreadful feeling. Gently you probe about what happens next. She says she cannot settle, paces the house and becomes irritable. You ask her what she thinks she could do to reduce them. She says that if her husband would help with the girls and sit with her, this would stop the thoughts. You put in place an action plan to ask her husband for help and company at night. You ask her to keep a diary and practise the action plan.

Psycho-dynamic counselling

Psycho-dynamic counselling is based upon the idea that experiences and past relationships are replayed and relived as if they are happening in the here and now. The counsellor from close listening to the patient may feel as if the patient is caught-up in past encounters. A link or a transfer of emotions encountered in the past is falsely connected to the present. This false connection occurs because the event from the past has elements connected to the present. Therefore the patient's difficulties are an indication of past distress, which now presents in the guise of the new symptom.

The counsellor has three important questions in mind when meeting the patient first: (1) Why does the patient fall ill when she does? (2) Why does she come to see the doctor now? (3) What sort of

person is this? It is from the answers to these questions that the cause of the patient's symptoms will be found (Halliday, 1948).

Case study

Let us return to Mrs Blue. You ask her what has been happening to make her feel this way. She is hesitant but says she fears she is dying. Her husband has little time to listen to her – "she is talking nonsense, and there is nothing wrong". He is irritable with her. She is frightened about what will happen to her girls. Gently you ask her why she has come along now. She starts to weep; her oldest daughter turned 5 years old 2 months ago. The fear started at the time of the birthday and increased. When she was 5 years old, her mother, then 35, who had always been healthy, died very suddenly in the night. She is terrified this will happen to her and that her daughters will grieve for her as she still does for her mother. Her husband will not manage – like her father – and he would just fall apart. How can we explain Mrs Blue's symptoms of anxiety and depression? Mrs Blue's distressful memories of her mother were reflected in her low mood, fears of separation and sleep disturbances. Mrs Blue fell ill now because a false connection had been made between her mother and her 5-year-old self and herself as a mother aged 35 with a daughter now also 5. Her sense of loss and a longing for her mother were unconsciously reactivated by her daughter's and her own birthday, as manifest in her presenting symptoms of depression and anxiety.

Counselling

- Counselling is an important alternative to psychotropic medication in general practice.
- It is effective in reducing mental health–related difficulties.
- Counselling includes (1) person-centred approach, (2) mutual-participative counsellor–patient interaction and (3) transference.
- Two major types of counselling include CBT and psycho-dynamic approaches.

67 | Urban nature, health and well-being

Over half of the world's population now live in cities. In England, alone, approximately 84% of the population lives in urban areas. Potential health-related advantages of urbanization include better sanitation, lower exposure to vector-borne diseases (e.g. mosquito-borne infections) and greater proximity to health care services. However, urban living also poses threats to health, including higher levels of air pollution and greater opportunities to live a sedentary lifestyle.

Some evidence suggests that growing detachment from the kinds of natural environments in which our ancestors evolved physically and culturally can have negative impacts on mental health and feelings of well-being. Cities can be modern, built of steel, concrete and glass (Fig. 67.1) and perhaps lonely places to work and live in, or old run-down and deprived. We are, perhaps, poorly adapted to the noisy, fast-paced aspects of urban life. Indeed, non-communicable diseases (NCDs), including cardiovascular disease (see pp. 104–105) and depression (see pp. 114–115), both of which are associated with inactivity and stress, are now the leading causes of disability and mortality in most developed countries (see spread Health: a global perspective, pp. 156–157). Furthermore brain imaging research suggests that growing up in a highly urban environment can negatively affect neural development. This has led to many, including governments, to call for a greater integration of nature into the urban environment and a reconnection of people to the natural world (Department of Environment, Food and Rural Affairs (DEFRA), 2011). These observations underpin a new movement referred to as *ecological public health*.

What is urban nature?

Urban nature, also referred to as 'urban greenspace' or 'urban green infrastructure', describes outdoor spaces in urban settings, including parks, allotments, playing fields, river/canal banks, ponds and gardens. Some observers also include more localized natural features such as green roofs, green walls and sustainable urban drainage systems. Others consider companion animals (e.g. dogs, cats etc.) and even indoor plants as helping connect humans to nature and thus potentially providing benefits to health and well-being.

Why might urban nature be good for health?

Several studies have reported positive associations between the amount of urban nature in a specific area and positive health outcomes. These include better mental health, higher birth weights and lower cardiovascular disease (Hartig et al., 2014). Results of experiments in Japan have suggested that spending even relatively short amounts of leisure time in urban woodlands (known as 'shinrin-yoku' or 'forest bathing') can lead to several positive health outcomes, principally related to lower levels of stress (see spread 'Anxiety', pp. 112–113).

Several potential pathways have been proposed to account for why urban nature can help promote health and well-being, including (1) reducing air pollution, (2) increasing exposure to health-enhancing microbiota, (3) encouraging physical activity, (4) helping to reduce stress, (5) encouraging social interactions and (6) promoting place attachment.

Can urban nature reduce health inequalities?

Urban areas exhibit particularly stark health inequalities. In London the difference in disability-free life expectancy for men from the richest and poorest boroughs (Richmond 70.3 years

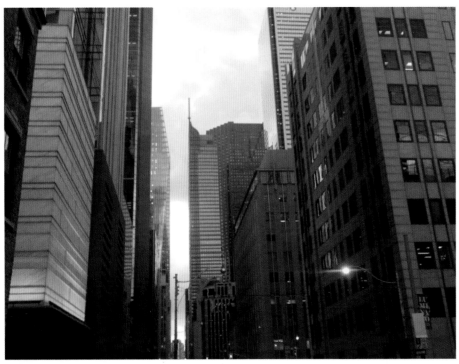

Fig. 67.1 The modern urban concrete, metal and glass built-up environment.

versus Newham 56.5 years, respectively) is nearly 14 years. Currently access to and use of green space is not equitably distributed. Moreover there is evidence that some social groups feel excluded from utilizing green spaces (see 'Unemployment and health', pp. 58–59). Despite this, two large-scale UK studies suggested that urban nature can help to reduce socio-economic–related health inequalities. The first showed differential mortality between the richest and poorest areas was significantly smaller in the greenest urban areas compared with the least green urban areas (Mitchell and Popham, 2008). The second study found that the difference in self-reported health between individuals living in richer and those in poorer areas was lower in urban coastal areas than in urban inland areas (Wheeler et al., 2012). The implication was that the coast, even in urban areas, might be another way of connecting with nature, encouraging physical activity and reducing stress. Given that over 8 million people live within three miles of the UK coast, the potential benefits to public health may be considerable and could be greater if more is done to support everyone's access to blue and green spaces.

There is increasing interest in the potential of nature to support health and well-being. A number of approaches have been introduced: for example, GPs and mental health practitioners may now 'prescribe' nature through linking patients, particularly those with long-term physical or mental health conditions (see spread 'Coping with illness and disability', pp. 140–141), with third-sector bodies and charities from the environmental, community and health sectors. Proposed activities range from walking, participating in conservation tasks, gardening or simply being in nature. The ways in which this is thought to help are varied and may be different for different groups of people engaging in different activities (see also spread 'Helping people to act on their intentions', pp. 74–75). Whilst physical activity is a well-recognised route to enhancing health, additional mechanisms are also noted such as an increased sense of connection to nature, mental restoration, the possibility of acquiring new knowledge and skills and improved self-confidence (Husk et al., 2015).

Bringing nature into health care settings

Some of the benefits of nature can also be enjoyed in health care settings. In one famous study, patients recovering from gall bladder surgery required less analgesics and left hospital sooner when the view from the window of their room was to trees and woodlands rather than the wall of another building (Ulrich, 1984). Paintings and photographs of natural scenes have been found to decrease stress and aggressive episodes in psychiatric wards and fish tanks, and plants are a fixture in many doctor and dental waiting rooms and surgeries. Some studies have suggested that even abstract representations of nature and the use of green paint may lead to more positive patient outcomes (see 'Patient experience', pp. 100–101). Bringing elements of nature into often sterile and stressful medical environments can help patients feel calmer and more positive about medical encounters.

Although many of the results from these strands of research are intuitively appealing, compared with other aspects of public health and medicine, the evidence base is still relatively small, and results are often mixed, with too few studies using the most robust study designs. For instance, although there is relatively good evidence that undertaking physical activity in urban green spaces is associated with more positive mental health outcomes than comparable activity indoors, the association between health outcomes such as obesity rates (see also pp. 106–107) and living near greener urban areas is far less clear. We also know little about dose–response relationships (e.g. how much nature is needed in urban areas, how often people need to visit it and for how long) or the importance of the type and quality of urban nature (e.g. open grassland versus woodlands).

Doctors will have to make a judgement on what is the appropriate recommendation regarding accessing urban nature for individual patients. Such advice needs to be tailored towards individual characteristics such as physical mobility or other impairments as well as socio-economic factors such as where the patient lives and their access to transport to get to green spaces.

Case study *Walking for health*

The 'Walking for Health' initiative was set up in 2000 by Natural England (part of the UK Department for Environment, Food and Rural Affairs) (Natural England, 2009). The aim was to increase levels of physical activity and thus improve health among people with sedentary lifestyles by supporting walks in natural environments, including in urban nature. As of 2015, there are around 3,000 different walks a week led by over 10,000 specially trained volunteers and a total of 70,000 regular walkers a year. In 2009 a cost–benefit analysis concluded that the savings to the health care budget (from the increased physical activity) was approximately £81 million a year and that the overall return on investment was about £7 of savings for every £1 spent. The Scheme is now supported by MacMillan Cancer Support and the Ramblers.

Stop and think

- Susan, a patient who has been overweight for several years, has visited you three times in the last few months feeling sad and low and complaining of stress at work and insomnia. After your previous suggestion, she joined a gym to try to get some exercise but said she felt uncomfortable and quit after a few weeks. She wonders whether anti-depressants might help but is worried about possible side-effects.

You have heard about a local all-female gardening group in the local park; do you mention it to her?

Urban nature, health and well-being

- Most people live in urban areas with potential disconnection from the natural world.
- Urban nature can help to reduce stress and encourage physical activity.
- Access to urban nature is currently unequally distributed but can reduce health inequalities.
- Nature can help improve patient experiences in medical contexts.
- Interventions involving urban nature can be highly cost-effective.
- There is much still to learn about urban nature, health and well-being.

68 | Coping and adaptation

There is a relationship between the way we adapt and cope with the external environment and our physical and mental health. This chapter explains the dynamics of coping and what the implications for our health might be. It also considers how people cope with and adapt to chronic illness.

Coping can mean any general adaptive process. It can also mean the mastery or control of major events. The behavioural sciences have developed two complementary ways of describing coping and adaptation – the first concerned with how people manage ordinary everyday things and the second with the way they deal with major life events. These two approaches have been brought together in what is called the *stress-coping paradigm*.

The stress-coping paradigm

The stress-coping paradigm was originally developed by Lazarus (1980). Lazarus started from the position that the social (and biological) worlds are ubiquitously stressful. People have to cope and adapt to different things, large and small, all the time. The degree to which this produces stress is determined by the extent to which these external stimuli exceed the ability of the person to deal with them and, therefore, to endanger well-being (see What is stress?, pp. 126–127).

Humans evolved to identify stressors or dangers in their environments. According to Lazarus, once a stimulus has been identified as potentially stressful, an individual engages in two processes of appraisal. These are called *primary* and *secondary* appraisals. Primary appraisal refers to the means whereby people determine whether a stimulus is dangerous or not. If individuals decide it is not dangerous, they may conclude that it is irrelevant to them. Alternatively, they may view it as benign or positive. If the stimulus is appraised as irrelevant, or benign or positive, it is not a stressor (Fig. 68.1).

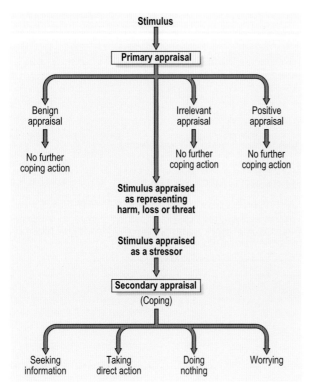

Fig. 68.1 The stress-coping paradigm *(from Kelly and Sullivan, 1992, with permission)*.

If a stimulus is regarded as stressful, this is because it is perceived to represent harm or loss or threat (anticipated harm or loss). The secondary appraisal process is about controlling harm or threat. This can take several forms: seeking out information; taking direct action to confront the stressor; doing nothing and attempting to ignore it; or just worrying about it (Fig. 68.1).

The importance of this model is that it recognizes that stimuli are not in themselves stressful. Stress arises as a consequence of the cognitive or thinking process that people bring to bear on particular stimuli (the appraisal processes) and on the extent to which they can control these stimuli by doing various things. It is when they are not able to control things because they do not have the resources to do so, that stress arises. It is important to note that researchers have observed that positive feelings can arise even in the most difficult and stressful of experiences. People find meaning and purpose in the difficulties they face, and this helps them deal with the problems they are trying to cope with (Folkman and Moscowitz, 2000; 2004). The observation of positive feelings is a relatively common, if somewhat surprising, finding in the case of people coping with illness, especially chronic illness. The stress-coping paradigm emphasizes, therefore, the social context within which coping takes place. A very important resource is social support from others. Social support may come from family, friends or the caring services. It seems that social support makes coping easier, although in itself social support will not solve all the problems a person has to deal with. Support can come in a variety of forms. It might include practical things such as minding children or providing aids and devices to make life easier around the home. The support might be emotional, in the form of talking and listening. There is no simple recipe, but where support networks are stronger, people seem to be able to deal with difficulties better than those without such support. Coping is, therefore, made easier or more difficult by the resources that people can bring to bear when they have difficult situations to deal with. In the absence of social support, life difficulties can be particularly damaging. A good deal of morbidity can be accounted for in terms of combinations of low self-esteem, lack of financial resources, experience of social disadvantage and absence of social support (Kelly, 2010a) (see Depression, pp. 114–115; Coping with illness and disability, pp. 141–141; Social class and health, pp. 42–43).

It has been noted that stress and, by implication, the failure to cope or adapt are responsible for the development of particular types of illness because certain biological responses to stress lead to tissue damage (Seyle, 1956). There is a good deal of evidence that describes the biological changes in the human body that follow the experience of stress. Research in epigenetics is particularly compelling in this respect (Relton and Davey Smith, 2012).

Strategies for adapting to chronic illness

The ways in which people deal with chronic illness is a good illustration of how coping works (Kelly, 2010b). A number of typical strategies have been observed. The responses are linked to the amount of threat their illness presents to them and what they are able to do about the threat.

Normalizing

Here the patient acknowledges the symptoms, for example, of asthma, but redefines them as part of normal experience and hence as nothing to worry about. By defining something abnormal as normal, the patient is neutralizing the threat. This can present particularly difficult clinical management problems because the more successful patients are in neutralizing the symptoms, the more likely they may be not to comply with treatment (see pp. 116–117).

Denial

Here the patient denies the existence of the illness altogether. This may have profoundly beneficial effects, especially in the early stages of a very worrying or threatening diagnosis. Denial may help the patient draw back, take stock and marshal help. In the longer run, however, denial prevents the patient from confronting the illness, will present particular difficulties for the treating doctor and may have considerable effects on the family or partner of the sufferer.

Avoidance

Patients who practise avoidance do not deny their problem. They set out to avoid those situations that might exacerbate their symptoms or lead to other problems. In this group of behaviours we find, for example, the person who suffers from claustrophobia and who therefore never lives or works anywhere where he or she may have to use a lift or get in an airplane. We find the reformed alcoholic who never goes to parties or social gatherings for fear of being tempted by the alcoholic drink. We find the person with epilepsy who never applies for a job where he or she might have to reveal the fact of this illness. Whilst individually each of these strategies is highly adaptive, they also contain within them certain maladaptive or potentially self-destructive elements. The person with claustrophobia or epilepsy may miss out on all sorts of opportunities, whilst the reformed alcoholic may be cut off from a great deal of social interaction.

Resignation

In resignation we find individuals who have totally embraced their illness and for whom the most important thing about their life is their illness. Their whole being is consumed by their disease. They resign themselves to their fate. The illness is defined in such a way that instead of being something threatening, it grants certain psychological rewards. At certain times in a serious and grave illness, resignation may be an entirely appropriate way to respond. However, in many less serious conditions, total resignation leads to invalidism. The problem that this type of behaviour presents for physicians is that their best efforts to get patients to attempt to take some control over their own life are resisted, as patients work hard to maintain their dependence on others.

Accommodation

Here patients acknowledge and deal with the problems their illness produces – whether this is managing their symptom manifestations such as pain or managing a self-administered drug regime. The everyday work of handling the disease is seen as part of normal living. No attempt is made to build a special status out of the illness. Instead people try to deal with others on the basis of their other characteristics such as being a keen gardener, a football fan, a member of the church, and so on. They do not make their illness central to their life.

Case study *Childhood diabetes*

It is important to avoid defining coping as either good or bad. The manner of people's response to stimuli will vary, and in some cases people may draw certain psychological or social rewards from the way they cope, even though others may regard their manner of coping as dangerous or self-destructive. This is sometimes observed in long-term chronic illness.

In childhood-onset diabetes, for example, the family has to cope with illness and the difficulties presented by the symptoms and managing the self-medication and diet. However, it is perfectly possible for the young child to come to enjoy some of the benefits of being a sick person in the family: being spoiled and receiving special privileges, for example. Moreover the family may come to adapt to the illness in ways that they too find rewarding. Parents may receive psychological rewards from taking on the role of carers. This may work quite well whilst the child is young, but as the child grows up and tries to free himself or herself from the parents' control, successful earlier coping may become highly maladaptive. The child's attempt to grow and be independent may be seen as a threat by the parents, who may insist on the adolescent remaining in the sick role. The individual with diabetes may respond by taking dietary risks in an effort to cope with parental control. Particular dynamics become established within the family, and these, in turn, may produce other problems that the family has to cope with.

Stop and think

Although many disorders have been linked directly or indirectly to coping, the precise mechanisms whereby human behaviour in the face of stress produces psychological and biological consequences are very complex, and compared with many branches of medicine, understanding of these mechanisms is limited.

- To what extent are coping and adaptation linked to psychological traits and psycho-sexual development on the one hand or to social factors, particularly availability of resources, on the other? Is it always going to be the case that what might be seen as maladaptive from a medical point of view would be bad for the patient?

Coping and adaptation

- *Adaptation* and *coping* refer to behaviours that involve dealing with everyday problems as well as major life events.
- It is the person who deals with these problems who defines them as everyday or major problems.
- Coping and adaptation are linked to a range of psychological variables and social support and resources.
- Stress results when the ability to deal with events is not equal to the events or stimuli.
- Failure to cope and adapt may have serious health consequences at both a physical and a psychological level.
- Some strategies of coping seem to be inherently unstable or potentially self-destructive.

69 | Cognitive–behavioural therapy

Cognitive–behavioural therapy (CBT) is a set of empirically grounded clinical interventions, applied in a systematic way to help people change their thoughts and behaviours so that they can function in a more adaptive and healthy way. The foundational model for CBT was outlined by Aaron Beck (1976), but as CBT has been applied to new clinical problems, there have been significant revisions.

CBT has become an increasingly popular approach for helping people with physical and mental health problems. The National Institute for Health and Care Excellence (NICE) recommends CBT as the 'treatment of choice' for most common mental health disorders, including depression and anxiety disorders. NICE guidance also highlights that people with long-term health conditions are much more likely to become depressed compared with people in good physical health. (NICE, 2009). Furthermore depression can adversely affect outcomes of physical illness, including increased mortality.

The rationale behind cognitive–behavioural therapy

The cognitive model emphasizes that people's emotions and behaviours are influenced by their perceptions of events and the meanings they attach to their experience. The way in which people *appraise* situations determines how they feel and behave (see pp. 126–127 and pp. 132–133). Depending on their unique development histories and temperaments, people process incoming information in ways that reflect their particular biases. Aspects of thinking may become distorted or maladaptive, leading to emotional and behavioural problems. For example, an individual whose parents were excessively preoccupied with the risks associated with illness may develop maladaptive beliefs about illness (e.g. 'Life with illness is unbearable'). These individuals may be hypervigilant for physical symptoms or signs of illness, repeatedly checking their bodies so that normal or minor fluctuations in bodily processes may be misinterpreted as evidence of illness. They may seek frequent reassurance from doctors and undergo unnecessary medical tests in their search for an explanation of symptoms.

CBT emphasizes the dynamic interactions between thoughts, moods and behaviours (see Case study). However, it gives primacy to the role of thinking in the development and maintenance of emotional disorders. The cognitive model proposes that there are different levels of thinking (see pp. 70–71). At the level closest to conscious awareness are the relatively rapid and involuntary thoughts we have in response to specific current situations. These are called *automatic thoughts*. At a deeper level, people develop *core beliefs* about themselves, others and their world. These are deeply felt, but often not easy to access or articulate. Between these two levels are *intermediate beliefs* that manifest in the rules, attitudes and assumptions that people live by.

Role of therapist

The role of the CBT therapist is, firstly, to assist individuals in identifying their current patterns of thinking and, secondly, to modify this thinking through a range of strategies that encourage individuals to take on a more rational or evidence-based view of their own experiences. Rather than the therapist acting as the expert, the therapist and the client collaborate to resolve problems. Treatment is conducted in a spirit of open-minded enquiry and *guided discovery* to help clients clarify and evaluate their thoughts and beliefs. An explicit goal of treatment is to teach clients coping strategies so that they can develop self-efficacy and the capacity to be their own therapist (for core CBT competencies, see http://www.ucl.ac.uk/clinical-psychology/CORE/CBT_Competences/CBT_Competence_List.pdf).

Structure of cognitive–behavioural therapy

CBT is a relatively short-term structured therapy. A typical course of CBT may last from 8 to 20 sessions, with follow-up sessions to ensure the maintenance of gains. Sessions are approached in a structured fashion and the therapist and client co-construct a shared plan or agenda for each session. Goals are clearly defined, measurable and specific. Progress in therapy is continually monitored.

CBT involves the mutual planning of therapeutic tasks. Homework exercises are performed by the client between sessions. Contemporary CBT approaches homework tasks as an opportunity for clients to test out existing dysfunctional beliefs and to learn new, more adaptive beliefs. For example, a client with health anxiety who engages in excessive reassurance-seeking might be asked to refrain from seeking medical reassurance for an agreed period to see the effect on anxiety.

Some basic techniques

Early stages of treatment focus on eliciting underlying negative automatic thoughts and beliefs, and identifying common themes and patterns. Clients are usually asked to keep a record of their thoughts in particular situations. For example, a client with health anxiety may be asked to record automatic thoughts, mood or actions when they notice new bodily signs or sensations (Fig. 69.1).

Clients may be asked to recount specific situations (e.g. a recent panic attack) in vivid detail to highlight automatic thoughts and appraisals. An effective way of eliciting negative automatic thoughts involves exploring the *worst-consequence scenario*. This usually takes the form of the question: '*What's the worst that could happen if …*'? Clients may be asked to engage in exposure tasks to activate fear and salient automatic thoughts. Exposure may be to external situations or internal bodily sensations and cues.

In the later stages of treatment, clients are helped to modify old beliefs and practise new behaviours. The choice of technique is guided by a *case formulation*, which is a working hypothesis about the cognitive and behavioural factors involved in the origins and maintenance of the client's difficulties. Case formulation usually includes several components: (1) formative early experiences (e.g. mother always worried about being ill); (2) related dysfunctional assumptions and beliefs (e.g. 'If there is pain there must be serious damage'); (3) critical trigger incidents (e.g. recent pain in

Situation	Thoughts	Mood and rating (0-10)	Behaviour
Got up in the morning and noticed lost of hairs on my pillow	Why is my hair falling out? I've never noticed it before. Could it be the start of alopecia? People with cancer lose their hair.	Worry 7	Checked other pillows to see if there were hairs. Combed hair to see if more hair was falling out. Pulled at hairs on head. Looked up alopecia on internet.

Fig. 69.1 Thought record showing links between thoughts, mood and behaviours.

lower abdomen); and (4) maintenance factors (e.g. frequent checking for bodily symptoms). The case formulation is openly discussed with the client and provides a basis for planning treatment interventions.

Clients may also be encouraged to identify and self-monitor common cognitive distortions or 'thinking errors' (e.g. *black-and-white thinking, personalizing and catastrophizing*) (see Counselling, pp. 132–133). Clients are encouraged to challenge these thinking errors and helped to develop alternative more rational and adaptive thought processes.

Applications of cognitive–behavioural therapy to physical health problems

Although CBT was established for the treatment of psychiatric problems, it has also proved effective in the treatment of physical health problems. Chronic medical conditions are frequently associated with psychological problems (see pp. 118–119 and pp. 120–121) and the effective treatment of psychological dysfunction is an important step in enabling patients to cope better with physical illness.

The thought processes relevant to treatments for most physical problems include patients' beliefs about bodily functioning and the causation of physical problems; misinterpretations of bodily symptoms and signs; evaluations of the threat to self and future well-being associated with illness; and changes in behaviour and mood after perceived impairment, which may increase emotional distress and the degree of handicap (Salkovskis, 1989). CBT is particularly useful in modifying thoughts and behaviours, which function to maintain physical problems, even when these originally had a physical cause. For example, excessive avoidance of physical exercise after a viral illness may eventually cause new fatigue symptoms unrelated to the original viral illness.

CBT has demonstrated effectiveness in the treatment of a wide range of chronic illnesses and disabilities. For example, there is promising evidence for the use of CBT in treating chronic fatigue syndrome and chronic pain (see pp. 146–147). There is also evidence to support the use of CBT to treat somatization and health anxiety. CBT for health problems is increasingly being offered through the internet-based interventions with promising effects and advantages in terms of cost and access.

Recent developments in cognitive–behavioural therapy

Recently a number of therapies have developed under the name of the third wave of CBT, including mindfulness-based cognitive therapy (MBCT), acceptance and commitment therapy (ACT) and dialectical behaviour therapy (DBT). These therapies are less concerned with changing negative thought content and more concerned with living in the present moment, acceptance and tolerance of distress and the development of greater self-compassion. A related CBT development has been a new focus on *metacognition* – that is, how people understand and relate to their own thoughts and thought processes (Wells, 2011). Metacognitive CBT aims to help people develop new ways of attending and relating to negative thoughts and beliefs and to modify maladaptive metacognitive beliefs.

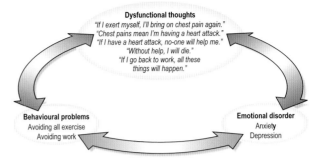

Fig. 69.2 Dysfunctional thoughts: the vicious circle.

On a note of caution, a systematic review of third wave therapies concluded that third wave therapies require further empirical support to prove they offer additional benefit to standard CBT (Ost, 2008).

Stop and think

- The next time you feel ill or have unexplained physical symptoms, try to note the effect of your feelings on your thoughts and mood. What beliefs about illness do you have, and what experiences in your life might have formed these beliefs?

Case study

A 47-year-old van driver suffered a heart attack 5 months ago while driving home from work. He had stopped the car and flagged down a passing motorist, who took him to hospital. On the day of his heart attack, he had felt unwell and had suffered chest pains when climbing stairs to make deliveries.

He made a full physical recovery and is not thought to be at great risk of another attack, but he is now depressed, will not walk uphill or take much exercise and thinks it unlikely that he will be able to return to work. Fig. 69.2 gives examples of the likely elements in the cognitive–behavioural cycle.

How would you begin to tackle this man's difficulties? What questions would you ask to enable him to examine his dysfunctional thoughts? Suppose that he agreed to try some gentle exercise and he did experience chest pain. Are there any possible psychological causes (see pp. 146–147)?

Cognitive–behavioural therapy

- CBT aims to identify, evaluate and test the beliefs and attitudes we hold about ourselves, others and the world around us.
- It aims to modify unhelpful and maladaptive beliefs and to generate more flexible, rational and adaptive beliefs.
- It emphasizes that the way we think about situations influences our mood and behaviour.
- CBT is a structured therapy that focusses on clearly identified and achievable treatment goals.
- It is a widely used treatment for physical and mental health problems with good evidence for its effectiveness.

70 | Role of carers

Health care professionals need to be aware of informal carers for two reasons because (1) enabling people to stay at home relies on family members being able to take on the role of carer and (2) caring for an older, chronically sick or disabled person can affect the health of the carer.

Roles of carers

The term (informal) *carer* generally refers to non-paid family carers, such as spouses, adult children or other relatives and friends. Whilst it is often assumed that carers are adults, there is a significant number of young people undertaking such roles for parents or siblings. Informal unpaid carers are integral to health and social care provision across the world: e.g. there are approximately 5.8 million people in England and Wales who provide unpaid care for family or friends; over a tenth of the population (Office for National Statistics, 2013b). Since 2000 there has been a significant increase in the number of people caring for 50 hours or more per week. It is estimated that the unpaid care is worth some £119 billion every year to the UK economy.

There is huge variation in carers' roles and responsibilities. They help maintain a sense of (1) continuity in the lives of those they care for and (2) identity of the person receiving care. Carers try to maintain their own sense of self, which can be challenging. Caring can range from helping with everyday tasks such as getting out of bed and dressing, to providing emotional support for someone living with symptoms of mental illness. Informal care can also mean providing personal care such as bathing and toileting. It can involve managing symptoms such as incontinence. Living with, and managing, such symptoms can contribute to the social isolation of both the carer and the person being cared for. This can be distressing for both people and being in a close relationship – e.g. being a partner – does not necessarily make attending to intimate care less problematic.

Four typologies of caring

Twigg and Atkin (1994) proposed a typology of caring, comprising four categories that seek to frame the diverse and complex nature of caring tasks and roles. These include:

- Carers as resources: This is the main model of caring representing the preferred source of care as family support, which is generally free and available. Within this model, carers are taken for granted and assumed to be available to step into the role. The focus of services is on the cared-for-person to maximize the provision of informal care.
- Carers as co-workers: This model also promotes informal care, but recognizes that carers themselves need to be supported. Within this model, carers work alongside professionals, conducting tasks that interlink with formal provision of support and formal services. Hence carers' needs are assessed and targeted to enable them to undertake their caring role.
- Carers as co-clients: Carers' needs and well-being are of equal importance to the person being cared for. Carers are supported in their own right by services to provide relief to the carer. The problems and needs of the carer are responded to even if this diverts attention from the person being cared for.
- Superseded carers: The last model focusses on the removal of the cared for person from informal carers, predominantly family carers, into independent living. The aim of services might be to start the process of separation: e.g. when services support a young person with special needs to transition from family care to independent living.

Where is this care given, and who does this care?

The role of a carer is disproportionately occupied by women (see pp. 44–45). However, it has been argued that gender should not be allowed to dominate the debate surrounding who conducts care. As highlighted previously, child carers are often less visible. Men's contribution to informal caring has long been ignored, and they make a larger contribution than has previously been recognized. Gay and Lesbian carers are also often invisible, and there are many gaps in our understanding of informal care practices within minority ethnic communities (see spread Ethnicity and health, pp. 48–49). With an increasing ageing population the majority of care is provided by older people. In 2000, one in six people over 65 years of age were providing some form of care to another older adult and often of 20 hours or more each week (Wanless et al., 2006). Experiences of informal caring roles are also influenced by geographical location that impact upon access to support services and compound social isolation. Caring is also affected by a person's socio-economic status, for example, co-resident care, which places greater constraint on carers' lives, is more frequently provided by those from more deprived socio-economic backgrounds (see pp. 42–43).

Impact of caring on the family

Evidence shows that people providing unpaid care are at an increased risk of psychological stress (Office for National Statistics, 2013b). Eighty-four percent of carers surveyed report that caring has had a negative impact on both their physical and mental health (Carers UK, 2013). Compared with the general population, carers are at significant risk of having a mental health problem, and the risk of a negative impact on a carer's mental health is more likely when caring for someone with a disability and higher care needs (see Physical disability, pp. 118–119 and Learning disability, pp. 120–121). Many carers juggle their caring responsibilities with work and other family commitments. Even where there is daytime support for carers, there is the invisibility of night-time caring, which has adverse effects on the carer's sleep; this is particularly true of carers who are co-residents or caring for someone with a life-limiting illness or dementia (Arber and Venn, 2011). Furthermore the carer's employment is negatively affected when unpaid care is provided for many hours a week (see spread Unemployment and health, pp. 58–59). Although under the Care Act (2014) local authorities have a duty to provide services and support to carers whose employment is at risk. General practitioners need to consider carer breaks to help support carers by giving them a break from caring. Giving carers a change to relax away from caring can help prevent burn-out in carers.

Stop and think

- Should relatives have the right to choose whether they should care for a dependant relative? And what happens, and who pays, if they choose not to take this care on?
- Should informal carers get paid for taking on this role? And how would this happen?

Increasing recognition of the role of carers

Caring for Carers in 1999 was the first UK strategy for carers, recognizing that carers need greater support than they had previously been given. Four priority areas to support carers were put forward in 2010: (1) early identification and recognition of carers; (2) enabling carers to fulfil their education and employment potential; (3)personalized support for carers and those being cared for; and (4) supporting carers to remain mentally and physically well (HMG, 2010:8). Most recently, in 2014 the introduction of the Care Act made it the legal responsibility of local authorities to assess any carer who needs support (see Assessing needs, pp. 150–151).

Carers and the organization of health and social care

Many carers want to be recognized for their role and respected as experts in care. They are a huge asset to health and social care services but often do not receive the recognition and support they deserve or need. The NHS has committed to doing more to 'help identify, support and recognize their vital roles'. The Royal College of General Practitioners (RCGP) argues that GPs and primary care teams are best placed to do this. GPs are often the first point of access for patients, many of whom are carers, and are, therefore, well placed to screen people undertaking a caring role to help detect those at risk of physical and mental health problems (RCGP, 2013). GP practices have many competing priorities, and unfortunately some, like the identification and support of carers, attract no payments (see Setting priorities and rationing, pp. 162–163).

The contested notion of caring

The term *carer* is increasingly viewed as an ineffective term, no longer describing the relationship between carers and those being

cared for. Debates continue about how to define a carer, their role and whether the term is useful for the development and provision of health and social care services (see Organizing and funding health care, pp. 148–149). Focussing primarily on the burden of care and the physical aspects of caring has meant that there has been far less attention to the cared-for person. The positive aspects of caring, in addition, have been relatively neglected (Nolan, Grant and Keady, 1996).

The RCGP and the NHS organised what they called Carers Evidence Summits in 2014 to find examples of good practice, what is working well for carers, resulting in several case studies on the NHS Improving Quality website http://www.nhsiq.nhs.uk/improvement-programmes/experience-of-care/commitment-for-carers/case-studies.aspx.

Stop and think

- As a GP, a family doctor, you are likely to look after more than one generation of the same family. Some of your patients might be carers for sick children or elderly relatives, some children might be carers for their parents. How do you manage your responsibility to your patient who needs care with your responsibility to the carer (who may also be your patient)?

Case study

Haydn Jones (age 79 years) lives with his wife Eileen (age 75 years) in a semi-detached house in a rural village. They have two daughters, who both work, have their own school-aged children, and live a 3-hour drive away; they visit as often as they can, given their work and own family commitments. Eileen was diagnosed with dementia. Recently Eileen has taken to wanting to go for walks outside at night and is restless. On one occasion, Eileen left the house at night and was found walking along a busy road, in her nightgown, miles away from home. Haydn is constantly tired because of sleep deprivation as a result of Eileen's restless nights. Door alarms were fitted, and Haydn checks that all doors and windows are locked each night; however, he worries about fires and not being able to get out of the house. Haydn used to go out regularly to watch the local football team and to meet friends at the local pub. However, he feels he cannot leave Eileen alone and therefore has very few opportunities to do the things that he used to like doing. Haydn worries about what would happen to Eileen if he could not look after her.

Box 70.1 Information and support for carers

Carers have certain rights and are able to access information and support through having an assessment carried out, anyone caring for a person is entitled to an assessment through the local authority. A person who spends at least 35 hours a week caring for a disabled person in the UK is entitled to certain benefits, for example, the Carer's Allowance. Furthermore a carer has the right to request flexible working arrangements. The carer assessment will cover:

- The caring role and how it affects your life and well-being
- Feelings and choices about caring
- The carer's health
- Work, study, training, leisure
- The need for carer breaks / respite care
- Relationships, social activities and the carer's goals
- Housing
- Planning for emergencies (e.g. carer emergency card schemes)

Role of carers

- Relatives and friends provide a considerable amount of care, saving our economy billions of pounds.
- Carers' backgrounds can impact on their experience of caring and contact with services.
- There are four models of care: carers as resources, co-workers, co-clients and superseded carers.
- Being a carer can have adverse effects on the carer's life in terms of physical and mental health, social isolation and employment.

71 | Palliative care

Development of palliative care

The main pioneer of the hospice (palliative care) movement in the UK was Dame Cicely Saunders, who worked as both a volunteer nurse and a social worker, and later as a doctor, at two of the first London hospices, St Joseph's and St Luke's. This experience made her aware of the need for a place of care that would specialize in pain and symptom control in the terminal stages of disease but that would also provide an environment that would allow people to adjust emotionally and spiritually to their approaching death (Saunders and Sykes, 1993). Her subsequent foundation of St Christopher's Hospice in London as a centre of excellence in palliative care provided the cornerstone of the modern hospice movement. Its rapid expansion over the past four decades has been accompanied by the recognition of palliative medicine as a medical specialty. Palliative care services are now being delivered in more than 150 countries, including the USA, and in Asia and Africa. Multi-national collaborations are developing to improve palliative care is worldwide (www.thewhpca.org). However, coverage is still patchy and some countries are not delivering palliative care at all (Wright et al., 2006). It is estimated that globally millions of people currently dying would benefit from a basic palliative care approach, and this number triples when including families and carers.

Defining palliative care

The World Health Organization (2002c) defined palliative care as 'the active care of patients with advanced progressive disease. Management of pain and other symptoms and provision of psychological, social and spiritual support is paramount. The goal of palliative care is achievement of the best quality of life for the patient.' In 1990 it first developed guiding principles for palliative care, namely, that palliative care:

- Affirms life and regards dying as a normal process
- Neither hastens nor postpones death
- Provides relief from pain and other distressing symptoms
- Integrates the psychological and spiritual aspects of patient care
- Offers a support system to help patients live as actively as possible until death
- Offers a support system to help the family cope during the patient's illness and their own bereavement

Although the advent of hospice care has dramatically improved the care of patients, particularly in the area of pain and symptom control, evidence suggests that these goals are still not being met in every setting in which palliative care is provided. There is, therefore, an increasing drive to make hospice standards of care available for all dying patients and not an exception for a small minority. New definitions now distinguish different levels of palliative care according to the setting in which it is provided and the expertize of care staff, although the number of levels is still being debated. At one level, the palliative care approach aims to promote both physical and psychosocial well-being as an integral part of all clinical practice, whatever the illness or stage, through a knowledge and practice of palliative care principles. At the other end of the spectrum, specialist palliative care is the active total care of patients with progressive far-advanced disease and limited prognosis, and their families, by a multi-professional team with recognized specialist palliative care training. More recently the definition of palliative care has been expanded to include early interventions that may incorporate life prolonging therapies, as well as supportive and end-of-life care, and an emphasis on a team approach as the discipline attempts to encompass the whole disease trajectory (www.who.int/cancer/palliative/definition/en).

Beyond the hospice

In the past, hospice care has largely been confined to those patients who were dying from cancer because most were funded by charitable contributions. An important consequence of the expansion of the hospice movement, however, has been the spread of its principles and goals to other places of care. Increasing demands are being made to improve the palliative care of people with other chronic non-malignant conditions (e.g. dementia or end stage renal disease) and to other sectors of the population (e.g. people with learning disabilities) who may have different disease trajectories. Palliative care services now exist in a wide variety of forms, ranging from autonomous inpatient units and day centres where patients can attend for medical or social care to multi-disciplinary hospital support teams that provide specialist palliative care advice to patients in large acute hospitals. Specialist palliative home care teams can also assist GPs in caring for patients at home.

Total pain

The philosophy of the hospice movement is the alleviation of total pain and the affirmation of the remaining quality of life. This means tackling not only physical pain (see pp. 146–147) but also any emotional, psychological, social or spiritual problems the patient has that might contribute to the patient's total distress.

Fig. 71.1 shows that the extent of a patient's pain may be affected by a whole range of physical, psychological, social and situational factors that may influence his or her ability to cope with it. Physical effects of disease and treatment (e.g. radiotherapy or surgery) may be exacerbated or precipitated by other complications. These may include anger at medical staff over unnecessary delays in diagnosis, lack of communication from them or failure to provide a cure, anxiety about other family members, finances, prognosis, and depression or loss of hope resulting from the loss of job, role or function as a result of illness. The degree to which individuals are free from total pain will, therefore, depend on the ability of their professional carers to understand and solve its many causes.

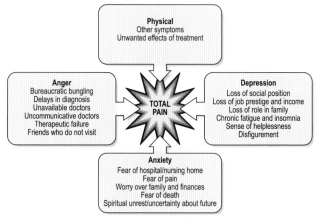

Fig. 71.1 Composition of total pain, and factors influencing sensitivity *(from Twycross, 1994, with permission).*

The multi-disciplinary team

The need for multi-disciplinary teams of health professionals who work together is essential to tackling total pain (Twycross, 1999), and increasingly team-working is seen as essential to the success of palliative care (see Case study). Core members will include medical and nursing staff, social workers, chaplains, physiotherapists and occupational therapists. However, the individual needs of the patient and the family will determine which team member plays a central role. For example, in the case of a patient with persistent nausea, it may be the doctor who directs the patient's care, a patient who is facing severe financial difficulties may need most help from the social worker, and a patient who has difficulty in coping may benefit from consultations with a psychologist. The team should delegate tasks amongst its members to ensure that its resources are mobilized effectively and care prioritized to meet individual needs. The effectiveness of the team will largely depend on good communication amongst members, other health professionals, and patients and their families (see also Clinical communication skills pp. 94–95).

Case study

Jane was a 49-year-old woman with cancer of the breast and bony metastasis. She was married to Adam, a lawyer, and had two teenage daughters. Her prognosis was poor, and after receiving a course of palliative radiotherapy, she had come home to spend her remaining time with her family. Neither daughter knew how serious their mother's condition was, although both suspected that it was not good because of the number of health professionals constantly visiting the house. Both Jane and her husband thought that in protecting their daughters from the truth, they were shielding them from unnecessary anxiety and grief. As a result, relationships in the family were strained, and both girls were doing badly at school. Jane was experiencing uncontrolled pain and nausea, which prevented her from sleeping and eating properly. At this point the GP, after consulting with the district nurse, decided to refer Jane to a specialist nurse for advice on pain control and help with improving communications among the family.

As the nurse's visits to the family progressed, Jane and Adam were encouraged to share Jane's prognosis with their daughters. Both learned that instead of protecting their daughters, they were, in fact, alienating them, causing them to feel confused and isolated. Gradually, through open communication, both daughters came to accept that their mother was dying but that, as a family, they could still make the most of the time that was left. Jane was also given a different form of pain relief: a syringe driver that administered analgesia continuously whilst allowing her to remain as mobile and unrestricted as possible. Jane died peacefully and comfortably at home surrounded by her family.

Measuring palliative care

As with every other medical specialty, practitioners of palliative care are increasingly accountable for care provision. Measuring palliative care can enable doctors and researchers to evaluate and improve the care patients receive, identify resources and requirements, and allow comparisons of care to be made across settings, between patients with different types of disease and between patients at different stages of the disease process. Standards and guidelines are now being developed to enable palliative care professionals to deliver and audit the structure, process and outcome of care. Although some people argue that the individual approach to providing palliative care means that it cannot, and should not, be measured, recognized goals of palliative care such as those of the World Health Organization (Johnston and Abraham, 1995) and concepts such as total pain have allowed the definition of measurable palliative care outcomes. These include pain and symptom control, communication and information, psychological well-being, social support, spiritual distress, quality of life and preference for place of care and death (Bausewein et al., 2011). Sometimes some of these factors are combined in a measure called *quality of life* (QoL). In palliative care, QoL can be used to measure and monitor results of care that go beyond the traditional end-points of tumour size, side-effects of treatment and survival (see spread QoL, pp. 50–51). QoL is usually measured by multi-dimensional instruments that assess the physical, functional, psychosocial and spiritual needs of patients. It is most accurately measured by patients themselves in self-reported measures. Measuring changes in the way patients report QoL over time can help doctors and organizations tailor the care they provide according to individual needs, which may change as the disease progresses. 'Optimising quality of life before a timely, dignified and peaceful death are the primary aims of palliative care' (Murray et al, 2005:1008).

Stop and think

- Consider the Case study: how do you think Jane's daughters felt when initially they were not told of the seriousness of her condition?
- Think how you would go about breaking down the barriers to communication between the family members. Imagine that you were the GP in this situation, and plan what you would say to Jane and Adam.
- Think how you might negotiate between them and their daughters.

Palliative care

- Provision of palliative care has been revolutionized by the modern hospice movement, particularly in the area of pain control.
- Recognition of the care of the dying as the medical specialty 'palliative medicine'.
- Philosophy of the hospice movement emphasizes the alleviation of total pain, and the patient and his or her carer as a unit of care.
- Palliative care is provided by a multi-disciplinary team of health professionals, including doctors and nurses, physiotherapists and occupational therapists, social workers, psychologists, pastoral staff and nurses specifically trained to be advisors in palliative care.
- Quality-of-life measures enable doctors and researchers to evaluate the physical and psychosocial well-being of patients.

72 | Complementary therapies

Why do people use complementary therapies?

Medical science has led the way in advancing the diagnostic and treatment expertise of the medical profession. In the past century more diseases have been cured or effectively managed than in the previous 2000 years combined. And yet the past decade has seen a dramatic rise in the numbers of people seeking complementary therapies to augment or replace their conventional medical treatment.

A reductionist scientific method of clinical medicine is now the norm. This approach divides the whole into objective measureable parts, and a given treatment tends to be evaluated in terms of quantifiable measures such as the presence or absence of disease symptoms (see The biopsychosocial model, pp. 2–3). In such an approach, health care providers can become overly centred on diagnosis and treatment. Often patients are left to their own devices to navigate emotional responses to their illness as reductionist methods pay little attention to the overall well-being, sense of meaning and quality of life of the patient, which are subjective measures of the person as opposed to the illness.

Complementary therapies, or Complementary and Alternative Medicine (CAM), in contrast, are health-promoting practices associated with whole medical systems such as Traditional Chinese Medicine (TCM) and Ayurvedic Medicine (AM) that function outside conventional medicine and embrace a more holistic view of health, aiming to treat the whole person rather than the illness.

What are complementary therapies?

Complementary therapies include medicinal herbs, natural supplements, vitamins and minerals, naturopathy, mindful meditation, visualization, reflexology, massage, yoga, qigong, therapeutic healing, homeopathy, acupuncture/acupressure and counselling. These are typically grouped into one of the following domains of practice: biologically based therapies, energy or bio-field therapies, mind–body therapies and manipulative body-based therapies. Energy-based practices such as homeopathy and reiki strive to restore the flow of energy throughout the body, enhancing a person's vitality to stimulate self-healing;

mind–body therapies such as mindful meditation, visualization, yoga, hypnosis, counselling (see pp. 132–133) and support groups (see pp. 49–50) are thought to restore a person's sense of harmony and balance, whilst, in contrast, manipulative body-based practices such as massage and reflexology stimulate circulatory and lymphatic systems to promote health and healing (National Center for Complementary and Alternative Medicine (NCCAM), 2015).

How does a CAM approach differ from conventional medicine?

Complementary therapies conceptualize a person in terms of the inseparability of the body, mind and spirit. Consequently, in a complementary medicine diagnosis and assessment, as much attention is given to the patient's emotional and psychological state as to the presenting physical symptoms. Generalities such as life situation and energy levels are also noted and the patient observed and understood in their entirety. By embracing the whole person, complementary therapists tailor their therapeutic approach to maximize the patient's wellness and quality of life (see pp. 50–51) and facilitate individuals' innate ability to heal themselves (Fig. 72.1). Good communication skills are vital in such approach requires (see pp. 94–95).

Do complementary therapies work?

The issue of whether complementary therapies can improve and resolve physical

symptoms remains largely unresolved, as assessed using 'gold standard' (randomized controlled trials (RCTs)). For example, although acupuncture is especially well researched, evaluations of this evidence vary in their conclusions depending on the medical condition being investigated (NCCAM; White, Rampes and Ernst, 2000).

Given that complementary therapies purport to treat the person rather than the disease, some researchers believe that subjective measures of the person (e.g. overall well-being and quality of life) may be usefully employed to evaluate effectiveness as opposed to physical symptoms (e.g. pain), which are a measure of the illness. Indeed, numerous studies attest to the benefits of various complementary practices on patient's psychological well-being and quality of life (see pp. 50–51). Given that a person's emotions and beliefs can affect the body's immune response, these interrelationships may account for the so-called healing response, which is thought to underlie the action of most complementary therapies.

Others point out that in 'real world scenarios' (especially with an ageing population increasingly living with multiple morbidities) complementary therapies are often taken in conjunction with conventional medicines (e.g. pain killers). RCTs designed to assess the impact of one intervention on a single medical condition cannot account for the individualized, synergistic and holistic effects of blended complementary and conventional treatments. A mixed method approach, combining quantitative and qualitative data, may be a more

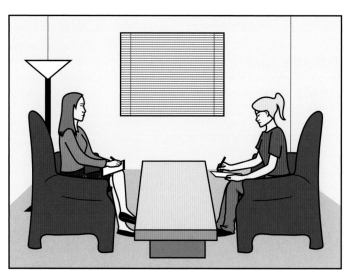

Fig. 72.1 Listening practitioner.

appropriate approach to evaluate the potential health and healing effects of such an integrated intervention (Bassman and Uellendahl, 2003).

Whole-person health care – the future of medicine?

Whole-person care combines the benefits of relevant complementary practices with effective medical interventions to optimize health by offering compassionate care tailored to the needs of the whole person. By facilitating a sense of meaning and well-being, complementary therapists may aid wellness in a way that health care professionals, working within the constraints of a conventional health care system, are currently unable to provide. There are valid concerns with complementary therapies regarding the possibility of drug interactions when the health care professionals are unaware of supplements or herbal medicines being taken alongside conventional medicines (see Case study; Fig. 72.3). Making complementary therapies an integral part of clinical practice would enable the needs of the whole person to be met while providing comprehensive care that is effective and safe.

Case study *St John's wort* (Hypericum perforatum)

Extracts of this herb (Fig. 72.2) have been used traditionally to treat depression and anxiety. It has been shown in RCTs to be an effective antidepressant for mild or moderate depression (Linde et al., 2005) and may be an appropriate alternative to conventional anti-depressants because it has fewer side effects. Psychologically the patient may feel more positive to receiving, in effect, a 'herbal' treatment, as opposed to a psycho-active drug. All recommendations will be subject, of course, to medical oversight, including herb/drug interactions (Fig. 72.3).

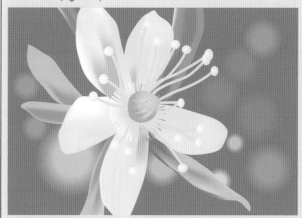

Fig. 72.2 St John's wort flower.

	R
Hypericin	H
Pseudohypericin	OH

Hyperforin

Fig. 72.3 Diagram of molecules of hypericin and hyperforin *(adapted from Mills and Bones, 2000, with permission)*.

Stop and think

A patient comes to you with a long-term chronic pain condition and associated sleeplessness and anxiety. He says he is keen to try a recommended complementary therapy in addition to the medications you are already prescribing him. His friend, who has a similar problem, says that it has helped her to cope with her pain and improve her sleep. The patient asks for your advice. The evidence base for this complementary therapy consists of a small number of RCTs with inconsistent results and no clear clinical benefit for physical pain. No adverse events have been found and no quantitative outcomes for sleep and anxiety have been assessed.

- Qualitative evidence suggests that the therapy improves overall well-being. What will you say to your patient?

Complementary therapies

- The number of people seeking complementary therapies is increasing.
- Complementary therapies are health-promoting practices that function outside conventional medicine. They aim to treat the whole person rather than the illness, maximizing the patient's psychological well-being and quality of life.
- Integrative medicine combines the benefits of relevant complementary practices with effective medical interventions.

73 | The management of pain

Pain is defined by the International Association for the Study of Pain as 'an unpleasant sensory and emotional experience associated with actual or potential tissue damage, or described in terms of such damage' (International Association for the Study of Pain (IASP), 1994). The experience of pain is subjective. We often associate pain with an acute injury or event that is assumed to signal harm or damage. This may be an appropriate interpretation where pain has an obvious cause or recent onset. However, many people's experience of pain is a more chronic picture. Chronic pain is defined as continuous pain that persists for 3 months and is unresponsive to medical treatment (IASP, 1994). Persistent pain can impact on people's quality of life and their capacity to engage in everyday activities. Severe pain is estimated to have a prevalence of 11% in the adult population (Price et al., 2012). Chronic pain is associated with demographic and socio-economic factors, including older age, female sex, poor housing and manual employment.

The way forward – a bio-psycho-social approach

There has been an historical shift from a biophysical focus on pain being a sensory experience, to pain being a complex psychological and social phenomenon (Hadjistavropoulos et al., 2011). The distinction between nociception and pain is important. Whilst nociception involves the stimulation of nociceptors conveying information about tissue damage, pain is the subjective perception that results from transmitted sensory information. However, this input may be filtered through an individual's genetic composition, prior learning history, current psychological status and socio-cultural influence.

A bio-psycho-social model (see Chapter 1, pp. 2–3) of pain highlights interaction among physiological, psychological and social factors in understanding how individual's pain is perceived and managed. Management of pain is complex and involves coordinated care from a range of health professionals. The inter-disciplinary treatment of pain involves physical treatment, along with cognitive, behavioural, environmental and emotional interventions.

Psychological factors: Health beliefs and misconceptions

The different psychological mechanisms used to manage pain can impact on how people cope with chronic pain. Patients' reactions to pain are guided by meaning systems (Higgins et al., 2015). For example, pain can be understood as externally located, difficult to control and fixed. Such beliefs are associated with passive coping strategies (hoping pain will get better) and predict psychological distress and disability. In contrast, individuals can also have strong self-efficacy beliefs and see pain as malleable. Believing that one's actions can improve chronic pain and adopting active coping strategies are associated with lower levels of pain, distress and disability. Individuals can also catastrophize their pain, which is associated with increased pain and psychological dysfunction.

Health beliefs can powerfully influence people's response to their symptoms and expectations of treatment (see pp. 36–37). If individuals with chronic pain believe that their pain is a signal of harm and damage, then they are likely to avoid doing things that encourage pain. This usually leads to a gradual reduction in physical mobility and can result in secondary problems, including postural changes, stiffness in joints or limited use of an affected limb. Individuals may be fearful of exercise and less compliant with advice, leading to anxiety and negative behavioural changes.

Social factors: Identity, interpersonal relationships and pain communication

People experience pain in a social context. An individual's experience of pain is mediated through communication. The way in which an experience of pain is expressed depends on a range of factors. For example, enduring illness in a silent or 'stoic' way is influenced by various socio-cultural factors such as generational attitudes, geographical environment and employment type. This can be related to maintaining a sense of identity over time. Pain can be misrepresented, both through exaggeration and suppression. For instance, a classic sociological study showed how organizational settings affect the character of interactions between patients who are in pain and the staff providing care (Fagerhaugh and Strauss, 1977). Patients balanced pride at not complaining (thereby maintaining a sense of identity) with the difficulty of enduring pain.

People's social identity incorporates their perceptions of how others see them. Individuals with chronic pain describe their activities being restricted. No longer being able to be active can challenge a person's self-identity if he or she is treated differently by others (Miles et al., 2005). People with chronic pain also describe being treated suspiciously, by family members, friends, colleagues and employers and health professionals. Being stigmatized means people are more likely to employ maladaptive coping strategies (e.g. concealing illnesses), hesitating to seek help and keeping a social distance from others. In contrast, strong social ties can serve as a resilience resource and aid with coping. Thus an individual's social context shapes how they experience pain and communicate this experience to others.

Cognitive–behavioural approaches

There are three linked components to the management of pain: dealing with unhelpful patterns of thinking, which can then lead to changes in behaviour and subsequent improvement in mood (see pp. 136–137). These psychological principles can be applied by all clinicians who have contact with pain patients. A more integrated and intensive approach is commonly used in pain management programmes.

Changes in cognitions

- Identify and help to reshape misconceptions about pain (Box 73.1) so that the patient understands the principles of pain mechanisms.

Box 73.1 Common misconceptions about pain

- 'I've been told my X-rays show wear and tear. This must mean that my bones are wearing away. I had better not do too much in case I wear things away even further.'
- 'If you have pain, it means that you have damaged and harmed something. I had better not do anything that gives me pain in case I harm myself.'
- 'It's best to avoid getting dependent on medication, so I'll go as long as possible without taking anything.'

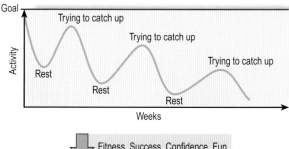

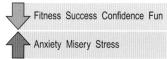

Fig. 73.1 The impact of pain on behaviour and behaviour on pain. The overactivity–rest cycle.

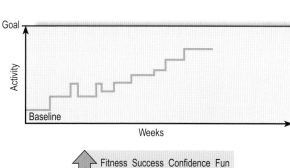

Fig. 73.2 Elements of pain management. Behavioural intervention: pacing, activity-scheduling and goal-setting.

- People often fear exercise and activity in case this causes a flare up, with the causal attribution of harm and damage. Mobility and fitness levels may decrease.
- Help patients to recognize and reframe unhelpful patterns of negative thoughts: e.g. 'I used to be able to decorate my house in no time – now I'm useless – there's no point in trying' could be changed to: 'If I get some help with the heavy bits, I could do this decorating in half an hour chunks'.

Changes in behaviour

Pain often leads to behaviour that is shaped by operant conditioning (see pp. 20–21):

- 'Good days' often lead to doing too much and trying to catch up. This usually results in 'bad days', when little can be done whilst waiting for the pain to settle. Mood is then often low, and frustration and anxiety are high (Fig. 73.1).
- This cycle can be broken by setting behavioural goals where a level of activity is found that does not cause pain to flare up. Levels are then gradually increased, which reduces the 'wind-up' pain effect and improves mood and confidence. (Fig. 73.2).
- Achievable levels of activity set as goals increases positive results and increases perceived control.
- Learning regular relaxation techniques can alter the vicious cycle where pain causes increasing frustration and irritability, raised adrenaline levels and increased spasm, leading to pain threshold changes.

Changes in mood and sense of control or self-efficacy

- As people accumulate skills and strategies to build up activity, they regain some of what was lost. This reduces frustration and improves mood.
- Correcting misconceptions and helping people to reframe negative patterns of thinking improves perceived control and mood.

What is the evidence?

A meta-analysis and systematic review of randomized controlled trials for cognitive–behavioural therapy for chronic pain by Morley et al. (1999) showed significant effects on pain experience, coping and behavioural expression of pain (see pp. 138–139). A comprehensive account of an interdisciplinary approach to chronic pain is found in Gatchel et al. (2014). Evidence also supports a whole systems approach to managing chronic pain (Phillips et al., 2008).

Stop and think

- Why is bed rest no longer recommended for people with back pain?

The management of pain

- Lack of findings on investigation does not mean that pain is not genuine.
- The mind/body split (i.e. all physical or all psychological) is an unhelpful conceptualization of pain.
- Injuries from accidents can lead to posttraumatic stress disorder or similar symptoms, which are frequently missed and maintain pain and disability.
- A cognitive–behavioural approach is effective in managing pain.
- Identify and correct patients' misconceptions.
- Help patients to reframe negative thinking.
- Help patients set achievable goals.
- Affirm patients' progress and improve their sense of control and self-efficacy of progress.
- Experiences of pain and their communication to others is shaped by people's social context.

Case study

John has had back and neck pain for 4 years after a road accident in which he suffered minor whiplash. An MRI scan showed some degenerative changes, not indicative for surgery. John was medically retired 1 year ago and reports disturbed sleep and poor concentration. His wife works full time, and he feels guilty about not working. He tends to push himself and then has to recover for the rest of the week. He has given up golf, is gaining weight, rarely sees friends, and is increasingly angry. Recently John was assessed in a multi-disciplinary pain clinic and given explanations about chronic pain and its effect on physical and psychological state. He began a pain management programme and initially found it difficult to shift from his pattern of over activity. However, with regular setting of activity and exercise goals he was able to gradually increase what he could do. He felt less anxious about harm, which has increased his confidence. He initially found relaxation difficult, but gradually built up skills, which has resulted in less irritability. He is now able to enjoy activities with his family and has started some voluntary work.

74 | Organizing and funding health care

The organization and funding of health care affect both patients and health care providers. For example, doctors may be restricted in ways of working because of the way health care is organized, or they may feel that their patients' access to certain expensive tests or interventions is restricted.

Health care systems all over the world seem to be facing a funding crisis. The main issue is the allocation of scarce resources. This is not simply a question of money but also of political decision-making and setting priorities. To understand the current organization and funding of health care, we have to look at historical developments and the underlying political systems.

We concentrate on three countries, the UK (with a predominantly state-run welfare system), the USA (with a predominantly free-market system), and Germany (with a mixed-health economy), representing the major ways health care is organized and funded (Table 74.1). Total expenditure per capita on health (including private and public health expenditure) in these three countries differs considerably, as does the proportion of the gross national product spent on health care.

UK

All citizens of the UK are included in the NHS. The NHS is a universal, tax-funded health care system. Doctors, nurses and hospitals are paid by the state. The NHS requires some additional payments from patients, for example, for prescriptions and dental check-ups, but the overwhelming majority of care provision is free of charge. Treatment is decided on (mostly) by doctors. GPs are gate-keepers in this system, selecting patients and referring patients to the appropriate specialist. Medical care is available to all and is, therefore, without stigma or significant financial cost to the poor. However, there is a problem of waiting lists (see pp. 152–153). This has stimulated an increase in the small but growing private health care sector. In the UK this includes sales of over-the-counter medicines and private payments for alternative therapies and hospital treatment. The latter is often provided by the same doctors in the same hospitals as the standard NHS care.

USA

The system in the USA is predominantly commercial insurance–based. Most people take out their own private health insurance, or are insured through their employer. These insurance companies reimburse doctors, hospitals and others for care provided. Most people have the freedom to go to the medical professional or hospital of their choice. A limited number of people are covered by state-run schemes such as Medicaid, which provides health care for the poor, but eligibility is incomplete and coverage usually excludes dental services and prescribed drugs. Medicare, for all people over 65 years of age, provides limited coverage. Some 45

million Americans are not insured or underinsured, and a national survey in 2016 suggested 4.5% of children were uninsured and 12.8% of adults aged 18 to 64 years (https://www.cdc.gov/nchs/nhis/releases.htm).

Germany

Most Germans are insured by one of 250 sick funds, which are funded by income-related contributions and are self-governing non-profit institutions. The average contribution rate is 15.5% of an employee's gross income. Just under half of the contributions are paid by employers and just over half by employees. Self-employed persons and employees earning over a certain ceiling (52,500 Euros in 2017) are allowed to opt out of the statutory insurance scheme and join one of the 50 or so private health insurance companies. As in the UK, family doctors are gate-keepers, selecting and referring patients to the appropriate specialist. Patients receive comprehensive coverage, which entitles them to primary and hospital care, but patients pay a small fee for the first doctor or dentist visit each quarter and for prescriptions. The sick funds reimburse the doctors, hospitals and pharmacists for delivery of their services. Privately insured people pay the doctor or pharmacist, and their insurance company reimburses the patient. Legal restrictions and government regulations limit the freedom of the sick funds to control cost, prices and the quantities and range of provisions.

What are the advantages of each system?

The German national insurance-funded and the British tax-funded systems have many similarities as predominantly universal and comprehensive systems. The two are more similar to each other than either is to the US system. Therefore the European collective system will be compared with the private system in the USA.

Box 74.1 lists some of the main advantages and disadvantages of collective health care systems. Some of the listed issues are political, others more clearly medical. For example, the first advantage is obviously political: it expresses ideals of shared citizenship and enhances social cohesiveness in society. The issue that 'free care encourages trivial complaints' has a direct impact on the doctor. If care is free for the patients we might expect that more people will come forward with relatively minor complaints.

Box 74.2 shows some of the main advantages and disadvantages of private health care. For example, in the first advantage, 'liberal citizenship/choice', Americans have the freedom to shop around for their health care; they can decide to have an all-inclusive insurance or only insure for hospital treatment. They are not told by the state what they must do; this is a very political argument. The first disadvantage, 'choice only for those who can pay', refers to the fact that many Americans do not have access to proper

Table 74.1 **Three different ways of funding and organizing health care (data for 2015)**		
UK	**USA**	**Germany**
• State-run national health service mainly funded through taxation	• Mainly private health insurance system with market-based health care provision	• National health insurance-based system with a market-based health care system
• Every citizen covered, but small fees paid on prescriptions	• 10% of the population not covered	• Every citizen covered, but small fees paid on use
• Per capita spending on health US$ 4,003	• Per capita spending on health US$ 9,451	• Per capita spending on health US$ 5,267
• 9.8% of gross domestic product (GDP) spent on health care	• 16.2% of GDP spent on health care	• 11.1% of GDP spent on health care
Source: Organisation for Economic Co-operation and Development (OECD), http://stats.oecd.org/index.aspx?DataSetCode=HEALTH_STAT.		

Advantages

- Social citizenship/cohesion
- Combats the inverse-care law*
- No fee results in less over-doctoring
- More scope for coordinated planning
- Bargaining-power economies of scale
- Tax revenue is cheap to collect
- Easier to meet emergencies (e.g. Ebolavirus and Zika virus outbreaks, war)

Disadvantages

- Reduces individual responsibility
- Increases deference towards the doctor
- Free care encourages trivial complaints
- Impedes search for market solutions
- Vote-catching discourages quality
- Higher public spending
- Makes health a political football

*The inverse-care law argues that the provision of health care in a market economy is inversely related to the need for it; in other words poor facilities are to be found in depressed areas characterized by high morbidity, and better facilities in affluent areas characterized by low morbidity (Tudor Hart, 1971: 405).

Advantages

- Liberal citizenship/choice
- Market: best mechanism for regulating any distribution
- Similar-quality care for low price; better care for higher price
- Direct service and short waiting lists
- Improvements stimulated by market
- Patients = consumers – i.e. know their rights

Disadvantages

- Choice only for those who can pay
- Health insurance market does not equate health care market
- Many cannot afford the higher price
- Inverse-care law: services concentrated
- Improvement stimulated by profit, not need
- Patients still depend on doctors' expertize

health care and, therefore, no choice at all. In the USA, only people with enough money or a good health insurance scheme can buy the best available medical care. Consequently people who have a good medical insurance cover have little incentive to seek lower prices for health care. This is one of the reasons why the system is so expensive. Finally, an issue concerning doctors directly is the extent to which patients have a choice. For example, someone with lower back pain can opt for physiotherapy, chiropractic or drug treatment. However, this is not a completely free choice, since most patients are unable to judge the quality and the usefulness of the services on offer (see pp. 86–87). Furthermore, the increase in patients' complaints and litigation indicates that patients are dissatisfied with the services provided. However, this is not completely a problem of private medicine, since the numbers of complaints and court cases in the UK are also on the increase.

Paying the doctor

These are observations of imperfections in the different ways of organizing health care, not judgements about these systems. Similarly, there is no right way of fixing the doctor's payment. Every method has significant disadvantages: a fee-for-service payment may have the effect of encouraging some doctors to advise more treatment than is really necessary, whereas payment on a capitation basis, i.e. number of patients on the roll, may mean that doctors are in too much of a hurry to give adequate individual attention to each patient, to be able to consult with as many as possible per day.

Convergence

There appears to be a tendency for the different models of health care provision to converge. In 2010 the USA reformed its health care system introducing the Patient Protection and Affordable Care Act, known as Obamacare (named after the then president Barack Obama). Obamacare extended health insurance coverage to many of the estimated 15% of the US citizens who lack it. At the same time, in countries with a national health care system (e.g. the UK) or a national health insurance system (e.g. Germany), governments are often trying to increase the role of the private health care and the market. In the UK we see more health services traditionally provided by the NHS now being provided by private health care orgnizations on behalf of the NHS.

What about prevention?

Apart from decisions around who organizes, provides and pays for health care, any health system also has to consider how much emphasis to place on dealing with current patients and how much on preventing illness and disease (see pp. 76–77). Regardless of the way the health system is organized, immediate expensive health care is expected to be on offer, whilst long-term preventative interventions are underfunded and perhaps unpopular. That prevention is often cost saving in the long-term does not seem to help in raising its share of health expenditure.

Stop and think

- In what ways is the government of your country involved in the provision of health care?

Stop and think

- What are the main differences for doctors in the way health care is delivered in the USA, Germany and the UK?

Organizing and funding health care

- The organization of a nation's health care system is closely related to the way it is funded.
- Both public and private health care and the ways we organize and fund our health systems have specific advantages and disadvantages.
- Different types of health care systems seem to be converging.

75 | Assessing needs

The health services are constantly in a state of flux resulting from alterations at the supply side of care, for example, the introduction of new drugs or medical technology, and attempts to make services more effective and efficient. Health services are also changing through alterations in demand, for example, as a result of an ageing population (see Social aspects of ageing, pp. 14–15), migration (see Ethnicity and health, pp. 48–49) or the appearance of 'new' diseases (Ebola) and changing preferences for and expectations of treatment options. Somewhere in this pool of conflicting interests we have to establish the needs of individuals, communities and populations whilst ensuring that each receives maximum benefit within the limits of available resources, including staff, buildings and funding (see web pages Health Management Specialist Library).

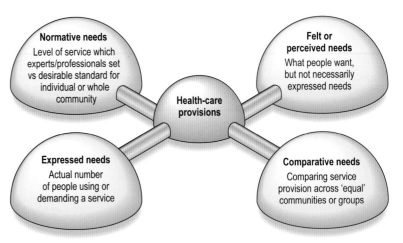

Fig. 75.1 Types of needs in health care provision *(from Bradshaw, 1972).*

Why needs assessment

Why does a service provider, a policy-maker, a doctor or a hospital manager try identifying the needs of people? Providers of health care need to know (1) what users need (and where and when) and (2) what is needed in a particular locality, to improve the health of the population. These two objectives are not the same. What potential or actual service users feel they need ('perceived needs' in Fig. 75.1) might only partially overlap with what policy-makers/experts consider to be the best possible range of services in an area that can improve the health of the people locally ('normative needs'). Both types have to be distinguished from 'expressed needs', the actual use or demand for a service, and 'comparative needs', which compares services across similar communities or client groups, for example, comparing the services for people with HIV and those with cancer, or comparing services available in Tasmania with those in New South Wales. Thus need is not a unified concept.

Needs assessment

It is difficult to assess all needs at the same time, since needs-assessment exercises require funding and can take time. Consequently needs assessments usually focus on a specific illness and a limited area of care, thus assessing the needs of a particular group of (potential) patients to

determine how their need might be met. When we consider the needs of the population in a given area we also have to ask questions such as 'Whose needs do we take into consideration?' and 'Are we looking at the present needs of ill people or the potential future needs of the total population?' The assessment of the needs of the local population should be performed regularly because a population changes over time, and their actual or perceived needs might change. Planning health care provision takes time, whether it be training of new doctors/nurses or building hospitals. Changing funding from one type of health service to another (e.g. from hospital care to community-based services) is often politically difficult and hence time consuming.

Thus the main issues are: 'How do we define, and secondly measure, need?' The next main questions are: 'Who should perform a needs assessment?' and 'Whose definition of 'needs' is it to be based on: (1) lay people, (2) professionals, (3) researchers, (4) politicians, (5) managers or (6) a combination of groups?'

Measuring health needs we can focus on all people (healthy and unhealthy) or only on those with the specific disease or illness. The former is the most equal way of assessing the overall need in a population, whilst the latter ensures that those who know what it is to have a particular illness help to establish an overview of the needs of its sufferers. Both approaches have drawbacks. Asking all people to identify needs will result in highlighting the need for provisions related to more common illnesses, and will under-represent specific needs for people with 'rarer' or less 'acceptable' conditions (Hopton and Dlugolecka, 1995). A needs assessment among people with specific

conditions will highlight their specific needs, but not to the general population or to people with other conditions. Although service users are likely to have a bias towards existing services, non-users are likely to lack experience and knowledge and will generally opt for provision for more common conditions.

The way a needs assessment is conducted can influence its findings. An uncritical social marketing approach may lead to more service for the general population, at the expense of specific services for those most in distress.

The Case study shows that the needs as assessed by different people all have a role to play in the provision of health services. It is important to remember that a prediction of more pregnancies in a certain area does not necessarily mean that more hospital beds and doctors are needed. Different conditions require different approaches to service provision, and the needs assessment itself might vary according to the illness in question. It is likely that service users have less input in a needs assessment of hospital-based orthopaedic surgery than in one of community-based mental health care.

Unmet and unlimited needs

There is a potential problem of unmet needs as well as unlimited needs. The former issue refers to missing out people in assessing needs, whilst the latter refers to whether we will be able to fulfil the needs we identify in a needs-assessment exercise. Asking people about their health problems to identify unmet needs might raise expectations about the service they expect to receive, but that society cannot provide.

In Fig. 75.2 three circles represent needs, demand and supply. Demand can be seen

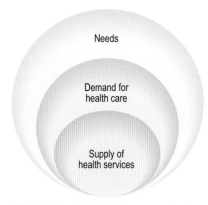

Fig. 75.2 The relationship between needs, demand and supply.

as the 'expressed needs' mentioned previously. Fig. 75.1 indicates that there might be needs that are not as such recognized by those who have them. This implies that people other than the users have conducted the needs assessment.

The realization that health needs are far more than demands from patients presented to the medical profession gave rise to the idea of a clinical iceberg or iceberg of disease (see Decision to consult, pp. 86–87). From a social science perspective the concept of an iceberg of disease is an indication that different perceived needs in different groups can lead to different reactions; some will result in seeking medical help while others will lead to self-medication (see Self-care, pp. 98–99) or are simply ignored (see Adherence, pp. 92–93).

Needs assessment and users

Needs assessment cannot be left completely to users: for example, recreational drug users might not feel that they have a drug problem, so a needs assessment would indicate that there is no need for a problem drug service. However, some drug users will develop problems and will need specific drug services (see: Illegal drug use, pp. 78–79). Or obese patients think they need gastric bands but your clinical opinion is they need lifestyle changes (see pp. 106–107).

Stop and think

- Can lay people assess their own health care needs?

Case study *Organizing maternity care*

Epidemiologists and policy-makers can establish the number of healthy babies that will be born in a certain locality. This estimate will be based on (1) the number of women of child-bearing age, and (2) the birth rate for that area, subtracting the likely number of mothers and babies needing specialist obstetric care before, during or after the delivery.

This information will not be sufficient to predict the local need for maternity services. We need to ask women and their partners how and where they want the maternity services to provide health care. Do women want a predominantly midwife-led care, or do they want obstetrician-led maternity care, or do they want shared care by doctors and midwives, or shared care by obstetricians and family doctors? A further question is: 'Where should these maternity services be based?' Answers may include: at home, in a freestanding midwifery unit, a midwifery-led unit attached to a large obstetric hospital or in a specialist obstetric hospital or all of these options, depending on the pregnant woman's preference.

Stop and think

- Considering maternity care, what would be the main needs identified by the following groups:
  - General practitioners
  - Obstetricians in hospital
  - Midwives based in hospital
  - Health administrators
  - Politicians
  - Community midwives
  - Pregnant women
  - Women of childbearing age but not currently pregnant

Remember to have another look at the spread, pregnancy and childbirth, on pages 4–5.

Assessing needs

- There are four ways of defining need: normative need, felt need, expressed need and comparative need.

- Needs assessment should include the views of different stakeholders, including service users (i.e. patients), as well as lay public, professionals, managers, politicians and researchers.

- Needs assessment runs the risk of raising people's expectations and of not having the resources to meet them.

Source: Powell, J. 2006. Health needs assessment: a systematic approach. Available online at: http://www.library.nhs.uk/HealthManagement/ViewResource.aspx?resID=29549&tabID=290&summaries=true&resultsPerPage=10&sort=TITLE&catID=4033.

76 | Setting priorities and rationing

The medical profession often has to prioritize treatment and ration services at the patient level. Any practising doctor can tell a personal story of having to choose between patients because resources are limited – whether staff, money, operating theatres or organ donors.

Rationing of health care has always taken place, however wealthy the country, but often this is done implicitly, not in the open inequitable (see pp. 148–149). As spending on health services has increased in most countries, discussion about priorities and rationing has become more explicit. Thus the question is not 'Will we have rationing?' but 'How should we organize rationing?'

Setting priorities

Setting priorities implies choosing a limited number of options from a wider range and ranking these in order of importance (Box 76.1). Following on from priority setting is a process of rationing. Rationing is often defined as allocating scarce resources by some criteria other than the price mechanism. This does not mean that the price is not an important consideration but that the cost (which may not be the same as the price) of a service, say, a hip replacement, is not the only factor in the decision whether or not a particular patient will receive treatment. Priority-setting is a dynamic process, and every year new technologies and information on health outcomes are taken into consideration in setting new priorities.

> **Box 76.1 Health decisions at national level too important to leave to health departments**
>
> Some countries have decided that health care is too important to leave to ministries of health and, therefore, made health care a priority for all government departments. Health in All Policies (HiAP), as this approach is called, was the focus of a cross-national study amongst Sweden, Québec and South Australia. One key conclusion was that 'allocating resources and making funding decisions regarding HiAP are inherently political acts that reflect tensions within government sectors' (Pinto et al., 2015).

Forms of rationing

Rationing is a trade-off between providing all services to a limited number of people or providing a limited number of services to all people. Rationing often involves a limitation of both the range and the volume of service provision. The process may attract opposition and/or media attention (Box 76.2). Decisions regarding rationing also have to be made at different levels: individual, local/regional and national.

A variety of rationing mechanisms exist (Klein et al., 1996):

- Denial: for example, refusing access to cosmetic surgery or refuse to treat older people for certain conditions
- Deterrence: putting up social, economic or psychological barriers

> **Box 76.2 Media headline**
>
> "Cancer drug X© too expensive for the NHS!"
> Media headlines like this one highlight the problem faced by funders and commissioners (see Media and health, pp. 52–53). These decision-makers may find that new drugs or treatments might be more effective but that they are nearly always also far more expensive. The latter may make them less cost-effective.

- Dilution: prescribing cheaper non-brand drugs, or reducing length of stay in hospital
- Delay: hospital waiting lists
- Deflection: having GPs as gate-keepers; or referring an elderly person for other non–health care services

Free-market provision of care is often not regarded as a form of rationing. Everybody who has enough money can buy any treatment (e.g. expensive operations) privately. However, many will not have the money either to buy the service directly or to take out comprehensive private insurance (see pp. 148–149). Hence, practically, the effect is similar to rationing.

Rationing: underlying principles

The key principle underpinning rationing is usually 'equity', but other principles are also important (see Harrison and Hunter, 1994):

- Equity: Everyone should have a fair opportunity to attain their full health potential. In other words, no one should be disadvantaged from achieving their potential if it can be avoided. Equity could refer not only to access to health care but also to healthy living conditions or equity of autonomy.
- Needs: The NHS was introduced on the principle that people should receive health services on the basis of their health and medical need rather than their 'ability to pay', but 'need' is not a simple, clear concept (see pp. 150–151).
- Equality: All individuals have an equal access to health care. Should a 70-year-old smoker and heavy drinker have the same chance of getting the next available donor kidney as a 21-year-old non-smoker and non-drinker?
- Effectiveness: the ability of an intervention to achieve its intended effect in those to whom it is offered (i.e. does it work?).
- Cost-effectiveness (efficiency): The effectiveness of an intervention in relation to the resources used (e.g. time, labour, equipment and materials).
- Quality-adjusted life-years (QALYs): A technique for estimating the extra years of life gained from particular interventions, adjusted for the quality of the extra years. They are often combined with costs to give a 'cost per additional QALY', but there are many assumptions built into their calculation (see also pp. 50–51).

Decision-making

In a democracy, we have to establish who should set priorities and ration services. Should priorities be decided by doctors, administrators, politicians, service users, pressure groups, courts or some sort of consensus group?

Commissioning is where decisions are being made by the purchasers of health care regarding the range, the quantity and the quality of health services for a specific population at a specific time. Commissioners are effectively taking decisions on the rationing. This is a case where decision-making about priority setting and rationing lies predominantly with the health care managers and, to a lesser extent, the medical profession, but certainly not the services users.

Internationally, two organizations illustrate good examples of the assessment of the clinical and cost effectiveness of drugs, treatments and medical technologies: the National Institute for Health and Care Excellence (NICE) in the UK and the Canadian

Agency for Drugs and Technology for Health (CADTH). Both are independent government agencies that pull together the best available information to help others to make funding decisions about health care. Their advice is usually adopted by decision-makers (See NICE: www.nice.org.uk and CADTH: www.cadth.ca/).

Consultation of users

The appeal of the Oregon experiment (see Case study 2) lies partly in its explicit approach to rationing and partly in community participation in priority setting. It is interesting to note that prevention comes high on the priority list. Fig. 76.1 shows the main forms of rationing whereby medical and economic considerations are taken in to account. The bottom left-hand corner is the situation often found in the UK, and the top right-hand corner is a serious possibility in countries with private medicine working for profit.

Consultations with users are not without problems. Users are likely to be biased towards patients like them who have similar conditions and diseases. For example, cancer patients may consider the needs of maternity care users or users based in cities might not understand the particular needs of rural patients (see pp. 158–159).

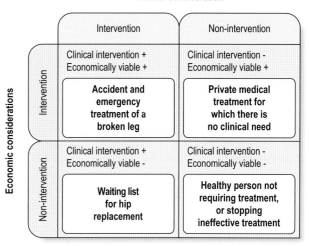

Fig. 76.1 Overview of medical and economic considerations in decision-making.

Stop and think

- What principles should guide a decision to spend more money on either (1) clinical psychology services for people with depression or (2) hip replacement surgery, both of which have 6-month waiting lists? What information would you need to make a decision?
- What effect would using different principles have on the decision?

Case study 1

During World War II, penicillin was scarce on the battlefields. Doctors had to make decisions on which soldiers would be treated and which not. The recovery rate of getting the soldiers back to the front was considerably higher among those with a sexually transmitted infection (STI) rather than those with serious shot and shrapnel wounds. However, medical considerations (i.e. best recovery rate) were overruled by political (what people at home might think) and ethical considerations such as 'soldiers with an STI are less deserving than those with bullet wounds' (see Labelling and stigma, pp. 60–61).

Setting priorities and rationing

- All countries and all care systems have some in-built form of rationing.
- Rationing takes different forms.
- Key principles of rationing care are equity, equality, effectiveness and cost-effectiveness. Needs and value are also important but difficult to operationalize.
- Much rationing and setting of priorities takes place implicitly. Explicit rationing forces people to make difficult choices. Who makes these choices and decisions is another key issue.

Case study 2 *The Oregon experiment*

The American state of Oregon pioneered a system for prioritizing health care in an attempt to address the widespread problem of the growing number of people who are without private health insurance and who are not eligible for federal assistance programmes. Most controversial of the reforms is the use by the legislature of a priority list of health services to determine benefit levels for the insurance programmes. In addition Oregon aimed to bring cover for the rationed services to everyone in the population. Priorities were set by a Health Services Commission, initially on the basis of a technical methodology similar to 'cost per QALY', and, subsequently, on broad-based consensus through public consultation. The Commission came up with the following priorities:

- Acute, fatal conditions where treatment prevents death and leads to full recovery
- Maternity care
- Acute, fatal conditions where treatment prevents death but does not lead to full recovery
- Preventive care for children
- Chronic, fatal conditions where treatment prolongs life and improves quality of care, comfort or palliative care

The next step was for politicians to determine how much could be funded. This clearly brought the provision of health care to the centre of the political arena, since an increase in the health budget meant an increase in taxation or a decrease in the provision of other state provisions, for example, in education. Thus the Oregon experiment introduced a rational plan for expanding services to the entire state, whilst acknowledging the limitations of funding resources.

Based on Kitzhaber, 1993.

77 | Community care

Community care is a broad, messy and contested concept. In its simplest articulation it is about enabling people to live independently. For at least 30 years, community care has been a cornerstone in the development of health and social care services, particularly in the UK, although various interpretations exist in most high-income countries, including the USA, Australia and Italy. It can be seen as a way of delivering much-needed support and services such as domiciliary care (help at home), meals, counselling, supported accommodation and day and respite care to people with illnesses, learning, physical, sensory or mental health issues. Yet, more recently, this needs-based provision (see pp. 150–151) and focus has moved to a language of 'participation', 'control', 'choice' and 'empowerment' as the following Case study highlights.

Case study *Tom's community care*

Tom (age 38 years) was born with cerebral palsy and until recently was cared for by his mother. Over the years Tom regularly had his needs assessed and has been provided with services to meet these needs (see pp. 150–151). Services from private social care and wider organizations were often purchased on his behalf by the local government, which assessed his needs. Services were targeted to allow 'for a range of options'; respond 'flexibly and sensitively' to his needs and those of his mother; and intervene no more than 'necessary to foster independence'.

However, because the health of Tom's mother deteriorated, they both realized that other provisions would have to be put in place. Over recent years, Tom had understood the calls for 'person-centred care', 'joint working' and the 'integration' of health, social care and wider services. Tom took this opportunity to express his desire to live independently. He wanted to shape his own care. Having choice and control over his care plan and the budget that goes with it has been a very empowering experience for him.

In time he was housed in a specially adapted flat through a supported housing project that provided carers to help with personal care and daily living tasks and a support worker to facilitate a social and personal life. Tom is learning computing skills that aid in his communication. He hopes these skills will help him gain employment. Tom now has a girlfriend he met through his computer classes. He has made many other friends through the internet, and he enjoys the freedom the internet gives. As time goes on he realizes others see him as an individual with a contribution to make to the community rather than as a passive recipient of aid for his needs.

At its broadest conception, community care involves service delivery, economic policy, political rhetoric and philosophical ideology. The development of community care throughout developed countries has come about through a variety of clinical, social and political influences (Fig. 77.1).

Influences on community care

The community

Two powerful beliefs are at work here. The first is that a community that cares and accepts people who are old, ill or cope with disabilities will treat them as equal and valued members of that community. This is about developing strong, inclusive communities. The second is that living in the community is, by definition, better than living in an institution. For those who receive good care and support and have appropriate housing and a good social network, living in the community empowers them to make choices over their lives, freed from the restrictions of institutions.

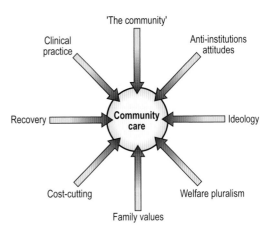

Fig. 77.1 Influences on community care.

Anti-institutions

Institutions are expensive, can be dehumanizing and provide an environment for abuse; loss of ability, independence and general apathy can be the outcomes for those involved (Goffman, 1968b). The true meaning of asylum as sanctuary has been forgotten, and with the number of beds being reduced, especially for patients with mental health problems, it can be difficult to admit patients in acute crises. As the population of long-stay psychiatric patients has diminished, their place has been taken by the numbers of elderly people with dementia (see also pp. 40–41).

Ideology

The political right supports the view that market forces should dictate all. Therefore services are needs-led not service-led. Consumers, customers or clients (formerly patients) have rights and are to be consulted about service delivery. The left supports consumerism more from a position of advocacy and empowerment (see pp. 98–99).

Welfare pluralism

In the move from the welfare state towards a mixed economy of care, services are provided by statutory agencies, voluntary organizations and the private sector. This can incorporate assessments for certain kinds of care.

Cost-cutting

The growing elderly population means that the cost of residential care is escalating for welfare-state countries. Community care can be seen a way of capping this cost by restricting residential care and moving costs to families. In continuing care of elderly people in England and Wales, distinctions are made between medical care, which requires hospitalization, and nursing care, which can take place in nursing homes and thus is not part of free health care. Scotland has an integrated health and social care system where this distinction has been removed, and personal care for the elderly is now funded (see also pp. 148–149).

Family values

A return to traditional 'family' values is a major political theme for conservative governments in, for example, the UK, Australia and North America. The family is promoted as the front line of care 'by' the community and services are directed at helping families care rather than care 'in' the community (e.g. state or private facilities) (see pp. 98–99).

Clinical practice

From the 1950s onwards new advances in treatment, including the introduction of phenothiazines, behaviour therapy, rehabilitation and psychosocial therapies, meant that custodial care for groups such as those with mental health issues became less relevant. Consequently more patients are being treated at home and/or in their own community.

Recovery

These changes have contributed to a change in emphasis on the types of services and outcomes. In mental health services, for example, there is now an emphasis on recovery. The focus is, therefore, less on the illness and more on developing a positive approach to tackling the adverse impact of having a mental health issue, with individuals seeing themselves as being able to have a positive life and being involved in their own recovery, rather than simply being passive recipients of services (Repper and Perkins, 2006).

Some of the problems in discussing community care come from translating what is a generic policy to services appropriate for different patient and client groups. Guiding users through a variety of different agencies and organizations, all of which should cooperate and interrelate with each other (Fig. 77.2), adds to the problem. Doctors can play a roll in guiding their patients towards appropriate agencies and support in the community.

Underlying problems

Coherence of vision

Community care requires multi-disciplinary cooperation at all levels: staff and policy in housing, social work, social security,

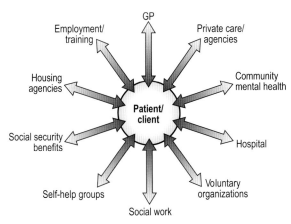

Fig. 77.2 Agencies with whom the patient/client may be involved.

medicine, nursing, occupational and physiotherapy, psychology and employment are all involved; in addition there are often self-help groups, too. Policy often requires joint planning and working between health and social services to provide seamless services in the community to clients. Different professional views, ways of working and priorities can cause practical problems. In mental illness, for example, the biomedical versus the social–environmental view requires radically different approaches to people and services (see pp. 2–3). A bio-psycho-social approach brings these together and is advocated by many. The reality of service delivery, however, can be difficult as many agencies that have to cooperate have different views and priorities.

The role of women

By and large female relatives and friends are expected to fill the gaps left by the shortage of public service resources and provide informal care at home (see pp. 44–45). Community services tend to be staffed by low-paid, predominantly female workers with poor conditions and terms of employment.

'Them' and 'us'

There is still stigma attached to many of the health problems that need community-based care, such as mental health, drug misuse, some disabilities (see pp. 60–61). The well-known NIMBY (Not In My Back Yard) syndrome means that communities are often not willing to accept people with problems. Plans to develop hostels, community-based drug rehabilitation units or sheltered housing are often met with local opposition.

Stop and think

- Is there a role for institutions?
- Instead of asking a patient 'What is the matter', think about asking, 'What matters to you'?

Community care

- Community care is a broad, messy and contested concept.
- It is about helping people live independently.
- It is both inter- and multi-disciplinary.
- It can be described as aiming to empower individuals to take control of their care.
- Therefore the individual, not the system or institution, should be at the centre of this.

78 | Health: a global perspective

The world has become a much smaller place as more people travel. Hence diseases spread much faster across national boundaries, as travellers are accompanied by 'bugs', bacteria and viruses. There were nearly 250 million international migrants (3% of global population) in 2016. Health scares about Ebola, Zika virus, bird flu and severe acute respiratory syndrome (SARS) outbreaks reflect this global mobility. Patterns in the prevalence of diseases vary by geographical location: e.g. the prevalence of HIV is significantly higher in sub-Saharan Africa than in other regions of the world.

Some use the term 'international health' others 'global health'. The word 'international' is defined in terms of crossing national borders, whereas the word 'global' encompasses the entire world. We study not only different patterns of disease but also ways of providing health care (see pp. 148–149), and health policy-making. Therefore, it is not just health *problems* that are common around the world; *solutions* can also cross borders, and countries can learn from each other and also share their own experiences and information.

We group countries into three categories by using health, education and economic indicators (also known as the *human development index*). The common practice is to group Japan, Canada, the USA, Australia, New Zealand and western Europe as 'developed' or industrialized regions, or 'first world'. All countries in South and Middle America, Africa and most in Asia are grouped as 'developing' countries or the 'third world', whilst Russia and the Eastern European countries are somewhere in between. The 'developing' countries are further subdivided into the 'least developed' (or 'fourth world') category. The World Bank uses three categories on the basis of gross national income (GNI) per capita per year: low-income ($1,045 or less); middle-income ($1,045–$12,736); and high-income (greater than $12,736).

A *developing country* tends to have the following features:

1. Agriculture is more important than manufacturing.
2. Economic specialization and exchange are limited.
3. There are not enough savings to finance investment.
4. Population is expanding too rapidly for available resources.
5. The standard of living is low.

Terms such as 'third world', 'low-income' or 'developed' country can create the illusion that nations are homogeneous with similar social, political and/or cultural circumstances and problems. Developing countries are not equally poor, and people in even the poorest countries are not equally poor. Moreover terms such as 'developing country', 'third world' or even 'Africa' may carry a notion of inferiority, poverty, disease, corruption and failure.

The level of development in countries has a direct effect on its population. Not only do five in six people live in developing countries, they are also young; in developed countries 16.4% is younger than 15, in less developed regions this is 28%. More young people mean a larger generation becoming sexually active (see pp. 28–29), leading to population growth.

International health issues

There are different patterns of disease between countries (Table 78.1). In high-income countries, two-thirds of people live beyond the age of 70, and the main causes of mortality are chronic and non-infectious diseases. In low-income countries, less than a quarter of people reach 70, and although the causes of mortality includes heart disease, infectious diseases (e.g. HIV) and complications of pregnancy and childbirth continue to be major

Table 78.1 **Leading causes of death by income group (2015)**

	Disease	Deaths (per 100,000 population)
High-income countries	Ischaemic heart disease	145
	Stroke	65
	Alzheimer disease & other dementias	60
	Trachea, bronchus, lung cancers	50
	Chronic obstructive pulmonary disease	43
Low-income countries	Lower respiratory infections	85
	Diarrhoeal diseases	57
	Stroke	50
	Ischaemic heart disease	49
	HIV/AIDS	34.5

Adapted from World Health Organization (2018). http://www.who.int/mediacentre/factsheets/fs310/en/index1.html.

Box 78.1 **Top 10 risks to global health**

1. Underweight
2. Unsafe sex
3. High blood pressure
4. Tobacco consumption
5. Alcohol consumption
6. Unsafe water, sanitation and hygiene
7. Iron deficiency
8. Indoor smoke from solid fuels
9. High cholesterol
10. Obesity

From www.who.int/whr/en/.

causes of death. Governments will need to prioritize (see pp. 152–153) differently to provide the health services needed to combat these different causes of death.

Box 78.1 suggests that malnutrition (largely resulting from poverty) is the single most important cause of death. The average person in a developed country will probably attribute this to famine and disasters as these get media attention (see pp. 52–53). However, for many, poverty means chronic malnutrition (see pp. 106–107). This does not make world news, but it is estimated that it takes many more lives than the famines we see in the media.

HIV is the second risk factor – unsafe sex. Globally some 35 million people are living with HIV. Sub-Saharan Africa is the worst affected region (see pp. 108–109). The AIDS epidemic impacts on households, education, workplaces and economies, not just health and health care.

Inequality

Whilst global health improves, inequalities in health remain and, in many instances, are increasing. This is the case not only within many countries but also between countries, so whilst life expectancy has been improving worldwide, in sub-Saharan Africa this improvement has been halted by HIV.

The poorest 20% of people in the world are 10 times more likely to die before age 14 compared with the richest 20% (DFID, 2000). Women in the poorest countries are 500 times more likely to die in childbirth than in developed countries. Developing countries account for 84% of the world population and 93% of the global burden of disease. However, they account for only 18% of global income and 11% of global health spending.

The same inequality exists in research, with less than 10% of global spending on health research used for diseases or conditions that account for 90% of the global disease burden – known as the *10/90 gap*. Poverty is the single biggest cause of preventable death in the world. It underscores lack of education, access to food, resources, medical services and adequate housing.

Globalization

Globalization refers to integration across the globe. It means that worldwide human interaction has become more intense in a range of fields including economics, health, politics, knowledge and technology transfer (Lee, 2003). It has positive and negative impacts on health and health care. New technologies and the development of health systems help reduce mortality and morbidity.

The globalization of pharmaceutical markets has increased the availability of drugs reaching some of the remotest areas of the world. However, pharmaceutical companies are nearly all large, multi-national companies that exist to make profits, but profits are much higher in countries where people have money. Therefore companies develop drugs for minor lifestyle issues in middle-class consumers rather than drugs for life-threatening diseases in poor populations without money. Moreover the pharmaceutical industry spends millions to convince doctors to prescribe their products. Commercial information provided by sales representatives of pharmaceutical companies has greater influence than scientific sources on doctors' prescribing behaviour in developing countries. The tobacco industry (as multi-nationals) have shifted their focus from markets in Western countries to developing countries, with major implications for health (see pp. 82–83).

Migration

Migration brings a number of health issues. Migrants who are refugees are often most at risk of range of diseases whilst least likely to have access to the necessary health care. There are 1 billion migrants globally, of whom 250 million are international migrants and 763 million internal migrants – one in seven of the world's population. Approximately 65 million migrants are forcibly displaced, according to the World Health Organization (2017). War, terror, natural disasters and disease epidemics can effect on large groups of people, either directly through disaster or war or indirectly because of displacement of people. Developing countries account for three-quarters of reported global deaths caused by conflicts and disasters.

There is a migration of trained health workers, mainly from developing countries to developed countries. Poor wages, economic instability, poorly funded health systems, the burden and risks of HIV and safety concerns are factors that 'push' staff to leave developing countries. Additional factors, including higher wages, better living and working conditions and opportunities for advancing their education and skills, 'pull' health workers to developed countries. Some countries, despite their domestic health care needs, cannot offer enough jobs for all health professionals they train, thus motivating them to emigrate. This loss of skilled personnel (brain drain) is a major concern for many countries. With fewer than two-thirds of UK registered doctors being trained in the UK, it may be affected by 'Brexit' (Fig. 78.1).

Sustainable Development Goals

To achieve long-term development goals, leading development, organizations and governments set global targets. For 2015–2030 world health policy is guided by the Sustainable Development Goals (SDGs). One of these 17 SDGs, namely, SDG3, focusses on health (Box 78.2) although several others such as SDG2 (nutrition) and SDG6 (reducing inequality) affect people's health.

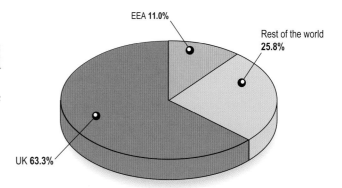

Fig. 78.1 UK registered doctors by country of qualification.

Stop and think

- What can you give to developing countries, and what can (or do) you learn from developing countries?

Health: a global perspective

- Globalization has made the world a smaller place, where diseases spread more easily over greater distances.
- Disease prevalence varies between high-, middle- and low-income countries.
- Health inequalities exist between countries affected by health worker migration, the way pharmaceutical companies operate and/or lack of research funding for problems specific to developing countries.

79 | Health: a rural perspective

Across the world more and more people live and work in urban areas (see Urban nature, health and well-being, pp. 134–135). There are advantages in terms of living and working in rural areas, but providing appropriate health care in sparsely populated and remote areas brings its own particular challenges as well as additional costs for members of the public and health care providers alike.

Health and health care needs

There are common characteristics relating to health and health care in remote and rural areas; however, it is important to remember that not all rural communities are the same. Remote and rural areas are geographically distant from urban centres and often sparsely populated, but rural areas have distinct demographic, geographical and socio-economic profiles. For example, a fishing community in Shetland will have a very different population from that of a deprived village in Wales where the main source of employment was a coal mine that closed down 3 decades ago. This in turn will determine health priorities and challenges.

Although the particular health needs will vary, rural communities in developed countries often have a relatively high ageing population. Social care needs and support services then become a priority. Injuries relating to certain occupations such as farming, fishing, game-keeping or forestry are also more common in rural areas. Rural communities in many industrial countries are becoming increasingly dependent on tourism, which brings seasonal variations in health care needs. This may be in the form of people with chronic conditions, injuries resulting from adventure sports or road traffic accidents. Research comparing the health of rural and urban populations in the UK is inconclusive and varies with type of condition. Canada and Australia, with many more remote and rural communities and generally greater travelling distances, have invested more in rural health research.

Access to health care is complex. Rural communities may benefit from improved access to primary care compared with cities but experience more difficulties accessing secondary and specialized care. There is consistent evidence that people in rural areas have lower levels of health service use and that they present later with medical problems (see Deciding to consult, pp. 86–87). The latter can have an impact on prognosis and morbidity and mortality.

Stop and think

- What difference do you expect as a doctor working in a small rural town compared with working in a big city practice?

Rural communities

Service provision is often less comprehensive in rural areas, with regard to not only health care but also education, libraries, financial services or entertainment. Service provision is poorer because of distance to (health) services, poorer public transport, poorer internet access and the fact that transport is at the mercy of the weather. Moreover in the past decades we have seen the decline of services in many rural areas in the UK, with closure of schools, garages, pharmacies, pubs and post offices and

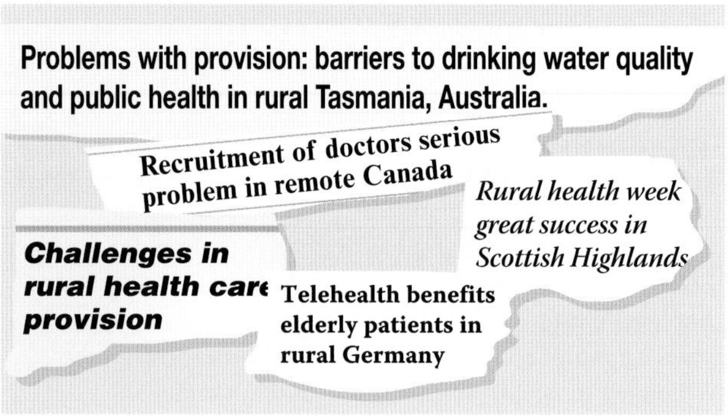

Fig. 79.1 Problems with rural health provision often hit media headlines.

discontinuation of local bus services. Local GP surgeries and community hospitals have suffered the same fate (Fig. 79.1). For example, in England the number of maternity units fell by 23.2% in a 14-year period from 341 in 1996 to 262 in 2010. Many of these disappearing units were located in rural England. It is impossible to have a full-scale academic hospital or an opera house in every single village for reasons of economies of scale (see pp. 152–153), but at the same time a decline in service provision may be less acceptable to local communities where services are often poorer to start with.

Rural patients do expect to have to travel; they do so to get to shop, sporting facilities, schooling, libraries, pubs or police stations. Although car ownership in rural areas of the UK is higher than in the cities, many people have no access to a car and have to rely on the poorer public transport. Rural poverty is not always recognized (see Social class and health, pp. 42–43). This means that services are even more difficult to access for vulnerable groups, often those most in need. People with young children, adolescents (especially those too young to drive), elderly people without their own transport (see pp. 14–15), those with disabilities (see pp. 70–71) and the poor (see pp. 42–43) may find it hard to attend clinics and hospital appointments.

Rural health care

People in small communities are more likely to know each other and each other's business. This may make it more difficult, for example, for a young person to obtain condoms in the local pharmacist or shop (see pp. 28–29) or to make an appointment with the local doctor to discuss drug misuse (see pp. 78–79). Anonymity and confidentiality are harder to maintain, and stigma (see pp. 60–61) is harder to avoid. People in rural areas may choose to travel to a more anonymous clinic in a city to receive screening, testing or treatment related to, for example, mental illness, domestic violence or sexually transmitted infections.

The closeness of communities also has advantages for health. It is possible to achieve greater continuity with health care professionals and establish better relationships (Farmer et al., 2006). GPs are more familiar with the wider context of their patients' lives, families and relationships, which can lead to a better understanding and the prescription of more effective psycho-social and medical interventions. However, changes in out-of-hour services in the UK may have an impact on continuity of care because out-of-hours duties will not necessarily be carried out by local GPs known to the community. This will have implications for patients and health care professionals.

Providing health services is more expensive in rural areas because of fewer patient consultations per health care worker (higher staff–patient ratios) and more staff time spent on travelling. Doctors and nurses having to travel to patients living far apart means increased travel costs also more time wasted on traveling, for the same reasons training and staff development costs are also higher. Health care is also more expensive for patients because of extra travel costs and having to take more time off work to attend hospital appointments, perhaps with overnight stays in a hotel.

Community-level initiatives such as voluntary hospital car services can help those who need it to access hospital care (see pp. 154–155) but this is then a cost borne by the individual and community rather than the health service. Centralization of services may result in greater efficiency for the health service (see Setting priorities and rationing, pp. 152–153), but may result in an increase in indirect costs such as travel.

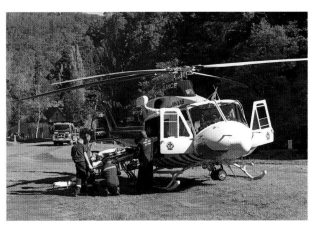

Fig. 79.2 Overcoming distances: The Royal Flying Doctors Service of Australia. *iStock.com/BeyondImages*.

Staffing problems

Recruitment and retention of health care staff in rural areas is a global problem. Extra incentives in terms of allowances or relocation packages can be offered to fill key posts. Medical students who do (part of) their training in rural areas are more likely to settle there as doctors (see Medical students' experience, pp. 160–161). It is harder to maintain certain skills in rural areas, especially around rarer health care problems. For example, if recommendations are that GPs need to attend at least 12 normal deliveries a year or do 25 minor surgical procedures, rural GPs simply might not see enough patients to get enough practice.

One possible solution to help community-based practitioners to keep up their skills is to rotate them in a central hospital for a short period each year. This has the disadvantage that the rural practitioner is away from the rural community where locum cover is more difficult to organize. Some posts have been specially created for rural roaming practitioners who regularly alternate between rural practices to allow permanent GPs to maintain training, and rural fellowships offer additional training to GPs (Siderfin, 2005).

One way of providing services is using mobile services (e.g. for dentistry or breast cancer screening), more care at home, or doctors (GPs or specialists) who may offer branch surgeries one morning per week or month. These services may be prone to disruption, especially when the weather is bad. Maintaining skills is a fundamental requirement, but there have been suggestions of professional snobbery amongst hospital-based specialists towards their more generalist rural colleagues.

Centralization of health services

Even with a highly centralized service we need to consider what we need to offer in rural areas in case of an emergency. For example, over the past 4 decades UK maternity services have been more centralised (see Pregnancy and childbirth, pp. 4–5). Many rural community maternity units have been closed. This means more women and/or their babies have to travel greater distances when something goes wrong. Moreover they need to travel earlier to avoid travelling in labour and, as a consequence, may end up waiting in the central obstetric units until labour starts. Women and their babies may be kept in hospital slightly longer after the delivery because of the long distance between where women live and their health care facility.

Similarly, services once provided by cottage hospitals such as dealing with minor injuries have now been centralized to urban hospitals. As travel is not always possible because of adverse weather conditions, we still need to have some kind of provision to deal with emergencies in rural areas. The UK sometimes uses flying squads, where hospital specialists come out by ambulance or air ambulance to provide emergency cover in case of, for example, road traffic accidents or obstetric emergencies. Other countries with vast rural areas and low population density, for example, Australia, have developed a flying-doctor service to reach patients in remote locations (Fig. 79.2).

Tele-health

One possible solution for remote and rural communities has been the use of the internet and computer-based technology. For example, a rural GP examining a patient with skin problems in her practice could have a video link with a dermatologist in a hospital 500 miles away. Rural practitioners can also use computer technology to update their skills, knowledge and competencies on a regular basis. Distance learning, whereby rural practitioners update their skills using video conferencing with trainers in central hospitals, has been promoted as a way forward. This has been helped by the extension and improvement of internet services into remote areas.

Health: a rural perspective

- Health care needs, expectations and facilities in rural areas can differ greatly from those in cities.
- Working as a rural doctor brings the advantages and disadvantages of living in a rural community.
- Anonymity and confidentiality are harder to maintain for patients and health care providers alike in rural areas.
- In many countries, health care facilities have been centralized over the past decades, leaving rural people with fewer (poorer) services and greater costs (time and money).
- Tele-medicine can improve rural health care as well as training rural practitioners.

80 | Medical students' experience

Wherever you train to be a doctor, there are some experiences common to all medical students, which may set you apart from other undergraduate students. Thinking about how you tackle challenges during this time will enable you to cope with the pressures of a career in medicine and facilitate an understanding of how doctors, other professionals and patients deal with their own difficulties (see The profession of medicine, pp. 164–165).

The need for ongoing curriculum evolution in response to developments in medicine and society is well-recognized worldwide. In the 1990s UK medical schools underwent several curriculum reforms. Research into students' experiences of newer curriculum models (e.g. early clinical exposure, a focus on clinical and communication skills and professionalism, integration of basic and clinical sciences content, small group and self-directed learning) and the resulting changes in students' knowledge, clinical and cognitive skills and professional behaviours have followed.

Where strong evidence exists, the impact of newer curriculum approaches has been generally positively reviewed. For example, one systematic literature review concluded that problem-based learning during medical school had positive effects on competency after graduation. Similarly, a questionnaire survey of all UK medical students who graduated between 1999 and 2005 showed that self-reported preparedness improved 1 year after graduation. In addition, initiatives such as student assistantships and shadowing schemes in the final year of medical school, changes to postgraduate training that aims to improve the working conditions for junior doctors (e.g. the European Working Time Directive) and strategies to improve supervision and feedback, all suggest a positive trajectory in terms of experience in medical school and early clinical practice.

Despite these encouraging developments, the challenges of preparing students for practice are still substantial, and high levels of anxiety and stress persist amongst doctors and medical students (see Life as a trainee doctor, pp. 162–163; The profession of medicine, pp. 164–165). The proportion of doctors and other health care professionals experiencing above threshold levels of stress is around 28% (see What is stress?, pp. 126–127). A recent systematic review (Hope and Henderson, 2014) suggested prevalence

rates of 7.7% to 65.5% for anxiety, 6% to 66.5% for depression and 12.2% to 96.7% for psychological distress for medical students outside North America.

What is different about medicine?

Many of the pressures on medical students are not qualitatively different from those on other students: they worry about coursework, exams, money and relationships. There are specific aspects of a medical degree that may cause additional pressure, however, and these can be categorized into individual, interpersonal, academic and clinical factors.

Individual factors include personality type, tolerance of ambiguity, health and finances. The personality traits of individuals choosing medicine as a career may differ and personality traits are recognized as predictors of well-being (see Personality and health, pp. 18–19). Ambiguous situations are commonplace in medicine, and some medical students are more intolerant of ambiguity than others, which can result in distress and may influence attitudes towards certain patient groups and career choice. The length of the course potentially increases the burden of financial debt and also means that statistically more students will experience personal illness as an undergraduate. Dyrbye et al. (2006) recognized the strong relationship between personal life events and professional burnout among US medical students.

Interpersonal factors leading to anxiety include competition and familial expectations (see Anxiety, pp. 112–113). The fact that medical students have been high achievers prior to medical school may lead to a competitive environment within medical school, which may be reinforced through assessment and the need to rank students for intercalation and training places. Familial context may add to the

pressure because parents may have high expectations of their offspring.

Academic factors include workload and the transition to medical school learning. Medical students' workloads may be heavier than other degrees, which can be a stressor (Dahlin et al., 2005), and students are sometimes unfamiliar with the approach to learning required for success within medical programme. Uncertainty about individual study behaviour, progress and aptitude when coming close to exam time was the main stressor.

Clinical factors include relationships with clinical supervisors and exposure to death and dying (see pp. 130–131). Swedish students were worried about their personal endurance and/or competence in the future and reported 'non-supportive climate' as an important stressor (Dahlin et al., 2005). Similarly, 18% of medical trainees across multiple hospital, community and mental health trusts in London responded yes to the question "In this post, have you been subjected to persistent behaviour by others, which has eroded your professional confidence or self-esteem?" and more junior trainees were more likely to respond yes (Paice et al., 2004). The perpetrators were mostly other doctors within the medical hierarchy. It is to be hoped that earlier and phased introduction to clinical experience and faculty development of clinical teachers will reduce these complaints, but there is little research evidence to support such a belief, and the challenges are likely to be cultural rather than individual. An encouraging development is the creation of validated scales that can unpick aspects of quality of instructional quality within clinical placements.

Coping strategies and student support

Grant et al. (2015) offer a conceptual model to differentiate the different stages

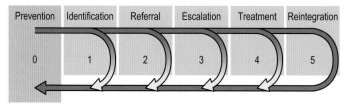

Fig. 80.1 Process model outlining different stages of medical students' mental ill-health *(from Grant, A., Rix, A., Winter, P., Mattick, K., Jones, D., 2015. Support for Medical Students with Mental Health Problems: a Conceptual Model Academic Psychiatry: 39 (1), 16–21. With permission from the General Medical Council).*

at which interventions can be targeted, including prevention, identification and treatment (Fig. 80.1). Clearly strategies aimed at prevention are most desirable.

There are several strategies that are helpful in preventing and managing anxiety and stress. It is important to try to deal with the source of the stress by managing the workload (prioritizing, delegating), ensuring the expectations made upon you (by yourself and by others) are realistic for your stage of medical training, keeping healthy (e.g. diet, sleep, exercise), scheduling in time to relax (e.g. sport, yoga, music) and seeking support from friends and family. A recent study of best practice in supporting medical students' well-being identified some curriculum interventions that successfully target whole student populations in the prevention of mental health issues. Grant (2013), for example, the use of health enhancement, including mindfulness, and the introduction of pass/fail grading.

There are also some well-known maladaptive coping strategies. One is avoidance, for example, by putting off work that is difficult. Similarly denial and dismissal of a negative event have been found to be coping strategies that increase stress levels, not reduce them. Alcohol abuse is another poor coping strategy (see Alcohol use, pp. 80–81), with prevalence of binge drinking reported at 58% recently in a private US Jesuit medical school (Trostler et al., 2014). Signs of psychological symptoms of anxiety and stress may include excessive worrying, difficulty sleeping or concentrating and/or an inability to relax. This may impact on performance in assessments at medical school.

Medical schools should offer support for students who are experiencing psychological distress. In the UK the General Medical Council (GMC) offers guidance to support medical schools in this task. The range of the support varies widely but often includes prevention strategies, peer-support initiatives, counselling, occupational health and avenues to explore such as interruption of medical studies and careers advice. Whilst many medical students perceive there to be a stigma (see Labelling and stigma, pp. 60–61) associated with help seeking, the GMC guidance aims to reassure students that they will be treated fairly and confidentially. There are many branches of medicine to consider as a specialty, not just general practice versus hospital medicine.

A career in medicine

Despite the demanding conditions of medical training, there are many rewards in the practice of medicine. Students and young doctors can have experience of different specialties and are likely to settle eventually in one that suits their personality and abilities. Those who derive most interest from science and research can move towards academic medicine, and those who enjoy the 'art' of medicine will go into specialties that include closer contact with patients. Although very different, both types of career can bring enormous personal satisfaction.

Case study

Ian, a third-year medical student, appeared before a faculty committee appealing to stay on despite having twice failed an assessment. He had fallen behind in studying but assured the committee that he would not do so again. When asked whether there were any relevant circumstances, he described a catalogue of misfortune. During his third year he had been off for several weeks with abdominal pain that eventually proved to be appendicitis and resulted in an appendectomy. Then his parents separated, and he kept going home at weekends to help his depressed mother. His landlord evicted him because a drunken flatmate had smashed the furniture. By the summer term, he was camping out in friends' flats and missing many days on clinical attachments. He was extremely anxious and unable to sleep or concentrate. Having failed the first assessment, he attempted to revise but had to earn money by working in a bar and made little progress. The committee took a sympathetic view but criticized him for not discussing his difficulties with a tutor and arranging to have time off officially, especially when he was ill. He was permitted to repeat his third year, but strongly advised to make contact with the accommodation service, the counselling service and his tutor.

Stop and think

There is evidence that levels of anxiety and depression in students are, to some extent, predetermined by personality. It has also been shown that teaching stress management to medical students enables them to control the symptoms of stress. Another view is that some experience of anxiety and depression may be helpful in working with patients who have those conditions. Given these various findings, and that lack of support from senior staff is a common complaint, should more be done for students? Interventions include stress management courses, regular meetings with members of staff or support groups across years.

- Is the stress of medical school perhaps part of the preparation for a challenging career that requires personal resilience? Remember to read also Life as a trainee doctor (pp. 162–163) and The profession of medicine (pp. 164–165).

Medical students' experience

- Medical students' experience of stress may differ from that of other students: at first in terms of workload and then later in terms of clinical contact.

- Personality traits may influence the choice of medicine as an undergraduate degree, performance in assessments at medical school and career choice. They may also influence the likelihood of experiencing psychological distress.

- Medical school is challenging, in terms of both academic workload and support in adapting to the clinical environment.

- A range of effective strategies for preventing and managing psychological distress in medical students have been reported and evaluated. The vast majority of medical students will overcome these difficulties and go on to be effective clinicians.

- Medical schools offer a wide range of avenues of student support, including careers counselling.

81 | Life as a trainee doctor

In spite of increased scrutiny of the profession and uncertainty in career progression, medicine continues to afford a challenging but rewarding career, which benefits from being the most trusted profession in society (see The profession of medicine, pp. 164–165).

Foundation years

After graduation, UK junior doctors begin work within a 2-year Foundation Programme. Adapting from life as a medical student to an essential member of the clinical team is one of the most exciting steps in your career. It is a unique time to experience different specialities both in hospital and in the community. The Foundation Programme provides wide opportunities with three or four different jobs each year.

As a Foundation year 1 doctor you take supervised responsibility for patient care. Completing this year and achieving the competencies leads to full (General Medical Council (GMC)) registration. The second year builds towards speciality training with increasing clinical responsibility. Foundation doctors are expected to evidence their progression against the curriculum, getting used to working in this way is essential for all training grades.

Starting work is daunting and a challenge. Every doctor will have clear memories of the start of their medical career. Everyone makes mistakes, but how you learn from them and reflect on them will define you as a person and as a clinician. Regular feedback from everyone you work with will help identify areas where you can develop and will also reassure you.

Support is necessary professionally and personally. Guidance can come from colleagues and supervisors. An active hospital mess will provide peer support, and usually social and sporting events that help balance the pressures of work. You have access to counsellors via occupational health, and further professional support may be available at the deanery level. There are also national bodies in the UK, for example, the British Medical Association (BMA), the Doctors Support Network and the Royal Medical Benevolent Fund, which can assist doctors in emotional or financial difficulties.

> **Stop and think**
>
> • What have I enjoyed in my years as a medical student, and can I see this as my career?

Career progression and supervision

Learning will continue throughout your career. The responsibility to identify aspects to develop and make you a more effective doctor increases as you progress through your training. With planning this could lead to the development of specialist interests such as research, management or educational expertise.

Career progression is standardized, and this can make you feel like you are on a treadmill from the foundation years through speciality training. Decision points such as the end of Foundation Training provide a chance to evaluate where you are going and provide career breaks. It is increasingly common to have a 'Gap' year allowing foreign work, volunteering or travel to gain extra experience in specific chosen areas.

Your portfolio is the on-going record of what you have achieved. Whilst it is used to assess you at annual appraisals, it is really your individual log of progress and a chance to show who you are as a clinician to those you have not worked alongside, for example, at interviews. There are guides on how to get the most from your portfolio (see links for BMA and NHS Careers in the following section).

Colleagues and supervisors (clinical and educational) are often the best source of advice. A clinical supervisor is usually the consultant for whom you work as a junior doctor. Their role is two-fold: (1) to maximize patient safety by guiding and reviewing your care and (2) to provide feedback on your clinical work. Educational supervision provides career guidance, direction and pastoral support. These roles are continued throughout the training grades in all specialities.

Speciality training

There are over 60 different specialities and sub-specialities within the NHS. Working experience in a speciality, which is a potential career choice, is often not possible prior to application to a training programme. Taster weeks and improvement projects are seen as valid experience and commitment to a speciality at the time of job application. During speciality training many doctors will undertake further study or research to gain an MSc or PhD degree. Out-of-Programme experience is diverse with options to volunteer, study, research or work either in the UK or abroad.

Approximately 50% of all UK medical school graduates will train to become general practitioners (GPs) (GP taskforce review, 2014). Entrance to GP training can come at completion of the Foundation Programme or via another speciality training scheme. Every speciality has a succession of examinations in any chosen field, usually allowing entrance to a speciality college such as the Royal College of Physicians.

The balance of service provision and education is extremely difficult. The increasing demands on health care make it difficult to find time for the trainee to fulfil everything that is required by their curriculum. Good planning, organization and patience will help achieve this goal. During your training you will learn by doing the job (experiential learning) and by preparing for examinations, through courses, conferences and self-learning (academic learning). Even if you are not in a training scheme, identifying individual learning needs is fundamental. A significant portion of today's accepted knowledge will be found to be false, so it is essential to embrace 'lifelong learning'.

Speciality training takes you from the Foundation Programme to the GP or consultant level. During this period decisions about speciality or special interest need to be developed. A key question to ask yourself as a trainee will be 'Do I want to do the job of consultant?' Others include 'What interests me? What aspects of the job do I not see as a junior doctor? What future opportunities are there in that role?'

The shape of training review looks to reform junior doctor training by adopting a broader base with more generalist roles. Currently there is no consensus on the shape of reform, but the effects will be seen over the next 10 years (Greenaway, shape of training).

> **Stop and think**
>
> • What do I need as a trainee, and where and how can I have this need met?

Key ideas

This amazing job can at times be overshadowed by the daily grind and relentless work pressures. Despite changes, being a junior doctor is exhausting; fatigue and stress are unfortunately common. Ultimately being allowed to be intimately included into the lives of strangers, to be told their life stories and to be able to offer the help they need, is both a privilege and a reward (see The profession of medicine, pp. 164–165).

Coping with pressure

A new Foundation doctor will find being on-call a stressful and challenging time. You can approach such stressful situations in the same way as other difficulties (see What is stress?, pp. 126–127). The stress and pressures of a life as a doctor never leave, but the ability to manage the pressure and continue to work effectively becomes as important as clinical acumen. All doctors have a pressured job, especially in times of increasing workloads and tighter resources. Taking time to establish individual mechanisms for coping with stress is essential. More generally, look after your own health. Try to rest when you can and to eat properly whenever possible. If you fall ill, despite the culture of working through illness, take time off and see a doctor if necessary. Really the approach to your own health should not be different from the health promotion advice you give your patients (see Health beliefs, motivation and behaviour, pp. 70–71).

Stop and think

How good are you at using your time effectively? How do you prioritize your work? How can you manage a decent work-life balance?

Useful websites

BMA careers advice, for every grade with workshops and webinars on most aspects of your career: http://bma.org.uk/developing-your-career

Foundation Programme website with curriculum and portfolio advice: http://www.foundationprogramme.nhs.uk/pages/home

The Doctors Support Network, an independent network to help doctors with mental health issues: http://www.dsn.org.uk

NHS Medical Careers, a useful guide to career paths and different specialties: https://www.healthcareers.nhs.uk/career-planning

Life as a trainee doctor

- Medicine offers a wide variety of careers.
- Reflection on what you enjoy and are good at will lead to specialty choice.
- Forming habits encouraging 'lifelong learning' is indispensable.
- Support and guidance from peers, supervisors and national bodies are essential.
- Take the time and opportunity to do what you enjoy.
- Stress management techniques can be helpful: focus on cognitions, feelings and behaviour.

Case study *Trainee doctors' organisations*

The British Medical Association (BMA) has a Junior Doctors Committee (JDC) which defends the rights of all junior doctors on education, training and contractual issues. It represent the views of junior doctors to the government and medico-political bodies including royal colleges and educational bodies.

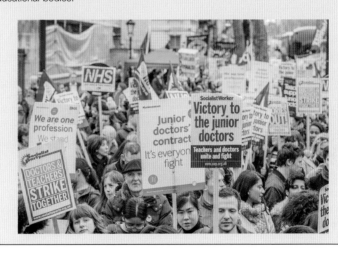

82 | The profession of medicine

Being a medical student means learning about the discipline of medicine (see Medical students' experience, pp. 160–161). However, more is learnt that is not part of the official medical curriculum. Implicit in medical training is showing students how to behave and act as doctors. Your medical education is a way of socialization into medicine. *Socialization* refers to a new recruit being exposed to the predominant norms (expected ways of behaving) and values of an occupation and gradually absorbing these ideas until they become 'natural'. Students, for example, learn to take decisions, to deal or cope with cutting up bodies in pathology practicals, to adhere to a dress code on the wards or to talk to patients and staff in a certain way. In other words, one learns to become a medical professional as much as a medical doctor.

The nature of professions

Professions are an important element in the organization of medical care and the structure of society. The former refers to the position that the medical profession has in the health services; the latter refers to the way professions are regarded as special occupations in society. We could ask, 'What do professionals such as doctors, clergy and lawyers have in common?' or 'What is the difference between doctors and rubbish collectors, two occupations we cannot really do without?' (Fig. 82.1).

There are two main perspectives on the origin and nature of professions. Professions, in the older of the two perspectives, represent the institutionalization of altruistic values because professions are seen as being committed to providing services for the common good. Thus stockbrokers and company directors differ from teachers, lawyers and doctors in that the former occupations consist of people working for an immediate personal gain, be it money, prestige or promotion. The latter occupations consist of people who are motivated not merely by personal interest or by financial gains. Those engaged in a profession are often said to have a *vocation*, or a *calling*. Sociologists who studied professions in the 1950s drew up lists of characteristics of professions as opposed to other occupations. Greenwood (1957) developed one such list:

1. Systematic theory
2. Authority recognized by its clientele
3. Broader community sanction

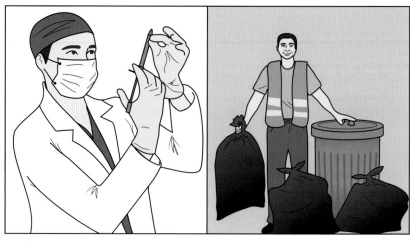

Fig. 82.1 Which is more important for public health?

4. Code of ethics
5. Professional culture sustained by formal sanctions

The medical profession incorporates all the features mentioned previously:

1. It has a theoretical basis.
2. Patients come to doctors for advice/help, and governments also come to the medical profession for advice/help.
3. No one is allowed to practise medicine without a licence.
4. The Hippocratic oath and the Declaration of Geneva (Box 82.1) form its code of ethics.
5. It has strong professional organizations that guard the quality of the work done by its members, leaving it relatively free of lay evaluation or legal contracts.

Continuous professional development, the doctor's obligation to keep up to date in both skills and knowledge, is part of this professional culture.

Professions and competition

More recent thinking approaches professions from the notion of *autonomy*, which is based on the profession being able to exercise power and control over, for example, other occupations, policy-makers and clients (Turner, 1995). Such approaches emphasize competition between different occupations. For example, the crucial feature of the division of labour in health care is the control that doctors exercise over their own work and that of allied occupations. The original function of nursing, for example, was to serve the doctor. Today nursing has developed to a more autonomous profession, with its own education (with professors of nursing in many universities), field of knowledge, control over its members and some power to exclude other occupations from its area of expertize. The maintenance of the medical profession requires the continuing exercise of dominance over allied and competing occupations. As a result the medical profession can be seen to possess an officially approved monopoly of the right to define health and illness and to treat illness. For example, in many countries it is illegal to practise medicine without a licence.

Depending on which approach one takes, a profession is defined as either an altruistic occupation serving the common good or a particularly successful competitor in the occupational arena. Perhaps we can see elements of both approaches at different times or in different types of doctors.

In many countries, doctors belong to the best-paid category of professionals. One way of being able to guarantee jobs for medical graduates is to limit the intake of students. Matching the supply of and demand for doctors maintains a sense of exclusiveness and enables the medical profession to claim a high remuneration.

Professions can be seen as occupations that somehow reduce risk and uncertainty in our lives. The priest, the lawyer and the doctor look after our souls, our rights and/or our bodies, respectively. Some have argued that this factor gives these occupations a higher status in society.

> **Stop and think**
>
> • What makes medicine a profession rather than just an occupation?

The organization of the medical profession

Doctors in nearly every country have a strong professional organization, which acts both as an advisory body to governments and the public and as a trade union. The medical view is often aired in prestigious medical journals, which are, in themselves, part of the organization of the profession. More significantly, such medical journals are regarded as important by the general population and government officials, and this makes them highly influential. The importance and influence of professions are not so much based on their claims as on society's reaction to these claims. Aromatherapists, clinical psychologists, kinesiologists and faith healers (see also Complementary therapies, pp. 144–145) make claims that are often not dissimilar to those made by doctors, but most people in industrialized societies put their faith most of the time in the medical profession and not in the other healers.

Challenges to medical autonomy

The medical profession is self-regulating in many countries, and in the UK it is regulated by the General Medical Council. Doctors often argue that the only person who can evaluate the work of a doctor is a fellow-doctor. However, medical autonomy has been increasingly challenged and eroded in recent years:

- The state has varying degrees of control over professionals such as regulating their income, training or the right to practise.
- Hospital administrators/managers and health insurance companies have a certain amount of control over doctors. Managers can direct funding from one medical specialty to another, or from hospital- to community-based practitioners, whilst insurance companies can influence the kind and amount of medical interventions conducted.
- Challenges have also come from the professionalization of other paramedical occupations, particularly nursing.

- Within medicine, there have been attempts to change the hierarchical structure of the profession and to embrace complementary therapies such as homeopathy and acupuncture.
- Consumers (and patients) have begun to question the kind of services they receive. In the UK the introduction of the Patient Charter has changed the balance towards the lay public. Moreover, the internet and social media has given patients easier access to medical information, guidelines, government reports and policy documents.
- The effectiveness of medical treatments has been challenged, and the number of complaints against doctors has increased; the number of court cases against doctors, especially in the USA, has made indemnity insurance very costly. The consequence of all these societal factors is that doctors have increasingly limited autonomy over medical issues.
- Negative media publicity has also led to calls for more control over the medical profession (see pp. 52–53).

> **Stop and think**
>
> • How altruistic is medicine as a profession?

> **Stop and think**
>
> • What does it mean to be a professional?

> **Case study** *The development of the medical profession in the UK*
>
> It was only as the 19th century progressed that doctors became the dominant group in treating illness. The British Medical Association was founded in 1832, and one of its roles was to transform the status of medicine into a profession ranking with other learned professions.
>
> After 15 unsuccessful attempts to convince parliament that doctors could be trusted with monopoly powers, the 1858 Medical Act unified the profession, combining surgeons, physicians and apothecaries, and created the General Medical Council, which was empowered to keep a register of qualified practitioners. As a result, employment positions were increasingly open only to registered doctors, particularly those posts controlled by the state's Poor Law hospitals and by the mutual Friendly Societies that provided insurance protection and medical care to working-class patients, often through trade unions. In 1911, again after successful political lobbying, the National Insurance Act brought the control of these Friendly Societies under local health committees with strong medical representation, thereby reducing the degree of external and lay control over these doctors' activities.

> **The profession of medicine**
>
> - Professionals are said to work towards professional standards, which are higher than the standards towards which other occupations work.
> - Professional standards combine an element of altruism with a well-developed system of quality control.
> - Students are socialized into the profession.
> - The state is the most limiting factor on professional freedom.
> - The rise in importance of managers, other health practitioners and patients has eroded the professional power of doctors.

References

Abraham, C., Sheeran, P., 2005. Health belief model. In: Conner, M., Norman, P. (Eds.), Predicting Health Behaviour: Research and Practice with Social Cognition Models, second ed. Open University Press, Buckingham, UK. pp. 28–80.

Ainsworth, M.D.S., Blehar, M.C., Waters, E., et al., 1978. Patterns of Attachment. Erlbaum, Hillsdale, NJ.

Ajzen, I., 1991. The theory of planned behavior. Org. Behav. Hum. Decision Process 50, 179–211.

Ajzen, I., Driver, B.L., 1991. Prediction of leisure participation from behavioural, normative, and control beliefs: An application of the theory of planned behavior. Leis. Sci. 13 (3), 185–204.

Albrecht, G.L., Devlieger, P.J., 1999. The disability paradox: high quality of life against all odds. Soc. Sci. Med. 48, 977–988.

Allen, M., Allen, J., Hogarth, S., Marmot, M., 2013. Working for Health Equity: The Role of Health Professionals. UCL Institute of Health Equity, London, UK.

Alonzo, A.A., Reynolds, N.R., 1995. Stigma, HIV, and AIDS: an exploration and elaboration of a stigma trajectory. Soc. Sci. Med. 41, 303–335.

American Association of Diabetes Educators, 2009. AADE Guidelines for the Practice of Diabetes Self-Management Education and Training (DSME/T). Diabetes Educ. 35 (3 Suppl.), 85S–107S. doi:10.1177/0145721709352436.

American Psychiatric Association, 2000. Diagnostic and Statistical Manual of Mental Disorders IV – Text Revision (DSM-IV-TR). American Psychiatric Association, Washington DC.

American Psychiatric Association, 2013. Diagnostic and Statistical Manual of Mental Disorders, fifth ed. American Psychiatric Publishing, Arlington, VA.

Andersen, B.L., Cacioppo, J.T., Roberts, D.C., 1995. Delay in seeking a cancer diagnosis: delay stages and psychophysiological comparison processes. Br. J. Soc. Psychol. 34, 33–52.

Anderson, P., Baumberg, B., 2006. Alcohol in Europe: a public health perspective. European Commission, Brussels, Belgium. http://ec.europa.eu/health-eu/news_alcoholineurope_en.htm/. (Accessed 15 May 2007).

Anionwu, E.N., 1993. Sickle cell and thalassaemia: community experiences and official response. In: Ahmad, W. (Ed.), 'Race' and Health in Contemporary Britain. Open University Press, Buckingham, UK.

Arber, S., Venn, S., 2011. Caregiving at night: understanding the impact on carers. J. Aging Studies 25 (2), 155–165.

ASH, 2014a. Smoking statistics—illness and death. ASH, London, UK. http://ash.org.uk/files/documents/ASH_107.pdf/.

ASH, 2014b. Secondhand smoke. ASH, London, UK. http://www.ash.org.uk/files/documents/ASH_113.pdf/.

ASH, 2014c. The economics of tobacco. ASH, London, UK. http://www.ash.org.uk/files/documents/ASH_121.pdf/.

ASH Scotland, 2011. Key statistics on smoking. ASH Scotland, Edinburgh, UK. http://www.ashscotland.org.uk/media/3815/Smcessstatsformedia.pdf/.

BACP, 2017. Training and educational resources. Ethical Framework for Counselling Professions. Accessed at: https://www.bacp.co.uk/events-and-resources/ethics-and-standards/ethical-framework-for-the-counselling-professions/training-and-education/.

Baird, B., Charles, A., Honeyman, M., et al., 2016. Understanding Pressures in General Practice, King's Fund, London, UK.

Bajekal, M., Primatesh, P., Prior, G., 2001. Health survey for England: disability. HMSO, Norwich, UK.

Bambra, C., Eikemo, T., 2008. Welfare regimes, unemployment and health: a comparative study of the relationship between unemployment and self-reported health in 23 European countries. J. Epidemiol. Community Health.

Bandura, A., 1986. Social Foundations of Thought and Action: A Social Cognitive Theory. Prentice-Hall, Englewood Cliffs, London, UK.

Barry, C.A., Bradley, C.P., Britten, N., et al., 2000. Patients' unvoiced agendas in general practice consultations: qualitative study. BMJ 320, 1246–1250.

Barsky, A.J., Saintfort, R., Rogers, M.P., et al., 2002. Nonspecific medication side effects and the nocebo phenomenon. JAMA 287, 622–627.

Bartholomew, L.K., Parcel, G.S., Kok, G., et al., 2006. Planning Health Promotion Programs. An Intervention Mapping Approach. Jossey-Bass, San Francisco, CA.

Bartlett, A., Smith, G., King, M., 2009. The response of mental health professionals to clients seeking help to change or redirect same-sex sexual orientation. BMC Psychiatry 9, 11.

Bartley, M., 2004. Health Inequality. Polity Press, Cambridge, UK.

Bartley, M., Blane, D., Davey Smith, G., 1998. The sociology of health inequalities. Blackwell, Oxford, UK.

Bassman, L.E., Uellendahl, G., 2003. Complementary/alternative medicine: ethical, professional, and practical challenges for psychologists. Prof. Psychol. Res. Pract. 34 (3), 264–270.

Bausewein, C., Daveson, B., Benalia, H., et al., 2011. Outcome measurement in palliative care. The essentials. PRISMA. www.prismafp7.eu/.

Beauvois, J.L., Joule, R.V., 1996. A Radical Theory of Dissonance. European Monographs in Social Psychology. Taylor and Francies, New York, USA.

Beck, A.T., 1976. Cognitive Therapy of the Emotional Disorders. New American Library, New York.

Becker, M.H., Rosenstok, I.M., 1987. Comparing social learning theory and the health belief model. Adv. Health Educ. Promot. 2, 245–249.

Berkman, L.F., Syme, S., 1979. Social networks, host resistance, and mortality: a nine year follow-up study of Alameda County residents. Am. J. Epidemiol. 109 (2), 186–203.

Bibace, R., Walsh, M.E., 1980. Development of children's concepts of illness. Pediatrics 66, 912–917.

Biesecker, B.B., Schwartz, M.D., Marteau, T.M., 2013. Enhancing informed choice to undergo health screening: a systematic review. Am. J. Health Behav. 37 (3), 351–359.

Biggs, S., 1999. The Mature Imagination: Dynamics of Identity in Midlife and Beyond. Open University Press, Buckingham, UK.

Birthplace in England Collaborative Group, 2011. Perinatal and maternal outcomes by planned place of birth for healthy women with low risk pregnancies: the Birthplace in England national prospective cohort study. BMJ 343, d7400.

Blaxter, M., Paterson, E., 1982. Mothers and Daughters: A Three-Generation Study of Health Attitudes and Behaviour. Heinemann, London, UK.

Blue, S., Shove, E., Carmona, C., Kelly, M.P., 2016. Theories of practice and public health: understanding (un)healthy practices. Crit. Public Health. 26 (1), 36–50.

Bogg, T., Roberts, B.W., 2013. The case for conscientiousness: evidence and implications for a personality trait marker of health and longevity. Anns Behav. Med. 45, 278–288.

Bowlby, J., 1969. Attachment and Loss, vol. 1. Hogarth Press, London, UK.

Bowlby, J., 1998. Attachment and Loss, vol. 3. Pimlico, London, UK.

Bowling, A., 2005. Measuring Health: A Review of Quality of Life Measurement Scales. Open University Press, Buckingham, UK.

Boyce, T., 2007. Health, Risk and News: The MMR Vaccine and the Media. Peter Lang, Oxford, UK.

Bradshaw, J., 1972. A taxonomy of social need. In: McLachlan, G. (Ed.), Problems and Progress in Medical Care, seventh series. Oxford University Press, Oxford, UK.

British Association of Counselling and Psychotherapy, 2013. Evidence for counselling and psychotherapy. http://www.bacp.co.uk/docs/pdf/12228_research%20evidence%20summary.pdf/.

British Association of Counselling and Psychotherapy, 2017. http://www.bacp.co.uk/research/resources/:additional information and training requirements/ http://www.bacp.co.uk/student/training.php/. (Accessed 20 February 2017).

BTS/SIGN British Guideline for the management of asthma, 2016, SIGN 153.

Buckman, R., 1992. How to Break Bad News. John Hopkins University Press, Baltimore, MD.

Bunton, R., Burrows, R., 1995. Consumption and health in the 'epidemiological' clinic of late modern medicine. In: Bunton, R., Nettleton, S., Burrows, R. (Eds.), The Sociology of Health Promotion. Routledge, London, UK.

Busseri, M.A., Sadava, S.W., 2011. A review of the tripartite structure of Subjective Wellbeing: implications for conceptualisation, operationalization, analysis and synthesis. Pers. Soc. Psychol. Rev. 15 (3), 290–314.

Butland, B., Jepp, S., Kopelman, P., et al., 2007. Foresight Tackling Obesities: Future Choices – Project Report, second ed. Government Office for Science London, UK.

Cannon, W.B., 1931. Again the James-Lange and the thalamic theories of emotion. Psychol. Rev. 38, 281–295. 10.1037/h0072957.

Carers UK, 2013. The State of Caring 2013 (online). https://www.carersuk.org/for-professionals/policy/policy-library/the-state-of-caring-2013/. (Accessed 23 December 2016).

Carpenter, M., Nagell, K., Tomasello, M., et al., 1998. Social cognition, joint attention, and communicative competence from 9 to 15 months of age. Monogr. Soc. Res. Child Dev. 63 (4), 1–143.

Carr, E.C.J., Thomas, V.N., Wilson-Barnet, J., 2005. Patient experiences of anxiety, depression and acute pain after surgery: a longitudinal perspective. Int. J. Nursing Studies. 42, 521–530.

Carver, C.S., Pozo, C., Harris, S.D., et al., 1993. How coping mediates the effect of optimism on distress: A study of women with early stage breast cancer. J. Pers. Soc. Psychol. 65, 375–390.

Carver, C.S., Scheier, M.F., 2014. Dispositional optimism. Trends Cognit. Sci. 18, 293–299.

Champion, V.L., 1994. Strategies to increase mammography utilization. Med. Care 32, 118–129.

Coker, N. (Ed.), 2002. Understanding Race and Racism. King's Fund Publishing, London, UK. Racism in Medicine. An Agenda for Change.

Coleman, J., Hendry, L., 1999. The Nature of Adolescence, third ed. Routledge, London, UK.

Coleman, P., Bond, J., Peace, S., 1993. Ageing in the twentieth century. In: Bond, J., Coleman, P., Peace, S. (Eds.), Ageing in Society: An Introduction to Social Gerontology, second ed. Sage, London, UK.

Committee on Health Promotion, 1996. Women and Coronary Heart Disease. Guidelines for Health Promotion no. 45. Faculty of Public Health Medicine, London, UK.

Cornwell, J., 1984. Hard-Earned Lives: Accounts of Health and Illness from East London. Tavistock, London, UK.

Coupland, N., Coupland, J., Giles, H., 1991. Language, Society and the Elderly. Blackwell, Oxford, UK.

Coyne, J.C., Stefanek, M., Palmer, S.C., 2007. Psychotherapy and survival in cancer: The conflict between hope and evidence. Psychol. Bull. 133 (3), 367–394.

Crawley, R., Lomax, S., Ayers, S., 2013. Recovering from stillbirth: the effects of making and sharing memories on maternal mental health. J. Reprod. Infant Psychol. 31 (2), 195–207.

Creighton, G.M., Oliffe, J.L., McMillan, A., Saewy, E.M., 2015. Living for the moment: men situating risk-taking after the death of a friend. Sociol. Health. Illness. 37 (3), 355–369.

Crisp, J., Ungerer, J.A., Goodnow, J.J., 1996. The impact of experience on children's understanding of illness. J. Pediatr. Psychol. 21, 57–72.

Crocker, T.F., Smith, J.K., Skevington, S.M., 2014. Family and professionals underestimate quality of life across diverse cultures and health conditions: Systematic review. J. Clin. Epidemiol. 68 (5), 584–595, (May). http://dx.doi.org/10.1016/j.jclinepi.2014.12.007.

Crowley, R., Wolfe, I., Lock, K., McKee, M., 2011. Improving the transition between paediatric and adult healthcare: a systematic review. Arch. Dis. Child. 96 (6), 548–553.

Cunningham-Burley, S., Boulton, M., 2000. The social context of the new genetics. In: Albrecht, G., Fitzpatrick, R., Scrimshaw, C. (Eds.), Handbook of Social Studies in Health and Medicine. Sage, London, UK.

D'Houtard, A., Field, M.G., 1984. The image of health: variations in perception by social class in a French population. Sociol. Health. Illness. 6, 30–60.

DAFNE Study Group, 2002. Training in flexible, intensive insulin management to enable dietary freedom in people with type 1 diabetes: dose adjustment for normal eating (DAFNE) randomized controlled trial. Br. Med. J. 325, 746–752.

Dahlgren, G., Whitehead, M., 1991. Policies and strategies to promote social equity in health. Institute for future studies, Stockholm, Sweden.

Dahlin, M., Joneborg, N., Runeson, B., 2005. Stress and depression among medical students: a cross-sectional study. Med. Educ. 39, 594–604.

Danaei, G., Vander Hoorn, S., Lopez, A.D., et al., 2005. Causes of cancer in the world: comparative risk assessment of nine behavioural and environmental factors. Lancet 366, 1784–1793.

Dansinger, M.L., Tatsioni, A., Wong, J.B., et al., 2007. Meta-analysis: the effect of dietary counseling for weight loss. Ann. Intern. Med. 147 (1), 41–50.

Data-Franco, J., Berk, M., 2013. The nocebo effect: a clinicians' guide. Austral. N. Z. J. Psychiat 47 (7), 617–623.

Daugirdaite, V., van den Akker, O., Purewal, S., 2015. Posttraumatic stress and posttraumatic stress disorder after termination of pregnancy and reproductive loss: a systematic review. J. Pregnancy doi:10.1155/2015/646345. [Epub 2015 Feb 5]; 646345.

Davey Smith, G., Hart, C., Blane, D., et al., 1997. Lifetime socioeconomic position and mortality:

prospective observational study. BMJ 314, 547–552.

Davison, C., Frankel, S., Smith, G.D., 1992. The limits of lifestyle: re-assessing 'fatalism' in the popular culture of illness prevention. Soc. Sci. and Med 34 (6), 675–685.

Deakin, T.A., Cade, J.E., Williams, R., Greenwood, D.C., 2006. Structured patient education: the Diabetes X-PERT Programme makes a difference. Dabet. Med. 23, 944–954. doi:10.1111/j.1464-5491.2006.01906.x.

de Beauvoir, S., 1960. The Second Sex. Four Square Books, London, UK.

Debate of the Age Health and Care Study Group, 1999. The Future of Health and Care for Older People: the Best is yet to Come. Age Concern, London.

Dennis, C.L., Dowswell, T., 2013. Psychosocial and psychological interventions for preventing postpartum depression. Cochrane Database Syst. Rev. 28(2), CD001134.

Dennis, M., Barbor, T.F., Roebuck, M.C., et al., 2002. Changing the focus: the case for recognizing the treatment of cannabis use disorders. Addiction 97 (Suppl. 1), 4–15.

Denollet, J., Sys, S.U., Stroobant, N., et al., 1996. Personality as independent predictor of long-term mortality in patients with coronary heart disease. Lancet 347, 417–421.

Department of Environment, Food and Rural Affairs (DEFRA), 2011. The natural choice: securing the value of nature. https://www.gov.uk/government/uploads/system/uploads/attachment_data/file/228842/8082.pdf/.

Department of Health, 1991. Drug Misuse and Dependence: Guidelines on Clinical Management. HMSO, London, UK.

Department of Health, 2001. Valuing People: A New Strategy for Learning Disability for the 21st Century. Cm 5086. The Stationery Office, London, UK.

Department of Work and Pensions, 2014. Labour Market Status by Ethnic Group: January 2014. Department of Work and Pensions, London, UK.

DFID, 2000. Better Health for Poor People. Department for International Development, London, UK.

Di Blasi, Z., Harkness, E., Ernst, E., et al., 2000. Influence of context effects on health outcomes: a systematic review. Lancet 357, 757–762.

Diabetes UK, 2014. Diabetes facts and stats. Available at: https://www.diabetes.org.uk/resources-s3/2017-11/diabetes-key-stats-guidelines-april2014.pdf. (Accessed 26 May 2018).

Diego, M.A., Field, T., Hernandez-Reif, M., 2005. Prepartum, postpartum and chronic depression effects on neonatal behaviour. Infant Behav. Develop. 28, 155–164.

Dieppe, P.A., 2004. Relationship between symptoms and structural changes in osteoarthritis. What are the important targets for osteoarthritis therapy? J. Rheumatol. 31 (Suppl. 70), 50–53.

DiMatteo, M.R., Haskard-Zolnierek, K.B., Martin, L.R., 2011. Improving patient adherence: a three-factor model to guide practice. Health Psychol. Rev. 6 (1), 74–91.

Dingemans, A.E., Bruna, M.J., van Furth, E.F., 2002. Binge-eating disorder: a review. Int. J. Obesity. 26, 299–307.

Ditton, J., Hammersley, R., 1996. A Very Greedy Drug: Cocaine in Context. Harwood, Reading, UK.

Doka, K.J. (Ed.), 2002. Disenfranchised Grief. New Directions, Challenges and Strategies in Practice. Research Press, Champaign, IL.

Dolan, A., 2010. 'You can't ask for a Dubonnet and lemonade!': working class masculinity and men's health practices. Sociol. Health Illness 33 (4), 586–601.

Doll, R., Peto, R., 1981. The causes of cancer—quantitative estimates of avoidable risks of

cancer in the United States today. J. Natl. Cancer Inst. 66 (6), 1191–1308.

Doll, R., Peto, R., Boreham, J., Sutherland, I., 2004. Mortality in relation to smoking: 50 years' observations on male British doctors. BMJ 328 (7455), 1519.

Dunkley, A.J., Bodicoat, D.H., Greaves, C.J., et al., 2014. Diabetes prevention in the real world: effectiveness of pragmatic lifestyle interventions for the prevention of type 2 diabetes and of the impact of adherence to guideline recommendations. A systematic review and meta-analysis. Diabetes Care 37, 922–933. doi:10.2337/dc13-2195.

Dunlosky, J., Rawson, K.A., Marsh, E.J., et al., 2013. Improving students' learning with effective learning techniques: promising directions from cognitive and educational psychology. Psychol. Sci. Public Interest 14 (1), 4–58.

Dunn, C., Deroo, L., Rivara, F.P., 2001. The use of brief interventions adapted from motivational interviewing across behavioral domains: a systematic review. Addiction 96, 1725–1742.

Dutton, E., van der Linden, D., Lynn, R., 2016. The negative Flynn Effect: a systematic literature review. Intelligence 59, 163–169.

Dyer, K.A., 2005. Jul-Aug. Identifying, understanding, and working with grieving parents in the NICU, part II: strategies. Neonatal Netw. 24 (4), 27–40.

Dyrbye, L.N., Thomas, M.R., Huntington, J.L., et al., 2006. Personal life events and medical student burnout: a multicenter study. Acad. Med. 81, 374–384.

Egbert, L.D., Battit, G.E., Welch, C.E., et al., 1964. Reduction of post-operative pain by encouragement and instruction of patients. New Engl. J. Med. 270, 825–827.

Eiser, C., Havermans, T., Casas, R., 1993. Healthy children's understanding of their blood: implications for explaining leukaemia to children. Br. J. Educ. Psychol. 63, 528–537.

Ekman, P., 1993. Facial expression and emotion. Am. Psychol. 48, 384–392.

Epstein, L.H., 1984. The direct effects of compliance on health outcome. Health Psychol. 3, 385–393.

Eriksen, M., Mackay, J., Ross, H., 2012. The Tobacco Atlas, fourth ed. American Cancer Society, Atlanta. http://www.tobaccoatlas.org/.

Erikson, E.H., 1968. Identity: Youth and Crisis. Norton, New York.

Etkin, A., Büchel, C., Gross, J.J., 2015. The neural bases of emotion regulation. Nature Rev. Neurosci. 16 (11), 693–700.

Eysenck, M., 1996. Simply Psychology. Psychology Press, Hove, UK.

Fagerhaugh, S.Y., Strauss, A., 1977. Politics of Pain Management: Staff-Patient Interaction. Addison-Wesley, Menlo Park, CA.

Falah-Hassani, K., Shiri, R., Vigod, S., Dennis, C.L., 2015. Prevalence of postpartum depression among immigrant women: a systematic review and meta-analysis. J. Psychiatr. Res. 70, 67–80.

Fallowfield, L., Jenkins, V., 2004. Communicating sad, bad and difficult news in medicine. Lancet 363, 312–319.

Farmer, J., Iverson, L., Campbell, N.C., et al., 2006. Rural/urban differences in accounts of patients' initial decisions to consult primary care. Health Place 12, 210–221.

Farrell, M., Boys, A., Bebbington, P., et al., 2002. Psychosis and drug dependence: results from a national survey of prisoners. Br. J. Psychiatry 181, 393–398.

Faulkner, A., 1995. Working with Bereaved People. Churchill Livingstone, Edinburgh, UK.

Faull, C., Woof, R., 2002. Palliative Care. Oxford University Press, Oxford, UK.

Ferguson, E., 2013. Personality is of central concern to understand health: towards a theoretical model for health psychology. Health Psychol. Rev. 7, S32–S70.

Ferrie, J.E., Martikainen, P., Shipley, M.J., et al., 2001. Employment status and health after privatization in white collar civil servants: prospective cohort study. BMJ 322, 1–7.

Festinger, L., 1957. A Theory of Cognitive Dissonance. Row Peterson, Evanston, IL.

Fielding, S., Porteous, T., Ferguson, J., et al., 2015. Estimating the burden of minor ailment consultations in general practices and emergency departments through retrospective review of routine data in North East Scotland. Fam. Pract. 32 (2), 165–172.

Finset, A., 2013. How Communication between Clinicians and Patients may Impact Pain Perception. In: Colloca, L., Flaten, M.A., Meissner, K. (Eds.), Placebo and Pain: From Bench to Bedside. Elsevier, Amsterdam, pp. 243–256.

Firth, S., 2001. Wider Horizons. Care of the Dying in a Multicultural Society. National Council for Hospice and Specialist Palliative Care Services, London, UK.

Fisher, K., Johnston, M., 1996. Experimental manipulation of perceived control and its effect on disability. Psychol. Health 11, 657–669.

Flynn, J.R., 1987. Massive IQ gains in 14 nations: what IQ tests really measure. Psychol. Bull. 101, 171–191.

Folkman, S., Moskowitz, J.T., 2000. Positive affect and the other side of coping. Am. Psychologist. 55, 647–654.

Folkman, S., Moskowitz, J.T., 2004. Coping: pitfalls and promise. Ann. Rev. Psychol. 55, 745–774.

Forrest Keenan, K., McKee, L., Miedzybrodzka, Z., 2015. Help or hindrance: young people's experiences of predictive testing for Huntington's disease. Clin. Genet. 87 (6), 563–569. doi:10.1111/cge.12439.

Frankel, S., Davison, C., Smith, G.D., 1991. Lay epidemiology and the rationality of responses to health education. Br. J. Gen. Pract. 41 (351), 428–430.

Frasure-Smith, N., Lesperance, F., Talajic, M., 1993. Depression following myocardial infarction. Impact on 6-month survival. JAMA 270, 1819–1825.

Freeman, G.K., Horder, J.P., Howie, J.G.R., et al., 2002. Evolving general practice consultations in Britain: issues of length and context. BMJ 324, 880–882.

Freidson, E., 1975. Profession of Medicine – a Study of the Sociology of Applied Knowledge. University of Chicago Press, London, UK.

Friedman, H.S., Tucker, J.S., Schwartz, J.E., et al., 1995. Childhood conscientiousness and longevity: Health behaviors and cause of death. J. Pers. Soc. Psychol. 68 (4), 696–703.

Friedman, H.S., 2000. Long-term relations of personality and health: dynamisms, mechanisms, tropisms. J. Pers. 68, 1089–1108.

Gardner, H., 2001. Intelligence Reframed: Multiple Intelligences for the 21st Century. Basic Books, New York.

Gaston, C.M., Mitchell, G., 2005. Information giving and decision-making in patients with advanced cancer: a systematic review. Soc. Sci. Med. 61, 2252–2264.

Gatchel, R.J., McGeary, D.D., McGeary, C.A., Lippe, B., 2014. Interdisciplinary chronic pain management: past, present and future. Am. Psychologist. 69 (2), 119–130.

General Medical Council, 2009. Tomorrow's Doctors. Outcomes and Standards for Undergraduate Medical Education. GMC, London, UK.

Ghosh, S., Shand, A., Ferguson, A., 2000. Ulcerative colitis. BMJ 320, 1119–1123.

Glasziou, P., Alexander, J., Beller, E., et al., 2007. Which health-related quality of life score? A comparison of alternative utility measures in patients with type 2 diabetes in the ADVANCE trial. Health Qual. Life Outcomes 5, 21.

Goffman, E., 1968a. Stigma. Penguin, London, UK.

Goffman, E., 1968b. Asylums. Penguin, Harmondsworth, UK.

Gollwitzer, P.M., 1999. Implementation intentions: strong effects of simple plans. Am. Psychologist. 54, 493–503.

Gomes, B., Calanzi, N., Higginson, I.J., 2011. Local Preferences and Place of Death in Regions within England 2010. Cicely Saunders Institute, London, UK.

Goodwin, R.D., Friedman, H.S., 2006. Health status and the five-factor personality traits in a nationally representative sample. J. Health Psychol. 11, 643–654.

Government Office for Science, 2007. Foresight Tackling Obesities: Future Choices – Project Report, second ed. The Stationary Office, London.

GP taskforce review. http://hee.nhs.uk/wp-content/uploads/sites/321/2014/07/GP-Taskforce-report.pdf/.

Graham, H., 1987. Women's smoking and family health. Soc. Sci. Med. 25 (1), 47–56.

Graham, C., Chattopadhyay, S., Picon, M., 2010. The Easterlin and other paradoxes: why both sides are correct. In: Diener, E., Helliwell, J.F., Kahneman, D. (Eds.), Oxford University Press, Oxford, pp. 247–290, (Chapter 9).

Grant, A., Rix, A., Mattick, K., et al., 2013. Identifying good practice among medical schools in the support of students with mental health concerns. A report for the General Medical Council. http://www.gmc-uk.org/Identifying_good_practice_among_medcal_schools_in_the_support_of_students_with_mental_health_concerns.pdf.52884825.pdf/.

Grant, A., Rix, A., Winter, P., et al., 2015. Support for medical students with mental health problems: a conceptual model. Acad. Psychiatry. 39, 16–21.

Grant, L., 1998. Remind Me Who I Am, Again. Granta Books, London, UK.

Greenaway, D., 2013. Shape of Training: securing the future of excellent medical care. Final report of the independent review led by Professor David Greenaway. General Medical Council. http://www.shapeoftraining.co.uk/static/documents/content/Shape_of_training_FINAL_Report.pdf.53977887.pdf.

Greenson, R.R., 1965. The working alliance and the transference neurosis. Psychoanalyt. Quart 34, 155–181.

Greenwood, E., 1957. Attributes of a profession. Soc. Work 2, 45–55.

Greer, S., Morris, T.E., Pettingale, K.W., 1979. Psychological responses to breast cancer: effect on outcome. Lancet ii, 785–787.

Groene, O., Arah, O.A., Klazinga, N.S., et al., 2015. Patient experience shows little relationship with hospital quality management strategies. PLoS ONE 10, e0131805.

Gross, J.J., 1998. The emerging field of emotion regulation: an integrative review. Rev. Gen. Psychol. 2, 271–299.

Guilford, J.P., 1967. The Nature of Human Intelligence. McGraw-Hill, New York.

Gyurak, A., Gross, J.J., Etkin, A., 2011. Explicit and implicit emotion regulation: a dual-process framework. Cognition Emotion. 25 (3), 400–412.

Hadjistavropoulos, T., Craig, K.D., Duck, S., et al., 2011. A biopsychosocial formulation of pain communication. Psychol. Bull. 137 (6), 910–939.

Halliday, J.L., 1948. Psycho-social Medicine: A Study of the Sick Society. W. W. Norton, Oxford, UK.

Hammen, C., Watkins, E., 2007. Depression. Psychology Press, Hove, UK.

Hammersley, R., Ditton, J., 2005. Binge or bout? Quantity and rate of drinking by young people in licensed premises. Drugs Educ. Prev. Policy. 12, 493–500.

Hampson, S.E., 2012. Personality processes: mechanisms by which personality traits 'get outside the skin'. Ann. Rev. Psychol. 63, 315–339.

Hannay, D., 1979. The Symptom Iceberg – a Study of Community Health. Routledge and Kegan Paul, London, UK.

Haran, J., Kitzinger, J., McNeil, M., et al., 2007. Human Cloning in the Media: From Science Fiction to Science Practice. Routledge, London, UK.

Harmon-Jones, E., Amodio, D.M., Harmon-Jones, C., 2009. Action -based model of dissonance: A review, integration, and expansion of conceptions of cognitive conflict. Adv. Exp. Soc. Psychol. 41, 119–166.

Harrison, S., Hunter, D.J., 1994. Rationing Health Care. Institute for Public Policy Research, London, UK.

Hartig, T., Mitchell, R., De Vries, S., Frumkin, H., 2014. Nature and health. Annu. Rev. Public Health 35, 207–228.

Health and Safety Executive, 2000. Revitalising Health and Safety. HSE, Suffolk, UK.

Health and Safety Executive, 2009. The health and safety of Great Britain: be part of the solution. http://www.hse.gov.uk/aboutus/strategiesandplans/strategy09.pdf.

Health and Safety Executive, 2014. European comparisons. http://www.hse.gov.uk/statistics/european/european-comparisons.pdf.

Health and Safety Executive, 2015. Health and safety statistics – annual report for Great Britain 2013/14. Available online.

Health Statistics Quarterly 43, 2009. Unemployment, mortality and the problem of health-related selection: Evidence from the Scottish and England and Wales (ONS) Longitudinal Studies. Office of National Statistics: London.

Heather, N., Robinson, I., 1983. Controlled Drinking. Routledge, London, UK.

Heather, N., Robinson, I., 1996. Let's Drink to Your Health! Routledge, Oxford, UK.

Henderson, L., Kitzinger, J., 1999. The human drama of genetics: 'hard' and 'soft' media representations of inherited breast cancer. Sociol. Health Illn. 21 (5), 560–578.

Henderson, L., Kitzinger, J., Green, J., 2000. Representing infant feeding: content analysis of British media portrayals of bottle feeding and breastfeeding. BMJ 321, 1196–1198.

Henry, C., Seymour, J., 2008. Advance care planning: a guide for health and social care staff. DoH. www.endoflifecareforadults.nhs.uk/.

Hepworth, M., 1995. Images of old age. In: Nussbaum, J.F., Coupland, J. (Eds.), Handbook of Communication and Ageing Research. Lawrence Erlbaum, Mahwah, NJ.

Heran, B.S., Chen, J.M., Egrahim, S., et al., 2011. Exercise-based cardiac rehabilitation for coronary heart disease. Cochrane Database Syst. Rev. (7), CD001800.

Her Majesty's Government, 2010. Carers Strategy: Second National Action Plan 2014–2016. Stationary Office, London, UK.

Higgins, N.C., Bailey, S.J., LaChapelle, D.L., et al., 2015. Coping styles, pain expressiveness, and implicit theories of chronic pain. J. Psychol. 149 (7), 737–750.

Hilts, P.J., 1995. Memory's Ghost. Simon & Schuster, New York.

Hing, E., Cherry, D.K., Woodwell, D.A., 2006. National ambulatory medical care survey: 2004 summary. http://www.cdc.gov/nchs/data/ad/ad374.pdf/.

Holmes, T.H., Rahe, R.H., 1967. The social readjustment scale. J. Psychosom. Res. 11, 213–218.

Holtedahl, R., Brox, J.I., Tjomsland, O., 2015. Placebo effects in trials evaluating 12 selected minimally invasive interventions: a systematic review and meta-analysis. BMJ Open. 5 (1), e007331.

Home Office, 2005 06. British crime survey. http://www.homeoffice.gov.uk/rds/bcs1.html/.

Hope, V., Henderson, M., 2014. Medical student depression, anxiety and distress outside North America: a systematic review. https://onlinelibrary.wiley.com/doi/abs/10.1111/medu.12512/.

Hopton, J.L., Dlugolecka, M., 1995. Patients' perceptions of need for primary health care services: useful for priority setting? BMJ 310, 1237–1240.

Horne, R., James, D., Petrie, K., et al., 2000. Patients' interpretation of symptoms as a cause of delay in reaching hospital during myocardial infarction. Heart 83, 388–393.

Househ, M., Grainger, R., Petersen, C., et al., 2018. Balancing Between Privacy and Patient Needs for Health Information in the Age of Participatory Health and Social Media: A Scoping Review. Yearb. Med. Inform. 29–36.

Howie, J.G.R., Heaney, D., Maxwell, M., et al., 1998. A comparison of a patient enablement instrument (PEI) against two established patient satisfaction scales as an outcome measure of primary care consultations. Fam. Pract. 15, 165–171.

Howie, J.G.R., Hopton, J.L., Heaney, D.J., et al., 1992. Attitudes to medical care, the organisation of work, and stress among general practitioners. Br. J. Gen. Pract. 42, 181–185.

http://hee.nhs.uk/wp-content/uploads/sites/321/2014/07/GP-Taskforce-report.pdf/.

https://www.cdc.gov/nchs/nhis/releases.htm/.

https://www.gov.uk/government/statistics/labour-market-status-by-ethnic-group. (Accessed 16 February 2015).

Hunt, S., 1997. Housing-related disorders. In: Charlton, J., Murphy, M. (Eds.), The Health of Adult Britain 1841–1994, vol. 1. Office for National Statistics. Decennial supplement no. 12. Stationery Office, London, UK, pp. 156–170.

Husk, K., Lovell, R., Cooper, C., Garside, R., 2015. Participation in environmental enhancement and conservation activities for health and well-being in adults: a systematic review of quantitative and qualitative evidence. Cochrane Database Syst. Rev.

International Association for the Study of Pain, 1994. Classification of Chronic Pain: Descriptions of Chronic Pain Syndromes and Definitions of Pain Terms, second ed. IASP Press, Seattle, WA.

Ioannou, S., 2005. Health logic and health-related behaviours. Crit. Public Health. 15 (3), 263–273.

James, W., 1884. What is an emotion? Mind 9, 188–205.

Jenkins, V., Fallowfield, L., Saul, J., 2001. Information needs of patients with cancer: results from a large study in UK cancer centres. Br. J. Cancer 84, 48–51.

Jerrome, D., 1992. Good Company: An Anthropological Study of Old People in Groups. Edinburgh University Press, Edinburgh, UK.

Johnson, M., 2003. Ethnic diversity in social context. In: Kai, J. (Ed.), Ethnicity, Health and Primary Care. Oxford University Press, Oxford, UK.

Johnson, S.R., 2004. The epidemiology of premenstrual syndrome. Prim. Psychiatry 11, 27–32.

Johnston, G., Abraham, C., 1995. The WHO objectives for palliative care: to what extent are we achieving them? Palliat. Med. 9 (2), 123–137.

Johnston, G., Abraham, C., 2000. Managing awareness: negotiating and coping with a terminal prognosis. Int. J. Palliat. Nurs. 6, 485–494.

Johnston, M., Dixon, D., 2013. Developing an integrated biomedical and behavioural theory of functioning and disability: adding models of

behaviour to the ICF framework. Health Psychol. Rev. 8 (4), 381–403.

Johnston, M., Pollard, B., Morrison, V., et al., 2005. Functional limitations and survival following stroke: psychological and clinical predictors of 3-year outcome. Int. J. Behav. Med. 11, 187–196.

Johnston, M., Vögele, C., 1993. Benefits of psychological preparation for surgery: a meta-analysis. Ann. Behav. Med. 15, 245–256.

Joseph-Williams, N., Elwyn, G., Edwards, A., 2014. Knowledge is not power for patients: a systematic review and thematic synthesis of patient-reported barriers and facilitators to shared decision making. Patient Educ. Couns. 94, 291–309.

Jutel, A., Dew, K., 2014. Social Issues in Diagnosis. John Hopkins University Press, Baltimore, MD.

Kai, J., 1996. Parents' difficulties and information needs in coping with acute illness in preschool children: a qualitative study. BMJ 313, 987–990.

Kai, J., Bhopal, R., 2003. Ethnic diversity in health and disease. In: Kai, J. (Ed.), Ethnicity, Health and Primary Care. Oxford University Press, Oxford, UK.

Kardas, P., Lewek, P., Matyjaszczyk, M., 2013. Determinants of patient adherence: a review of systematic reviews. Front. Pharmacol. 4, 91.

Karsten, I.P., Moser, K., 2009. Unemployment impairs mental health: meta-analyses. J. Vocation. Behav 74, 264–282.

Katz, A.H., Bender, E.I. (Eds.), 1976. The Strength in Us: Self-Help Groups in the Modern World. Franklin Watts, New York.

Keller, M.B., McCullough, J.P., Klein, D.N., et al., 2000. A comparison of nefazodone, the cognitive behavioral-analysis system of psychotherapy, and their combination for the treatment of chronic depression. New Engl. J. Med. 342, 1462–1470.

Kelly, M., 1991. Coping with an ileostomy. Soc. Sci. Med. 33, 115–125.

Kelly, M., 1992. Colitis. Routledge, London, UK.

Kelly, M.P., 2010a. A theoretical model of assets: the link between biology and the social structure. In: Morgan, A., Davies, M., Ziglio, E. (Eds.), Health Assets in a Global Context: Theory, Methods, Action. Springer, New York, pp. 41–58.

Kelly, M.P., 2010b. Chronic illness, labelling and stigma and pre-diabetes, London, UK. http://www.nice.org.uk/guidance/ph35/evidence/ep-2-illness-labelling-and-illness-experience2/.

Kelly, M.P., Sullivan, F., 1992. The productive use of threat in primary care: behavioural responses to health promotion. Fam. Pract. 9, 476–480.

Kerse, N.M., Flicker, L., Jolley, D., et al., 1999. Improving the health behaviours of elderly people: randomised controlled trial of a general practice education programme. BMJ 319, 683–687.

Kiecolt-Glaser, J.K., Marucha, P.T., Marlakey, W.B., et al., 1995. Slowing of wound healing by psychological stress. Lancet 346, 1194–1196.

Kinmonth, A., Woodcock, A., Griffin, S., et al., 1998. Randomised controlled trial of patient centred care of diabetes in general practice: impact on current well-being and future disease risk. BMJ 317, 1202–1208.

Kister, M.C., Patterson, C.J., 1980. Children's conceptions of the causes of illness: understanding of contagion and use of immanent justice. Child Develop. 51, 839–846.

Kitwood, T., 1997. Dementia Reconsidered: The Person Comes First. Open University Press, Buckingham, UK.

Kitzhaber, J.A., 1993. Prioritising health services in an era of limits: the Oregon experience. BMJ 307, 373–376.

Klass, D., Silverman, P.R., Nickman, S. (Eds.), 1996. Continuing Bonds. New Understandings of Grief. Taylor and Francis, London, UK.

Klein, R., Day, P., Redmayne, S., 1996. Managing scarcity. Open University Press, Buckingham, UK.

Kleinman, A., 1985. Indigenous systems of healing: questions for professional, popular and folk care. In: Salmon, J. (Ed.), Alternative Medicines: Popular and Policy Perspectives. Tavistock, London, UK.

Kleinman, A., 1986. Social Origins of Distress and Disease: Depression, Neurasthenia, and Pain in Modern China. Yale University Press, New Haven, CT.

Kraschnewski, J.L., Boan, J., Esposito, J., et al., 2010. Long-term weight loss maintenance in the United States. Int. J. Obes. (Lond) 34 (11), 1644–1654.

Krohne, H.W., Slangen, K.E., 2005. The influence of social support on adaptation to surgery. Health Psychol. 24, 101–105.

Kübler-Ross, E., 1969. On Death and Dying. Collier Macmillan, London, UK.

Kübler-Ross, E., 1970. On Death and Dying. Tavistock Publications, London, UK.

Kulik, J.A., Mahler, H.I., Moore, P.J., 1996. Social comparison and affiliation under threat: effects on recovery from major surgery. J. Personality Soc. Psychol 71, 967–979.

Kuper, H., Marmot, M., 2003. Job strain, job demands, decision latitude, and risk of coronary heart disease within the Whitehall II study. J. Epidemiol. Commun. Health. 57 (2), 147–153.

Kwasnicka, D., Presseau, J., White, M., Sniehotta, F.F., 2013. Does planning how to cope with anticipated barriers facilitate health-related behaviour change? A systematic review. Health Psychol. Rev. 7 (2), 129–145.

Lader, D., Meltzer, H., 2001. Drinking: Adults' Behaviour and Knowledge in 2000. Office for National Statistics, London, UK.

Lazarus, R.S., Folkman, S., 1984. Stress, Appraisal and Coping. Springer, New York.

LeDoux, J.E., 2000. Emotion circuits in the brain. Ann. Rev. Neurosci. 23, 155–184.

Lee, K., 2003. Globalisation and Health: An Introduction. Palgrave Macmillan, London, UK.

Leeson, J., Gray, L., 1978. Women and Health. Tavistock, London, UK.

Leka, S., Griffiths, A., Cox, T., 2004. Work Organisation and Stress: Systematic Approaches for Employers, Managers and Trade Union Representatives. World Health Organization, Geneva, Switzerland.

Lemert, E., 1951. Social Pathology. McGraw Hill, New York.

Leventhal, H., Phillips, L.A., Burns, E., 2016. The common-sense model of self-regulation (CSM): a dynamic framework for understanding illness self-management. J. Behav. Med. 39, 935–946.

Levine, J.D., Gordon, N.C., Fields, H.L., 1978. The mechanisms of placebo analgesia. Lancet 23 (2), 654–657.

Lieberman, M.D., Eisenberger, N.I., Crockett, M.J., et al., 2007. Putting feelings into words: affect labeling disrupts amygdala activity in response to affective stimuli. Psychol. Sci. 18 (5), 421–428.

Linde, K., Berner, M., Egger, M., Mulrow, C., 2005. St John's wort for depression: meta-analysis of randomised controlled trials. Br. J. Psychiatry 186 (2), 99–107.

Lok, I.H., Neugebauer, R., 2007. Psychological morbidity following miscarriage. Best Pract. Res. Clin. Obstet. Gynaecol. 21, 229–247.

Love, R.R., Leventhal, H., Easterling, D.V., Nerenz, D., 1989. Side effects and emotional distress during cancer chemotherapy. Cancer 63 (3), 604–612.

Low, J.T.S., Payne, S., 1996. The good and bad death perceptions of health professionals in palliative care. Eur. J. Cancer Care (Engl.) 5, 237–241.

Luebbert, K., Dahme, B., Hasenbring, M., 2001. The effectiveness of relaxation training in reducing treatment-related symptoms and improving emotional adjustment in acute non-surgical cancer treatment: A meta-analytic review. Psychooncology 10, 490–502.

Lundin, A., Lundberg, I., Hallsten, L., et al., 2010. Unemployment and mortality – a longitudinal prospective study on selection and causation in 49321 Swedish middle-aged men. J. Epidemiol. Commun. Health. 64, 22–28.

Luria, A.R., 1969. The Mind of a Mnemonist: A Little Book About a Vast Memory. Cape, London, UK.

Lutgendorf, S., Sood, A., 2011. Biobehavioral Factors and Cancer Progression: Physiological Pathways and Mechanisms. Invited review. Psychosom. Med. 73, 724–730.

Luty, S.E., Carter, J.D., McKenzie, J.M., et al., 2007. Randomised controlled trial of interpersonal psychotherapy and cognitive-behavioural therapy for depression. Br. J. Psychiatry 190, 496–502.

Lydeard, S., Jones, R., 1989. Factors affecting the decision to consult with dyspepsia: comparison of consulters and non-consulters. J. R. Coll. Gen. Pract. 39, 495–498.

Maguire, E.A., Burgess, N., Donnett, J.G., et al., 1998. Knowing where and getting there: a human navigation network. Science 280, 921–924.

Makoul, G., Zick, A., Green, M., 2007. An evidence-based perspective on greetings in medical encounters. Arch. Intern. Med. 167, 1172–1176.

Manary, M.P., Boulding, W., Staelin, R., Glickman, S.W., 2013. The patient experience and health outcomes. New Engl. J. Med. 368, 201–203.

Marmot, M.G., Davey Smith, G., Stanfeld, S.A., et al., 1991. Health inequalities among British civil servants: the Whitehall II study. Lancet 337, 1387–1393.

Marmot Review, 2010. Fair Society, Healthy Lives: Strategic Review of Health Inequalities in England Post 2010. Institute of Health Equity, London, UK.

Marmot, M., Geddes, I., Bloomer, E., et al., 2011. The health impacts of cold homes and fuel poverty. Friends of the Earth/Marmot Review Team.

Marteau, T.M., Dormandy, E., Michie, S., 2001. A measure of informed choice. Health Expect. 4 (2), 99–108.

Martin, L.R., Haskard-Zolnierek, K.B., DiMatteo, M.R., 2010. Health Behaviour Change and Treatment Adherence. Oxford University Press, Oxford, UK, pp. 19–20, (Chapter 1).

Matarazzo, J., 1984. Behavioural immunogens and pathogens in health and illness. In: Hammonds, B., Scheirer, C. (Eds.), Psychology and Health. American Psychological Society, Washington, USA, pp. 201–203.

Mayou, R., Farmer, A., 2002. Trauma. BMJ 325, 426–429.

McCrae, R.R., Costa, P.T., Jr., 1987. Validation of the five-factor model of personality across instruments and observers. J. Pers. Soc. Psychol. 52, 81–90.

McGuffin, P., Katz, R., Watkins, S., et al., 1996. A hospital-based twin register of the heritability of DSM-IV unipolar depression. Arch. Gen. Psychiatry 53, 129–136.

McKeown, T., 1979. The Role of Medicine: Dream, Mirage or Nemesis? Blackwell, Oxford, UK.

McKinlay, J.B., 1973. Social networks, lay consultation and help seeking behaviour. Soc. Forces 51, 279–292.

McLauchlan, C.A.J., 1990. Handling distressed relatives and breaking bad news. BMJ 301, 1145–1149.

Mead, N., Bower, P., Hann, M., 2002. The impact of general practitioners' patient-centredness on patients' post-consultation satisfaction and enablement. Soc. Sci. Med. 55, 283–299.

Measham, F., 2006. The new policy mix: alcohol, harm minimisation, and determined drunkenness in contemporary society. Int. J. Drug Policy 17, 258–268.

Meyer, I.H., 1995. Minority stress and mental health in gay men. J. Health Soc. Behav. 36, 38–56.

Miles, A., 1991. Women, Health and Medicine. Open University Press, Buckingham, UK.

Miles, A., Curran, H.V., Pearce, S., et al., 2005. Managing constraint: The experience of people with chronic pain. Soc. Sci. Med. 61 (2), 431–441.

Miller, D., Kitzinger, J., Eilliams, K., et al., 1998. The Circuit of Mass Communication: Media Strategies, Representation and Audience Reception in the AIDS Crisis. Sage, London, UK.

Miller, G.E., Cohen, S., 2001. Psychological interventions and the immune system: a meta-analytic review and critique. Health Psychol. 20 (1), 47–63.

Miller, W.R., Rollnick, S., 1991. Motivational Interviewing: Preparing People to Change Addictive Behaviour. Guilford Press, London, UK.

Mills, S., Bone, K., 2000. Principles and Practice of Phytotherapy. Modern Herbal Medicine. Churchill Livingstone, Edinburgh, UK, p. 544.

Mills, T., Paul, J., Stall, R., et al., 2004. Distress and depression in men who have sex with men: the urban men's health study. Am. J. Psychiatry 161, 278–285.

Mitchell, R., Popham, F., 2008. Effect of exposure to natural environment on health inequalities: an observational population study. Lancet 372 (9650), 1655–1660.

Molfino, N.A., Nannini, L.J., Rebuck, A.S., et al., 1992. The fatality-prone asthmatic patient. Follow-up study after near-fatal attacks. Chest 101, 621–623.

Montesi, L., Turchese Caletti, M., Marchesini, G., 2016. Diabetes in migrants and ethnic minorities in a changing world. World J. Diabetes. 7 (3), 34–44.

Montoya, P., Pauli, P., Batra, A., et al., 2005. Altered processing of pain-related information in patients with fibromyalgia. Eur. J. Pain 9, 293–303.

Morley, S., Greer, S., Bliss, J., et al., 1999. Systematic review and meta-analysis of randomised controlled trials of cognitive behaviour therapy and behaviour therapy for chronic pain in adults, excluding headaches. Pain 80, 1–13.

Morris, C.J., Cantrill, J.A., Weiss, M.C., 2003. Minor ailment consultations: a mismatch of perceptions between patients and GPs. Primary Health Care Res. Develop 4, 365–370.

Mulley, A.G., Trimble, C., Elwyn, G., 2012. Stop the silent misdiagnosis: patients' preferences matter. BMJ 345, e6572.

Murray, L., Cooper, P.J., 1997. Postpartum depression and child development. Psychol. Med. 27, 253–260.

Murray, L., Fiori-Cowley, A., Hooper, R., et al., 1996. The impact of postnatal depression and associated adversity on early mother infant interactions and later infant outcome. Child Develop. 67, 2512–2516.

Murray, S.A., Kendall, M., Boyd, K., Sheikh, A., 2005. Illness trajectories and palliative care. BMJ 330, 1007–1011.

Mustanski, B., Birkett, M., Kuhns, L.M., et al., 2014. The role of geographic and network factors in racial disparities in HIV among young men who have sex with men: an egocentric network study. AIDS Behav. 19 (6), 1037–1047.

Myant, K.A., Williams, J.M., 2005. Children's concepts of health and illness: understanding of contagious illnesses, non-contagious illnesses and injuries. J. Health Psychol. 10, 805–819.

Myant, K.A., Williams, J.M., 2008. What do children learn about biology from factual information? A comparison of interventions to improve understanding of contagious illnesses. Br. J. Educ. Psychol. 78, 223–244.

Narayanan, V., Bista, B., Koshy, C., 2010. 'BREAKS': protocol for breaking bad news. Indian J. Palliat. Care. 16 (2), 61–65.

Narayanasamy, A., White, E., 2005. A review of transcultural nursing. Nurse Educ. Today 25, 102–111.

National Alcohol Strategy, 2017. Safe, sensible, social. The next steps in the national alcohol strategy. http://www.dh.gov.uk/en/Publicationsandstatistics/Publications/PublicationsPolicyAndGuidance/DH_075218/.

National Records of Scotland, 2013. Key results on Population, Ethnicity, Identity, Language, Religion, Health, Housing and Accommodation in Scotland – Release 2A. https://www.nrsscotland.gov.uk/news/2013/census-2011-release-2a#footnote2. (Accessed 28 August 2018).

National Institute for Health and Clinical Excellence, 2009. Depression in adults with a chronic physical health problem. NICE guidelines (CG91).

Natural England, 2009. An estimate of the economic and health value and cost effectiveness of the expanded Walking to Health Initiative Scheme 2009.

Naughton, F., Eborall, H., Sutton, S., 2013. Dissonance and disengagement in pregnant smokers: a qualitative study. J. Smoking Cessation. 8 (1), 24–32.

Nazroo, J.Y., 2003. The structuring of ethnic inequalities in health: economic position, racial discrimination, and racism. Am. J. Public Health 93, 277–284.

NCCAM. What is CAM. National Center for Complementary and Alternative Medicine. http://nccam.nih.gov/health/whatiscam/.

Neisser, U., Boodoo, G., Bouchard, T.J., et al., 1996. Intelligence: knowns and unknowns. Am. Psychologist. 51, 77–101.

Nerenz, D.R., Leventhal, H., Love, R.R., 1982. Factors contributing to emotional distress during cancer chemotherapy. Cancer 50 (5), 1020–1027.

NHS Health Scotland, ASH Scotland, RCGP, 2010. A guide to smoking cessation in Scotland. NHS Health Scotland and ASH Scotland, Edinburgh. http://www.healthscotland.com/documents/4661.aspx/.

NICE, 2005. Post-traumatic Stress Disorder (PTSD) – the Management of PTSD in Adults and Children in Primary and Secondary Care. National Institute for Clinical Excellence, London, UK.

NICE, 2007. Depression (amended) – Management of Depression in Primary and Secondary Care. National Institute for Health and Clinical Excellence, London, UK.

NICE, 2009. Clinical Guideline 91. National Institute for Health and Clinical Excellence, London, UK.

NICE, 2011. Colorectal cancer prevention: colonoscopic surveillance in adults with ulcerative colitis, Crohn's disease or adenomas. https://www.nice.org.uk/guidance/cg118.

NICE, 2013. Ulcerative Colitis: Management. https://www.nice.org.uk/guidance/cg166/.

NICE, 2014. www.nice.org.uk/guidance/qs53/.

Nolan, M., Grant, G., Keady, J., 1996. Understanding family care: a multidimensional model of caring and coping. Open University.

Nuffield Council on Bioethics, 1993. Genetic Screening. Ethical issues. Nuffield Council on Bioethics, London, UK.

NS-SEC, 2007. The National Statistics Socio-economic classification (NS-SEC). Office for National Statistics, London.

O'Connor, D.B., Conner, M., Jones, F., et al., 2009. Exploring the benefits of conscientiousness: An investigation of daily stressors and health behaviors. Anns Behav. Med. 37, 184–196.

O'Donnell, K.J., Glover, V., Barker, E.D., O'Connor, T.G., 2014. The persisting effect of maternal mood in pregnancy on childhood psychopathology. Develop. Psychopathol 26 (2), 393–403.

Office for National Statistics, 2013a. Statistical bulletin: labour market statistics, June, 2013. http://www.ons.gov.uk/ons/rel/lms/. (Accessed 16 September 2014).

Office for National Statistics, 2013b. 2011 Census analysis: unpaid care in England and Wales, 2011 and comparison with 2001 (online). http://www.ons.gov.uk/ons/dcp171766_300039.pdf/. (Accessed 17 October 2016).

Office for National Statistics, 2014. Adult smoking habits in Great Britain, 2013. ONS. http://www.ons.gov.uk/ons/dcp171778_386291.pdf/.

Ogden, J., 2012. Health Psychology. McGraw-Hill Education, Maidenhead, UK.

Olshansky, B., 2007. Placebo and nocebo cardiovascular health. Implications for healthcare, research and doctor-patient relationship. J. Am. Coll. Cardiologists 49 (4), 415–421.

Ontario Society of Nutrition Professionals in Public Health (OSNPPH), 2015. https://www.osnpph.on.ca/upload/membership/document/2016-02/position-statement-2015-final.pdf#upload/membership/document/position-statement-2015-final.pdf/.

Orford, J., 2000. Excessive Appetites: A Psychological View of Addiction, second ed. Wiley, Chichester, UK.

Organisation and Service Department, 2011. How Unions Make a difference to Health and Safety. Trades Union Congress, London, UK.

Ost, L.G., 2008. Efficacy of the third wave of behavioural therapies: a systematic review and meat-analysis. Behav. Res. Ther. 46 (3), 296–321.

Paice, E., Aitken, M., Houghton, A., et al., 2004. Bullying among doctors in training: cross sectional questionnaire survey. BMJ 329, 658.

Parkes, C.M., 1975. Bereavement. Studies of Grief in Adult Life. Penguin Books, Harmondsworth, UK.

Parkes, C.M., 1996. Bereavement. Studies of Grief in Adult Life, third ed. Tavistock Publications, London, UK.

Parkes, C.M., 2006. Love and Loss. The Root of Grief and its Complications. Routledge, Hove, UK.

Peplau, L.A., Frederick, D.A., Yee, C., et al., 2009. Body image satisfaction in heterosexual, gay, and lesbian adults. Arch. Sexual Behav. 38 (5), 713–725.

Petticrew, M., Bell, R., Hunter, D., 2002. Influence of psychological coping on survival and recurrence in people with cancer: Systematic review. Br. Med. J. 325, 1066–1069.

Petty, R.E., Cacioppo, J.T., 1986. The elaboration Likelihood Model of Persuasion. Communication and Persuasion. Springer, New York, USA.

Peveler, R., Carson, A., Rodin, G., 2002. ABC of psychological medicine: Depression in medical patients. BMJ 325, 149–152.

Phillips, C., Main, C., Buck, R., et al., 2008. Prioritising pain in policy making: the need for a whole systems perspective. Health Policy (New York) 88 (2–3), 166–175.

Phillips, C., Thompson, G., 2001. What is a QALY?, vol. 1, (6). Hayward Medical Communications, Aventis Pharma, pp. 1–6. www.evidence-based-medicine.co.uk.

Philo, G., 1999. Media and mental illness. In: Philo, G. (Ed.), Message Received. Longman, London, UK.

Pinto, A.D., Molnar, A., Shankardass, K., et al., 2015. Economic considerations and health in all policies initiatives: evidence from interviews with key informants in Sweden, Quebec and South Australia. BMC Public Health 18 (15), 171.

Pogosova, N., Saner, H., Pedersen, S.S., et al., 2015. Psychosocial aspects in cardiac rehabilitation: from theory to practice. A position paper from the Cardiac Rehabilitation Section of the European Association of Cardiovascular Prevention and Rehabilitation of the European Society of Cardiology. Eur. J. Prev. Cardiol. 22 (10), 1290–1306.

Powell, J., 2006. Health needs assessment: a systematic approach. http://www.library.nhs.uk/HealthManagement/ViewResource.aspx?resID=29549&tabID=290&summaries=true&resultsPerPage=10&sort=TITLE&catID=4033/.

Powell, R., McKee, L., Bruce, J., 2009. Information and behavioural instruction along the health-care pathway: the perspective of people undergoing hernia repair surgery and the role of formal and informal information sources. Health Expectations. 12, 149–159.

Powell, R., Scott, N.W., Manyande, A., et al., 2016. Psychological preparation and postoperative outcomes for adults undergoing surgery under general anaesthesia. Cochrane Database Syst. Rev. (5), CD008646.

Price, C., Hoggart, B., Olukoga, O., et al., 2012. National pain audit final report, Dr Foster Research Ltd., London, UK. http://www.nationalpainaudit.org/media/files/NationalPainAudit-2012.pdf/.

Public Health England, 2014. Improving Young People's Health and Wellbeing. A Framework for Public Health. Public Health England, London, UK.

Public Health England, 2015. Public Health England: children and young people benchmarking tool. http://fingertips.phe.org.uk/profile/cyphof/.

Puri, B., Laking, P.J., Treasaden, I.H., 1996. Textbook of Psychiatry. Churchill Livingstone, Edinburg, UK.

Qureshi, K., Salway, S., Chowbey, P., Platt, L., 2014. Long-term ill health and the social embeddedness of work: a study in a post-industrial, multi-ethnic locality in the UK. Sociol. Health Illness. 36 (7), 955–969.

Ramchandani, P., Stein, A., Evans, J., et al., 2005. Paternal depression in the postnatal period and child development: a prospective population study. Lancet 365, 2201–2205.

Reid, K.M., Taylor, M.G., 2015. Social support, stress, and maternal postpartum depression: a comparison of supportive relationships. Soc. Sci. Res. 54, 246–262.

Relf, M., Machin, L., Archer, N., 2010. Guidance for Bereavement Needs Assessment in Palliative Care, second ed. Help the Hospices.

Relton, C.L., Davey Smith, G., 2012. Is epidemiology ready for epigenetics? Int. J. Epidemiol. 41 (1), 5–9.

Repper, J., Perkins, R., 2006. Social Inclusion and Recovery: A Model for Mental Health Services. Baillière Tindall, London, UK.

RCGP, 2013. http://www.rcgp.org.uk/~/media/EFE191B727514B66909FEED20FF23E1F.ashx.

Richards, H.M., Reid, M.E., Watt, G.C.M., 2002. Socioeconomic variations in response to chest pain: qualitative study. BMJ 324, 1308–1312.

Richards, M., 1993. The new genetics: some issues for social scientists. Sociol. Health Illness. 15, 567–586.

Rogers, R.W., 1975. A protection motivation theory of fear appeals and attitude change. J. Psychol. Interdisciplinary Applied 91 (1), 93–114.

Romano, J.M., Turner, J.A., Jensen, M.P., et al., 1995. Chronic pain patient spouse behavioral interactions predict patient disability. Pain 63, 353–360.

Rose, D., Fleischmann, P., Wykes, T., et al., 2003. Patients' perspectives on electroconvulsive therapy: systematic review. BMJ 326, 1363.

Rosenstock, I.M., 1974. The health belief model and preventive health behavior. Health Educ. Monogr. 2 (4), 354–386.

Rost, K., Nutting, P., Smith, J.L., et al., 2002. Managing depression as a chronic disease: a randomised trial of ongoing treatment in primary care. BMJ 325, 934.

Royal College of Paediatrics and Child Health and University College London, 2013. Overview of Child Deaths in the Four UK Counties. RCPCH, London, UK.

Royal College of Physicians, 2010. Passive Smoking and Children. A Report of the Tobacco Advisory Group of the Royal College of Physicians. RCP, London, UK.

RSA, 2007. Drugs – Facing Facts: The Report of the RSA Commission on Illegal Drugs, Communities and Public Policy. Royal Society for the Encouragement of Arts, Manufactures and Commerce, London, UK.

Rudd, P., Price, M.G., Graham, L.E., et al., 1986. Consequences of worksite hypertension screening: differential changes in psychosocial function. Am. J. Med. 80, 853–861.

Ruiz, J.G., Mintzer, M.J., Leipzig, R.M., 2006. The impact of E learning in medical education. Acad. Med. 81, 207–212.

Runnymede Trust, 2012. Runnymede blog – who are we? Census 2011 reports on ethnicity in the UK. http://www.runnymedetrust.org/blog/188/359/Who-are-we-Census-2011-reports-on-ethnicity-in-the-UK.html/. (Accessed 16 February 2015).

Ruston, A., Clayton, J., Calnan, M., 1998. Patients' actions during their cardiac event: qualitative study exploring differences and modifiable factors. BMJ 316, 1060–1065.

Rynn, M.A., Brawman-Mintzer, O., 2004. Generalized anxiety disorder: acute and chronic treatment. CNS Spectr. 9 (10), 716–723.

Sabat, S.R., Harré, R., 1992. The construction and deconstruction of self in Alzheimer's disease. Ageing Soc. 12, 443–461.

Sacks, O., 1986. The Man Who Mistook His Wife for a Hat. Picador, London, UK.

Saile, H., Burgemeir, R., Schmidt, L.R., 1988. A meta-analysis of studies on psychological preparation of children facing medical procedures. Psychol. Health 2, 107–132.

Salkovskis, P.M., 1989. Somatic problems. In: Hawton, K., Salkovskis, P.M., Kirk, J., et al. (Eds.), Cognitive Behaviour Therapy for Psychiatric Problems: A Practical Guide. Oxford University Press, New York, pp. 235–276.

Samuel, G., Kitzinger, J., 2013. Reporting consciousness in coma: media framing of neuro-scientific research, hope, and the response of families with relatives in vegetative and minimally conscious states. JOMEC J. 3, DOI: http://doi.org/10.18573/j.2013.10244.

Sargent, R.P., Shepard, R.M., Glantz, S.A., 2004. Reduced incidence of admissions for myocardial infarction associated with public smoking ban: before and after study. BMJ 328, 977–980.

Saunders, C., Sykes, N., 1993. The Management of Terminal Malignant Disease, third ed. Edward Arnold, London, UK.

Savage, M., Dumas, A., Stuart, S., 2013. Fatalism and short-termism as cultural barriers to cardiac rehabilitation among underprivileged men. Sociol. Health Illness. 35 (8), 1211–1226.

Sawyer, S., Drew, S., Yeo, M., et al., 2007. Adolescents with a chronic condition: challenges living, challenges treating. Lancet 369, 1481–1489.

Scambler, G., Hopkins, A., 1986. Being epileptic: coming to terms with stigma. Sociol. Health Illness. 8, 26–43.

Schaie, K.W., 1996. Intellectual development in adulthood. In: Birren, J.E., Schaie, K.W. (Eds.), Handbook of the Psychology of Aging. Academic Press, London, UK.

Schapira, K., McClelland, H.A., Griffiths, N.R., Newell, D.J., 1970. Study on the effects of tablet colour in the treatment of anxiety states. BMJ 23 (5707), 446–449.

Schenker, S., 2003. Undernutrition in the UK (briefing paper): British Nutrition Foundation. Nutr. Bull. 28, 87–120.

Schwartz, G.E., 1980. Testing the biopsychosocial model: the ultimate challenge facing behavioural medicine? J. Consult. Clin. Psychol. 50, 1040–1053.

Schwarzer, R., 1992. Self-efficacy: Thought Control of Action. Hemisphere Pub. Corp., Washington, DC; London, UK.

Scottish Executive, 2000. Same as You. The Scottish Executive, Edinburgh, UK.

Scottish Executive, 2000. The same as you? A Review of Services for People with Learning Disabilities, Edinburgh: Scottish Executive. http://www.scotland.gov.uk/Resource/Doc/1095/0001661.pdf.

Seale, C., 2003. Health and the Media. Sage, London.

Segerstrom, S.C., Miller, G.E., 2004. Psychological stress and the human immune system: a meta-analytic study of 30 years of inquiry. Psychol. Bull. 130 (4), 601–630.

Seyle, H., 1956. The Stress of Life. McGraw-Hill, New York.

Shalev, A.Y., 2001. Post-traumatic stress disorder. Disorder takes away human dignity and character. BMJ 322 (1301), 1303–1304.

Shalev, A.Y., Schreiber, S., Galai, T., et al., 1993. Post-traumatic stress disorder following medical events. Br. J. Clin. Psychol. 32, 247–253.

Shaw, M., Davey Smith, G., Dorling, D., 2005. Health inequalities and New Labour: how the promises compare with real progress. BMJ 330, 1016–1021.

Sheeran, P., Orbell, S., 2000. Using implementation intentions to increase attendance for cervical cancer screening. Health Psychol. 19 (3), 283–289.

Shepperd, J.A., Klein, W.M.P., Waters, E.A., Weinstein, N.D., 2013. Taking stock of unrealistic optimism. Perspect. Psychol. Sci. 8 (4), 395–411.

Shipley, B.A., Weiss, A., Der, G., et al., 2007. Neuroticism, extraversion, and mortality in the UK health and lifestyle survey: A 21-year prospective cohort study. Psychosom. Med. 69, 923–931.

Siderfin, C., 2005. Remote and rural general practice in Scotland. BMJ Career Focus. 331, 135–136.

Sikorski, J., Renfrew, M., Pindoria, S., et al., 2003. Support for breastfeeding mothers; a systematic review. Paediatr. Perinatal Epidemiol. 17, 407–417.

Silverman, J., Kurtz, S., Draper, J., 2013. Skills for Communication with Patients, third ed. Radcliffe Publishing Ltd, London, UK.

Slack, M.K., Brooks, A.J., 1995. Medication management issues for adolescents with asthma. Am. J. Health-Syst. Pharmacy 52, 1417–1421.

Skevington, S.M., Sartorius, N., Amir, M., the WHOQOL Group, 2004. Developing methods for assessing quality of life in different cultural settings: the history of the WHOQOL instruments. Social Psychiatry & Psychiatric Epidemiology 39 (1), 1–8.

Skevington, S.M., Boehnke, J.M., 2018. How is subjective wellbeing related to quality of life? Do we need two constructs and both measures? Soc. Sci. Med. (Accepted 4thApril). 206, 22–30, ISSN 0277-9536,1873-5347. doi:10.1016/j.socscimed.2018 04.005.

Sniehotta, F.F., Araújo Soares, V., Dombrowski, S.U., 2007. Randomized controlled trial of a one-minute intervention changing oral self-care behavior. J. Dent. Res. 86 (7), 641–645.

Sniehotta, F.F., Presseau, J., Araujo-Soares, V., 2014. Time to retire the theory of planned behaviour. Health Psychol. Rev. 8 (1), 1–7.

Sorce, J.F., Emde, R.N., Campos, J., et al., 1985. Maternal emotional signaling: its effect on the visual cliff behavior of 1-year-olds. Develop. Psychol. 21, 195–200.

Spiegel, D., Bloom, J.R., Kraemer, H.C., Gottheil, E., 1989. Effect of psychosocial treatment on survival of patients with metastatic breast cancer. Lancet 2, 888–891.

Steinberg, L., 2007. Risk taking in adolescence: new perspectives from brain and behavioral science. Curr. Direct. Psychol. Sci. 16, 55–59.

Sterba, R., 1934. The fate of the ego in analytic therapy. Int. J. Psychoanal. 15, 117–126.

Sternberg, R.J., 1996. Successful Intelligence. Simon & Schuster, New York.

Stewart, M., 2001. Towards a global definition of patient centred care. BMJ 322, 444–445.

Stewart-Williams, S., 2004. The placebo puzzle: putting together the pieces. Health Psychol. 23, 198–206.

Stone, J., Aronson, E., Crain, A.L., et al., 1994. Inducing hypocrisy as a means of encouraging young adults to use condoms. Personality Soc. Psychol. Bull. 20, 116–128.

Street, R.L., Jr., 2013. How clinician-patient communication contributes to health improvement: modeling pathways from talk to outcome. Patient Educ. Couns. 92, 286–291.

Stroebe, M., Schut, H., 1999. The dual process model of coping with bereavement; rationale and description. Death Stud. 23, 197–224.

Stroebe, W., Stroebe, M.S., 1987. Bereavement and Health: The Psychological and Physical Consequences of Partner Loss. Cambridge University Press, Cambridge, UK.

Stuart-Hamilton, I., 1994. The Psychology of Ageing. Jessica Kingsley, London, UK.

Summerfield, D., 2001. The invention of post-traumatic stress disorder and the social usefulness of a psychiatric category. BMJ 322, 95–98.

Symon, A., Williams, B., Adelasoye, Q.A., Cheyne, H., 2015. Nocebo and the potential harm of 'high risk' labelling: a scoping review. J. Adv. Nursing. 71 (7), 1518–1529.

Talge, N.M., Neal, C., Glover, V., 2007. Antenatal maternal stress and long-term effects on child neurodevelopment: how and why? J. Child Psychol. Psychiatry 48, 245–261.

Tassicker, R.J., Teltscher, B., Trembath, M.K., et al., 2009. Problems assessing uptake of Huntington disease predictive testing and a proposed solution. Eur. J. Hum. Genet. 17 (1), 66–70. doi:10.1038/ejhg.2008.142. [Epub 2008 Jul 30].

Tew, M., 1990. Safer Childbirth? A Critical History of Maternity Care. Chapman & Hall, London, UK.

Thorpe, G., 1993. Enabling more dying people to remain at home. BMJ 307, 915–918.

Thurstone, L.L., 1938. Primary Mental Abilities. University of Chicago Press, Chicago, IL.

Tillin, T., Hughes, A.D., Godsland, I.F., et al., 2013. Insulin resistance and truncal obesity as important determinants of the greater incidence of diabetes in Indian Asians and African Caribbeans compared with Europeans: the Southall And Brent REvisited (SABRE) cohort. Diabetes Care 36, 383–393.

Tincoff, R., Jusczyk, P.W., 1999. Some beginnings of word comprehension in 6-month-olds. Psychol. Sci. 10, 172–175.

Townsend, P., Davidson, N., Whitehead, M. (Eds.), 1992. Inequalities in Health: The Black Report and the Health Divide. Penguin, Harmondsworth, UK.

Trace, S.E., Baker, J.H., Peñas-Lledó, E., et al., 2013. The genetics of eating disorders. Ann. Rev. Clin. Psychol. 9, 589–620.

Trostler, M., Li, Y., Plankey, M.W., 2014. Prevalence of binge drinking and associated co-factors among medical students in a US Jesuit University. Am. J. Drug Alcohol Abuse 40 (4), 336–341.

Tuckett, D., Boulton, M., Olsen, C., et al., 1985. Meetings between Experts: An Approach to Sharing Ideas in Medical Consultations. Tavistock, London, UK.

Tuckman, B.W., 1965. Developmental sequence in small groups. Psychol. Bull. 63 (6), 384–399.

Tuomilehto, J., Lindström, J., Eriksson, J., et al., 2001. Prevention of type 2 diabetes mellitus by changes in lifestyle among subjects with impaired glucose tolerance. N Engl J Med 344, 1343–1350. doi:10.1056/NEJM20010503 3441801.

Turner, B., 1995. Medical Power and Social Knowledge, second ed. Sage, London, UK.

Twigg, J., Atkin, K., 1994. Carers Perceived: Policy and Practice in Informal Care. McGraw-Hill Education, London, UK.

Twycross, R., 1994. Pain Relief in Advanced Cancer. Churchill Livingstone, Edinburgh, UK.

Twycross, R., 1999. Introducing Palliative Care, third ed. Radcliffe Medical Press, Oxford, UK.

Ulrich, R., 1984. View through a window may influence recovery. Science 224 (4647), 224–225.

UN General Assembly, 2007. Convention on the Rights of Persons with Disabilities: Resolution/Adopted by the General Assembly. UN, New York.

van der Klink, J.L., Blonk, R.W.B., Schene, A.H., et al., 2001. The benefits of interventions for work-related stress. Am. J. Public Health 91, 270–276.

Vartiainen, E., Paavola, M., McAlister, A., et al., 1998. Fifteen-year follow-up of smoking prevention effects in the North Karelia Youth Project. Am. J. Public Health 88, 81–85.

Vasey, P., Bartlett, N., 2007. What can the Samoan "Fa'afafine" teach us about the Western concept of gender identity disorder in childhood? Perspect. Biol. Med. 50 (4), 481–490.

Waddell, G., Burton, A.K., 2006. Is Work Good for Your Health and Well-Being? TSO, London, UK.

Wadsworth, M.E.J., Montgomery, S.M., Bartley, M.J., 1999. The persisting effect of unemployment on health and social well-being in men in early working life. Soc. Sci. Med. 48, 1491–1499.

Wallace, S., Nazroo, J., Becares, L., 2016. Culmulative effect of racial discrimination on the mental health of ethnic minorities in the United Kingdom. Am. J. Public Health 106 (7), 1294–1300.

Walter, T., 1999. On Bereavement: The Culture of Grief. Open University Press, Buckingham, UK.

Wanless, D., Forder, J., Fernández, J.L., et al., 2006. Wanless Social Care Review: Securing Good Care for Older People, Taking a Long-Term View. King's Fund, London, UK.

Warr, P., 1987. Work, Unemployment and Mental Health. Oxford University Press, Oxford, UK.

Watson, J.B., Raynor, R., 1920. Conditioned emotional responses. J. Experiment. Psycho 3, 1–14.

Watson, M., Lucas, C., Hoy, A., 2006. Adult Palliative Care Guidance, second ed. Mount Vernon and Sussex Cancer Networks and Northern Ireland Palliative Medicine Group, South West London, Surrey, West Sussex and Hampshire, UK.

Watts, T., 2013. The media critique of the Liverpool Care Pathway: some implications for nursing education. Int. J. Palliat. Nurs. 19 (6), 275–280.

Webster, R.K., Weinman, J., Rubin, G., James, A., 2016. Systematic review of factors that contribute to nocebo effects. Health Psychol. 35 (12), 1334–1355.

Weevers, H., Van de Beek, A.J., Anema, J.R., et al., 2005. Work-related disease in general practice: a systematic review. Fam. Pract. 22 (2), 197–204.

Wegner, D.M., 1987. Transactive memory: a contemporary analysis of the group mind. In: Mullen, B., Goethals, G. (Eds.), Theories of Group Behaviour. Springer, New York.

Weich, S., Lewis, G., 1998. Poverty, unemployment and common mental disorders: population based cohort study. BMJ 317, 115–119.

Weinstein, N.D., 1980. Unrealistic optimism about future life events. J. Personality Soc. Psychol 39, 806–820.

Weinstein, N.D., 1987. Unrealistic optimism about susceptibility to health problems: conclusions from a community wide sample. J. Behav. Med. 10, 481–500.

Weinstein, N.D., 2000. Perceived probability, perceived severity, and health-protective behaviour. Health Psychol. 19 (1), 65–74.

Weinstein, N.D., Lyon, J.E., 1999. Mindset, optimistic bias about personal risk and health-protective behaviour. Br. J. Health Psychol. 4, 289–300.

Weinstein, N.D., Slovic, P., Gibson, G., 2004. Accuracy and optimism in smokers' beliefs about quitting. Nicotine Tobacco Res. 6 (S3), S375–S380.

Wellings, K., Wadsworth, J., Johnson, A.M., et al., 1995. Provision of sex education and early sexual experience: the relation examined. BMJ 311, 417–420.

Wenger, E., 1998. Communities of Practice: Learning, Meaning and Identity. Cambridge University Press, New York.

Wells, A., 2011. Metacognitive Therapy for Anxiety and Depression. Guildford Press, New York.

West, M., Markiewicz, L., 2004. Building Team-Based Working. Blackwells, Oxford, UK.

Whalley, L.J., Deary, I.J., 2001. Longitudinal cohort study of childhood IQ and survival up to age 76. BMJ 322, 1–5.

Wheeler, B.W., White, M., Stahl-Timmins, W., Depledge, M.H., 2012. Does living by the coast improve health and wellbeing? Health Place 18 (5), 1198–1201.

White, A.R., Rampes, H., Ernst, E., 2000. Acupuncture for smoking cessation. Cochrane Database Syst. Rev. (2), CD000009.

WHOQOL Group, 1998. The World Health Organization quality of life assessment (WHOQOL): development and general psychometric properties. Soc. Sci. Med. 46, 1569–1585.

Wight, D., Henderson, M., Raab, G., et al., 2000. Extent of regretted sexual intercourse among young teenagers in Scotland: a cross-sectional survey. BMJ 320, 1243–1244.

Wilkinson, R., Pickett, K., 2009. The Spirit Level: Why More Equal Societies Almost Always Do Better. Allen Lane, London, UK.

Williams, A., Gajevic, S., 2013. Selling science: source struggles, public relations, and UK press coverage of animal–human hybrid embryos. J. Stud. 14 (4), 507–522.

Williams, C., Kitzinger, J., Henderson, L., 2003. Envisaging the embryo in stem cell research: rhetorical strategies and media reporting of the ethical debates. Sociol. Health Illness. 25, 793–814.

Williams, K.E., Chambless, D.L., Ahrens, A., 1997. Are emotions frightening? An extension of the fear of fear construct. Behav. Res. Ther. 35, 229–248.

Williams, L., O'Connor, R.C., Howard, S., et al., 2008. Type D personality mechanisms of effect: the role of health-related behaviour and social support. J. Psychosom. Res. 64, 63–69.

Willis, E., 2002. Public health and the 'new' genetics: balancing individual and collective outcomes. Crit. Public Health. 12, 119–138.

Wing, R.R., Tate, D.F., Gorin, A.A., et al., 2006. A self-regulation program for maintenance of weight loss. New Eng. J. Med. 355 (15), 1563–1571.

Winterton Report, 1992. Maternity Services Second Report, vol. 1. HMSO, London, UK.

Wood, W., Kallgren, C.A., Priesler, R.M., 1985. Access to attitude-relevant information in memory as a determinant of persuasion: the role of message attributes. J. Exper. Soc. Psychol. 21, 73–85.

Worden, J.W., 1991. Grief Counselling and Grief Therapy. A Handbook for the Mental Health Practitioner. Routledge, London, UK.

World Health Organization, 2002a. Infant and young child nutrition; global strategy for infant and young child feeding. WHO, Geneva, Switzerland.

World Health Organization, 2002b. Towards a common language for functioning, disability and health: ICF. WHO, Geneva, Switzerland.

World Health Organization, 2002c. National cancer control programmes: policies and guidelines. WHO, Geneva, Switzerland.

World Health Organization, 2008. http://www.who.int/whosis/database/core/core_select.cfm/.

World Health Organization, 2009. Infant and Young Child Feeding: Model Chapter for Textbooks for Medical Students and Allied Health Professionals. World Health Organization, Geneva.

World Health Organization, 2012. Risks to mental health: an overview of vulnerabilities and risk factors. Background paper by WHO secretariat for the development of a comprehensive mental health action plan. WHO, Geneva, Switzerland.

World Health Organization, 2014. http://www.who.int/mediacentre/factsheets/fs310/en/.

World Health Organization, 2017. Refugee and migrant health. http://www.who.int/migrants/en/.

World Health Organization Commission on Social Determinants of Health, World Health Organization, 2008. Closing the gap in a generation: health equity through action on the social determinants of health: Commission on Social Determinants of Health final report. World Health Organization. (CSD WHO 2006). WHO, Geneva, Switzerland.

World Health Organization, 2009. Infant and young child feeding: Model chapter for textbooks for medical students and allied health professionals. World Health Organization, Geneva.

Wright, M., Wood, J., Lynch, T., Clark, D., 2006. Mapping levels of palliative care development: a global view. International Observatory on End of life Care. Help the Hospices and National Palliative Care Organisation. London, UK.

Yang, C.L., Tan, Y.H., Jiang, X.X., et al., 2012. Pre-operative education and counselling are associated with reduced anxiety symptoms following carotid endarterectomy: a randomized and open-label study. Eur. J. Cardiovasc. Nursing. 11, 284–288.

Yuan, S., Freeman, R., 2011. Can social support in the guise of an oral health education intervention promote mother–infant bonding in Chinese immigrant mothers and their infants? Health Educ. J. 70 (1), 57–66.

Zamora, A., Romo, L.F., Au, T.K., 2006. Using biology to teach adolescents about STD transmission and self-protective behaviors. Appl. Develop. Psychol. 27, 109–124.

Zellner, D.A., Garriga-Trillo, A., Centeno, S., et al., 2004. Chocolate craving and the menstrual cycle. Appetite 42, 119–121.

Zigler, E., Valentine, J., 1979. Project Head Start: A Legacy of the War on Poverty. Free Press, New York.

Zimmermann, C., Del Piccolo, L., Finset, A., 2007. Cues and concerns by patients in medical consultations: a literature review. Psychol. Bull. 133 (3), 438–463.

Weblinks

www.anxietyuk.org.uk/.
www.breakingbadnews.org/.
www.dyingmatters.org/.
www.nice.org.uk/.
www.thewhpca.org/.
www.who.int/cancer/palliative/definition/en/.
www.who.int/whr/en/.

Index

Page numbers followed by "*f*" indicate figures, "*t*" indicate tables, and "*b*" indicate boxes.